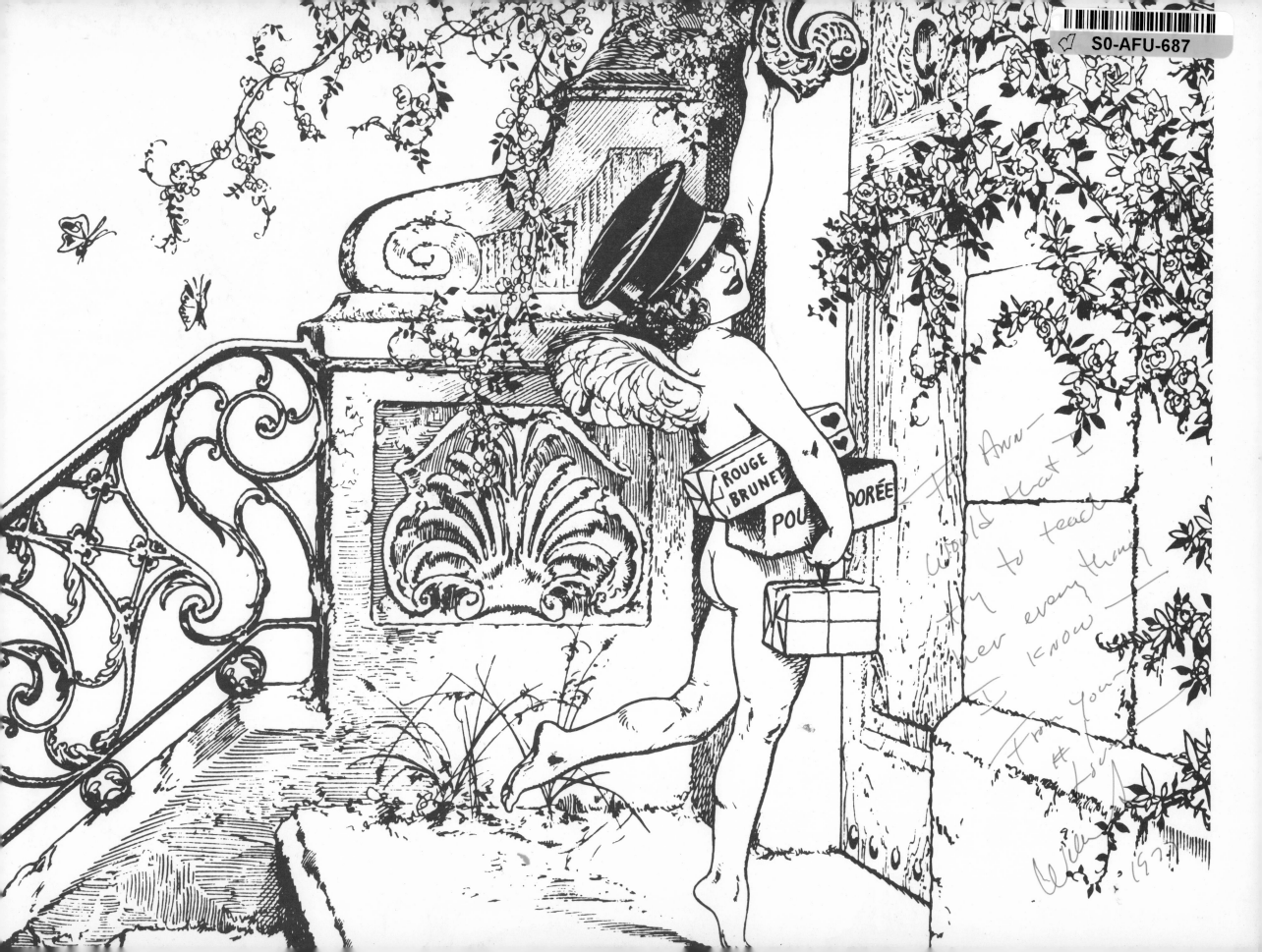

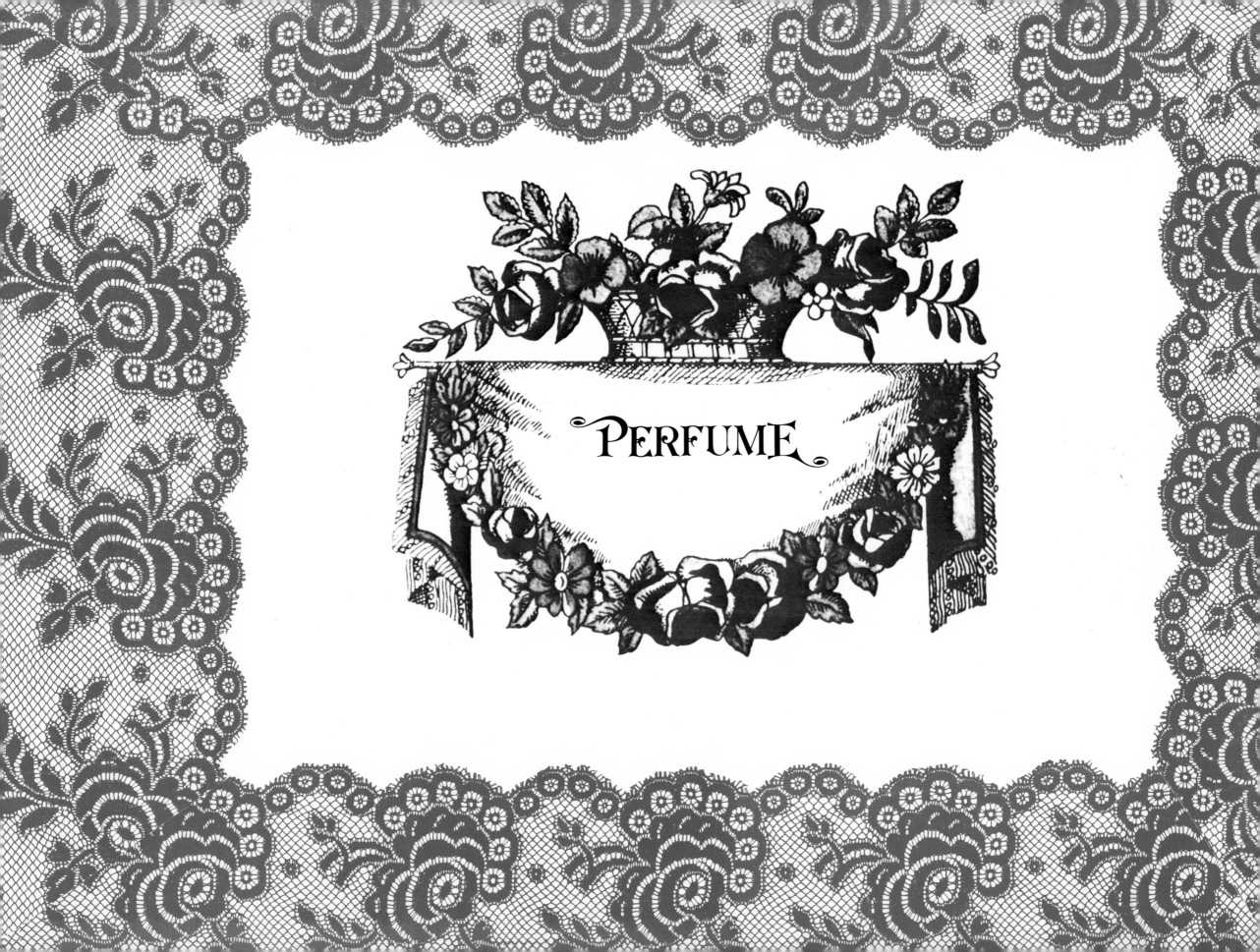

PERFUME

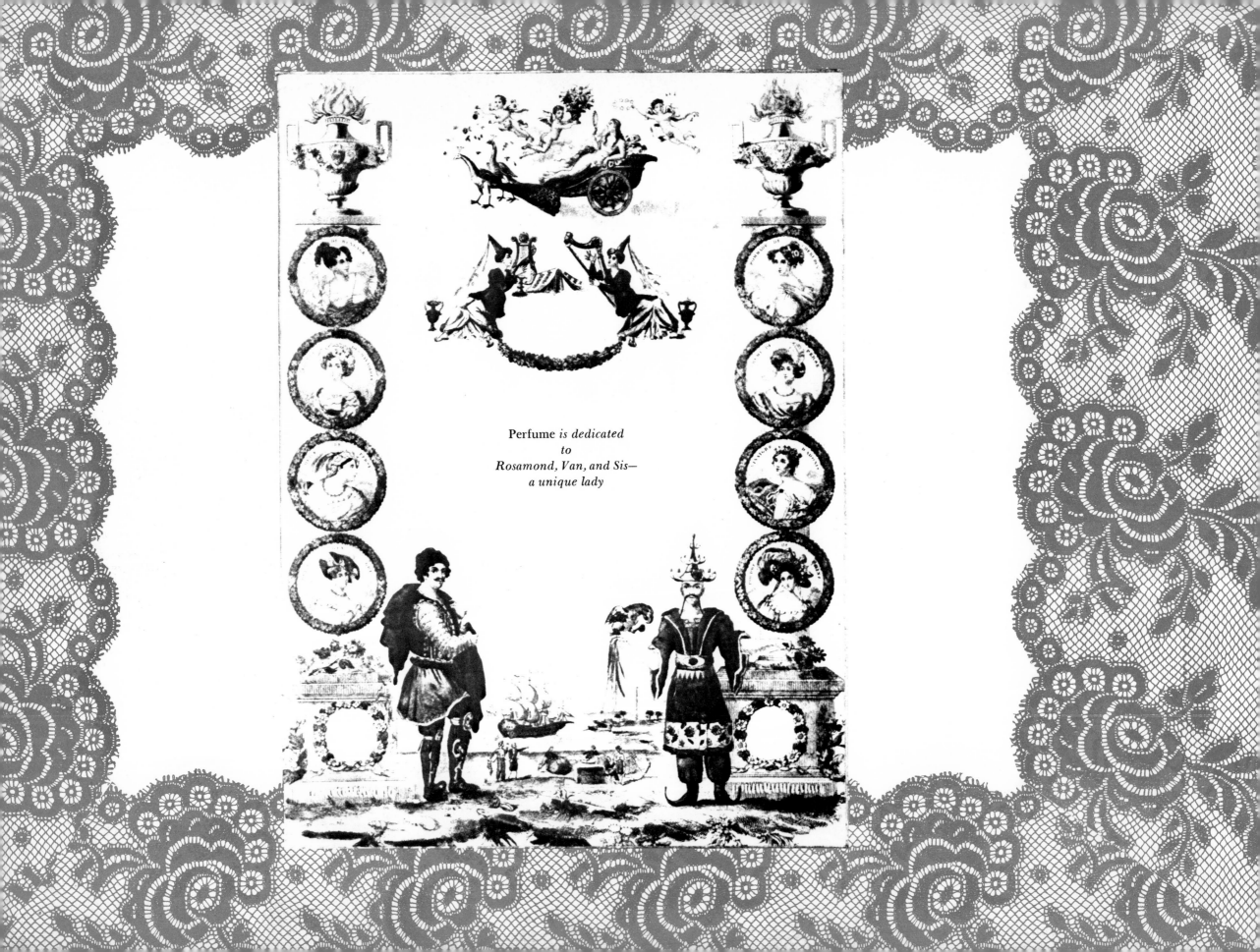

Perfume *is dedicated*
*to*
*Rosamond, Van, and Sis—*
*a unique lady*

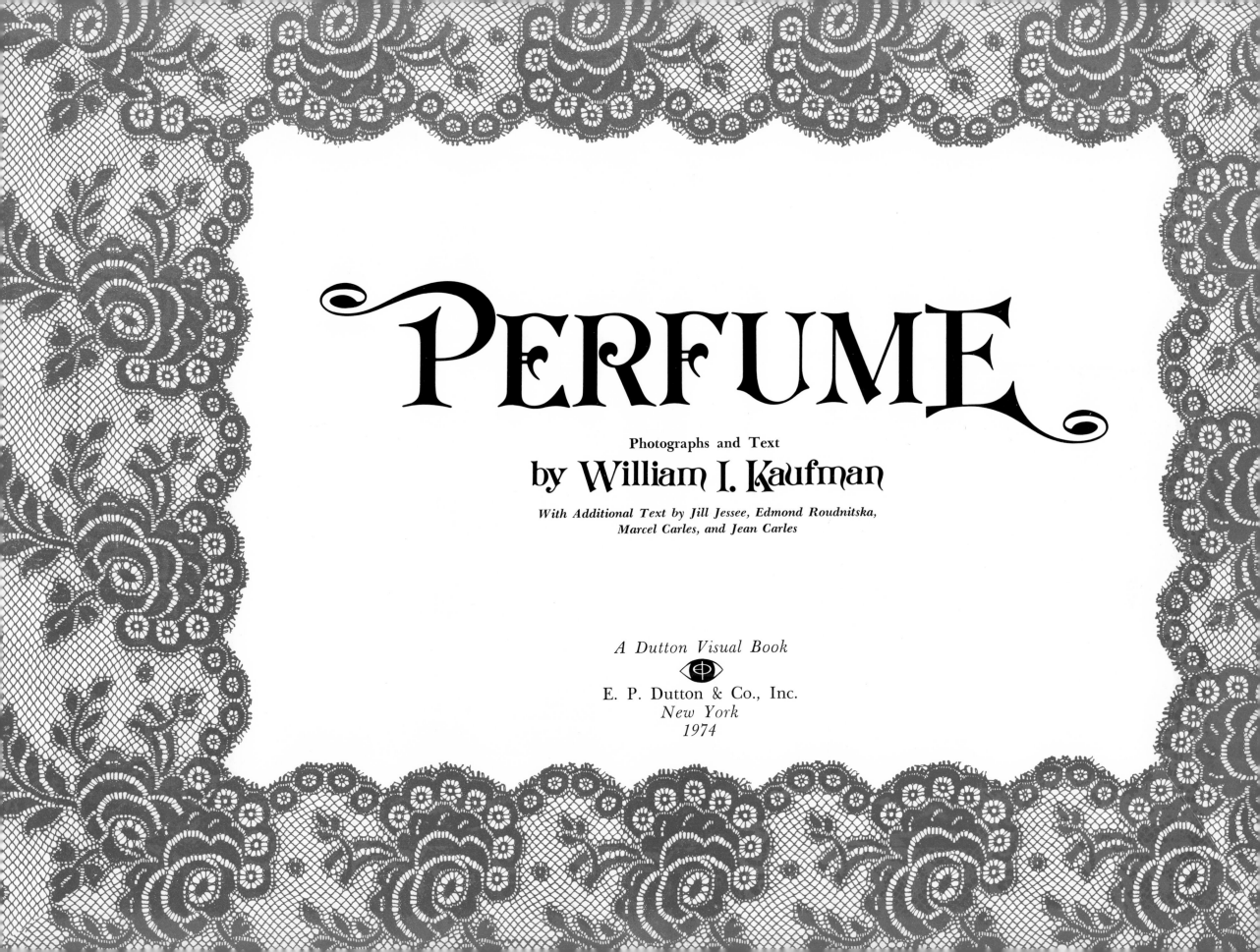

# PERFUME

Photographs and Text
### by William I. Kaufman

*With Additional Text by Jill Jessee, Edmond Roudnitska,*
*Marcel Carles, and Jean Carles*

*A Dutton Visual Book*

E. P. Dutton & Co., Inc.
*New York*
*1974*

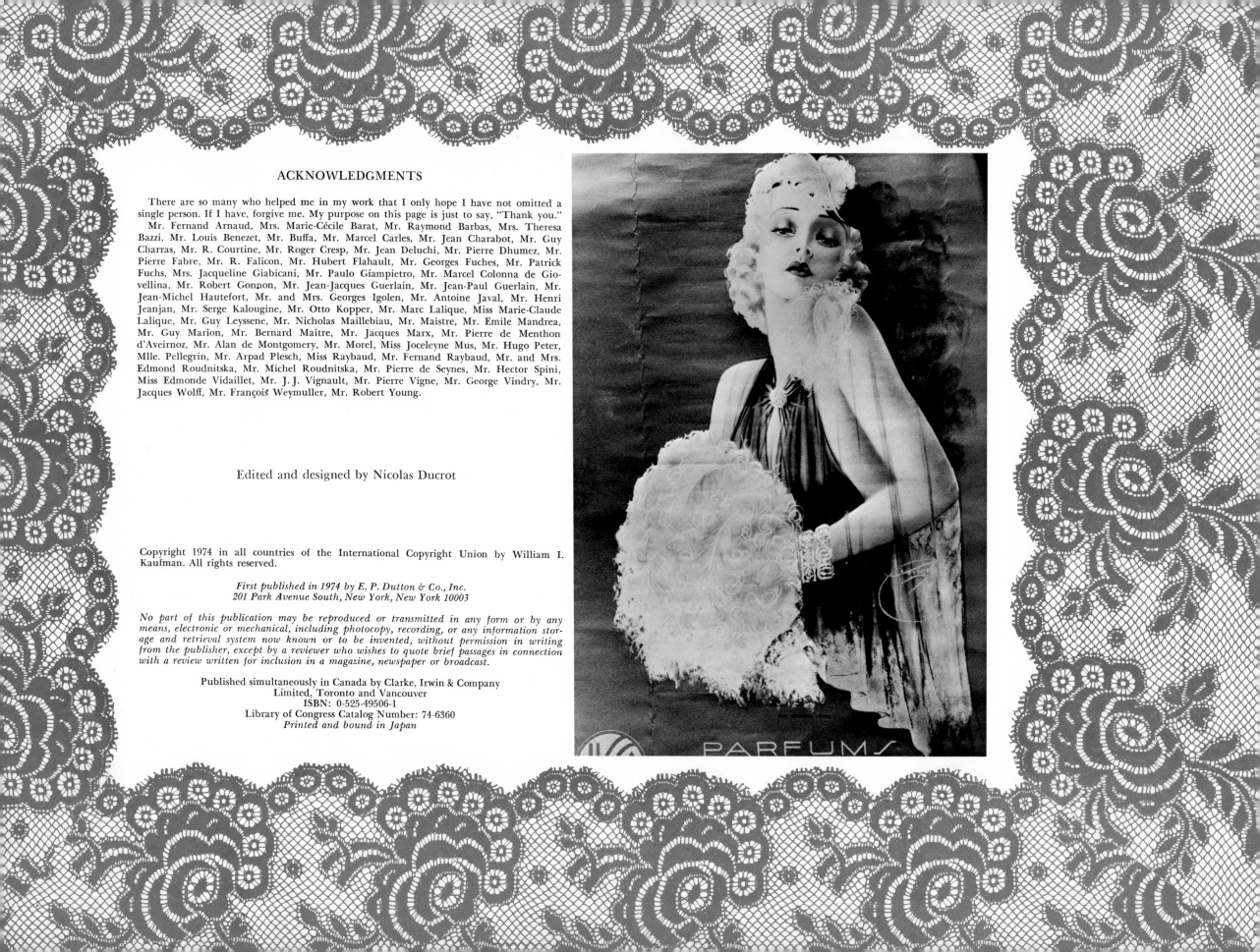

## ACKNOWLEDGMENTS

There are so many who helped me in my work that I only hope I have not omitted a single person. If I have, forgive me. My purpose on this page is just to say, "Thank you."

Mr. Fernand Arnaud, Mrs. Marie-Cécile Barat, Mr. Raymond Barbas, Mrs. Theresa Bazzi, Mr. Louis Benezet, Mr. Buffa, Mr. Marcel Carles, Mr. Jean Charabot, Mr. Guy Charras, Mr. R. Courtine, Mr. Roger Cresp, Mr. Jean Deluchi, Mr. Pierre Dhumez, Mr. Pierre Fabre, Mr. R. Falicon, Mr. Hubert Flahault, Mr. Georges Fuches, Mr. Patrick Fuchs, Mrs. Jacqueline Giabicani, Mr. Paulo Giampietro, Mr. Marcel Colonna de Giovellina, Mr. Robert Gonnon, Mr. Jean-Jacques Guerlain, Mr. Jean-Paul Guerlain, Mr. Jean-Michel Hautefort, Mr. and Mrs. Georges Igolen, Mr. Antoine Javal, Mr. Henri Jeanjan, Mr. Serge Kalougine, Mr. Otto Kopper, Mr. Marc Lalique, Miss Marie-Claude Lalique, Mr. Guy Leyssene, Mr. Nicholas Maillebiau, Mr. Maistre, Mr. Emile Mandrea, Mr. Guy Marion, Mr. Bernard Maitre, Mr. Jacques Marx, Mr. Pierre de Menthon d'Aveirnoz, Mr. Alan de Montgomery, Mr. Morel, Miss Joceleyne Mus, Mr. Hugo Peter, Mlle. Pellegrin, Mr. Arpad Plesch, Miss Raybaud, Mr. Fernand Raybaud, Mr. and Mrs. Edmond Roudnitska, Mr. Michel Roudnitska, Mr. Pierre de Seynes, Mr. Hector Spini, Miss Edmonde Vidaillet, Mr. J. J. Vignault, Mr. Pierre Vigne, Mr. George Vindry, Mr. Jacques Wolff, Mr. François Weymuller, Mr. Robert Young.

Edited and designed by Nicolas Ducrot

Published simultaneously in Canada by Clarke, Irwin & Company
Limited, Toronto and Vancouver
ISBN: 0-525-49506-1
Library of Congress Catalog Number: 74-6360
Printed and bound in Japan

# CONTENTS

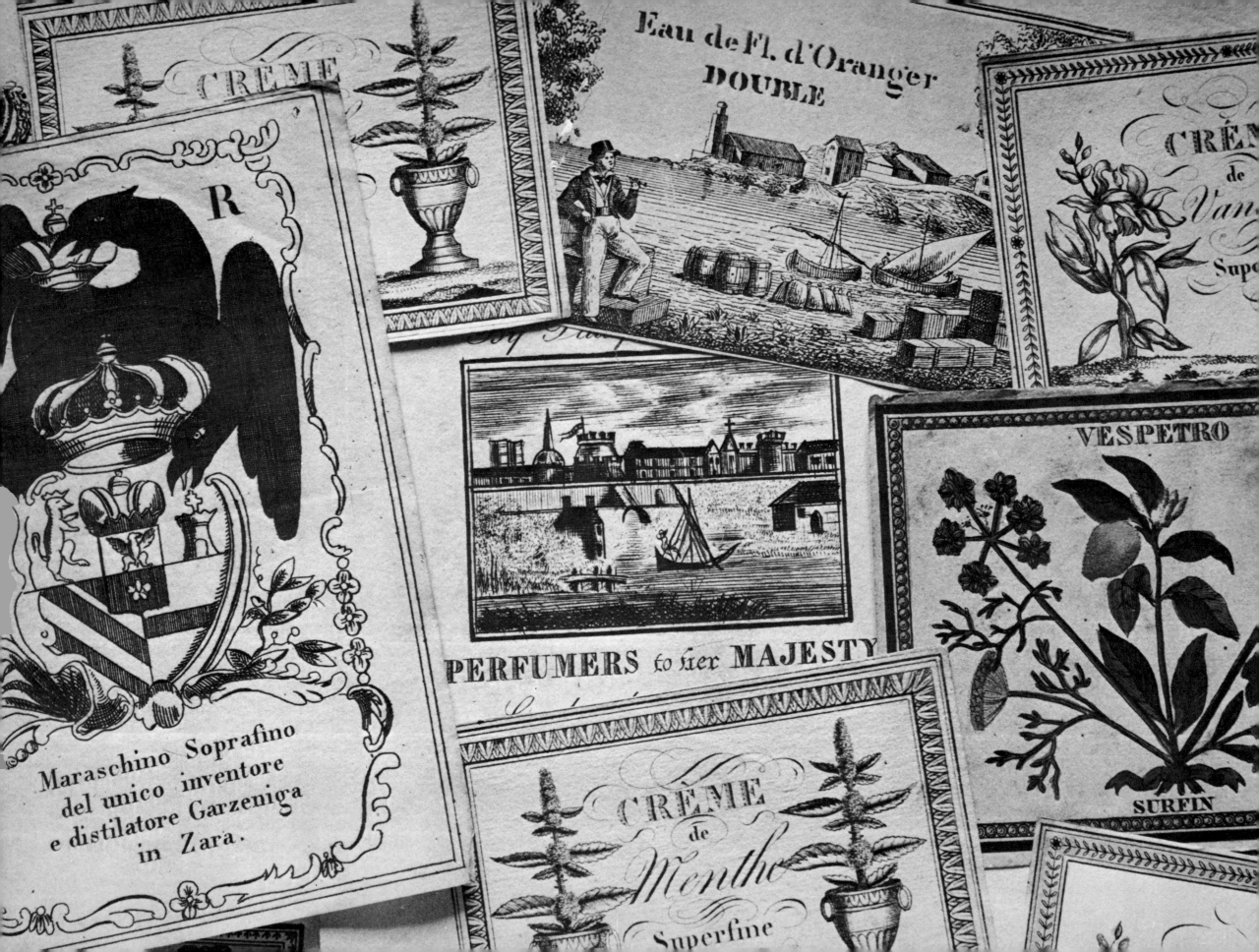

# INTRODUCTION

*A caravan from China comes.*
*For miles it sweetens all the air*
*With fragrant silks and stealing gums,*
*Attar and myrrh—*

*A caravan from China comes.*
*Oh, Merchant, tell me what you bring,*
*With music sweet of camel bells.*
*How long have you been traveling*
*With these sweet smells?*
*Oh, Merchant, tell me what you bring.*

Perfume—a magical, mystical word that conjures in the mind all the romance of life. It has been thus since the dawn of history.

Perfume—the smell of herbs, spices, wild grass, flowers; the smell of fluids of fish, of animals, of trees—is one of the secrets of the universe. Why the ambergris of the whale, the civet of the cat, the musk of the Florida alligator? Why the oils from the petals of *some* flowers and the leaves of *others,* and not from all? Perhaps it is best to leave the mysterious undefined and the unsolvable unsolved, but that is not the way of man. Questions must be answered, and so the quest goes on.

The perfumer—a modern-day alchemist—takes a note from here and a note from there. He is a trader in romance, and he brings together the exotic, the sweet, the pure, the piquant—ilang-ilang from the Philippines, woods and grasses from Africa, blossoms from Provence in France, spices from Grenada, to mention only a few.

The creation of perfume, like the composition of a musical score, is the result of complete artistic and professional dedication, and when the scent has been born, the forces of the world of art contribute to its refinement—the flacon, the box, each another note on the scale, another tone on the canvas.

In the words of one great perfumer, "Perfume is a weapon." But it is a weapon of peace, of love, of beauty. Through perfume one man touches the soul of another. Plutarch said, "The soul of man? A man in love is full of perfumes and sweet odors." Perfume seems to be the essence, the soul of the flower, as the spirit of man seems to be the essence of his body. We say nothing smells as sweet as the child in sleep, and no adult can explain the unique, warm, joyful odor that emanates from a child who is being caressed. Perhaps it is the purity of a new human, undefiled, whose spirit is yet untouched by the world's vulgarities, that causes the divinity of the child to reach us in a "cloud of perfume."

Through the ages perfume that reaches us through the most discriminating of human senses has been a "divine attribute." It is thus natural that priests were the first perfumers, and as you read in the pages of this book our notes on the history and development and tradition of this precious liquid, I hope you will be as fascinated as I with the unfolding of the universe of perfume.

Too many of our dreams are shattered in a lifetime, and I think that herein lodges the reason for my creating this book. It has been a challenge to show how the worlds of nature, of science, and of art have combined to produce the pleasure of perfume, which stimulates while it comforts, which excites the imagination and awakens all our senses to the beauty and the mystery and the romance that lie within our reach.

WILLIAM I. KAUFMAN

Grasse, France
1974

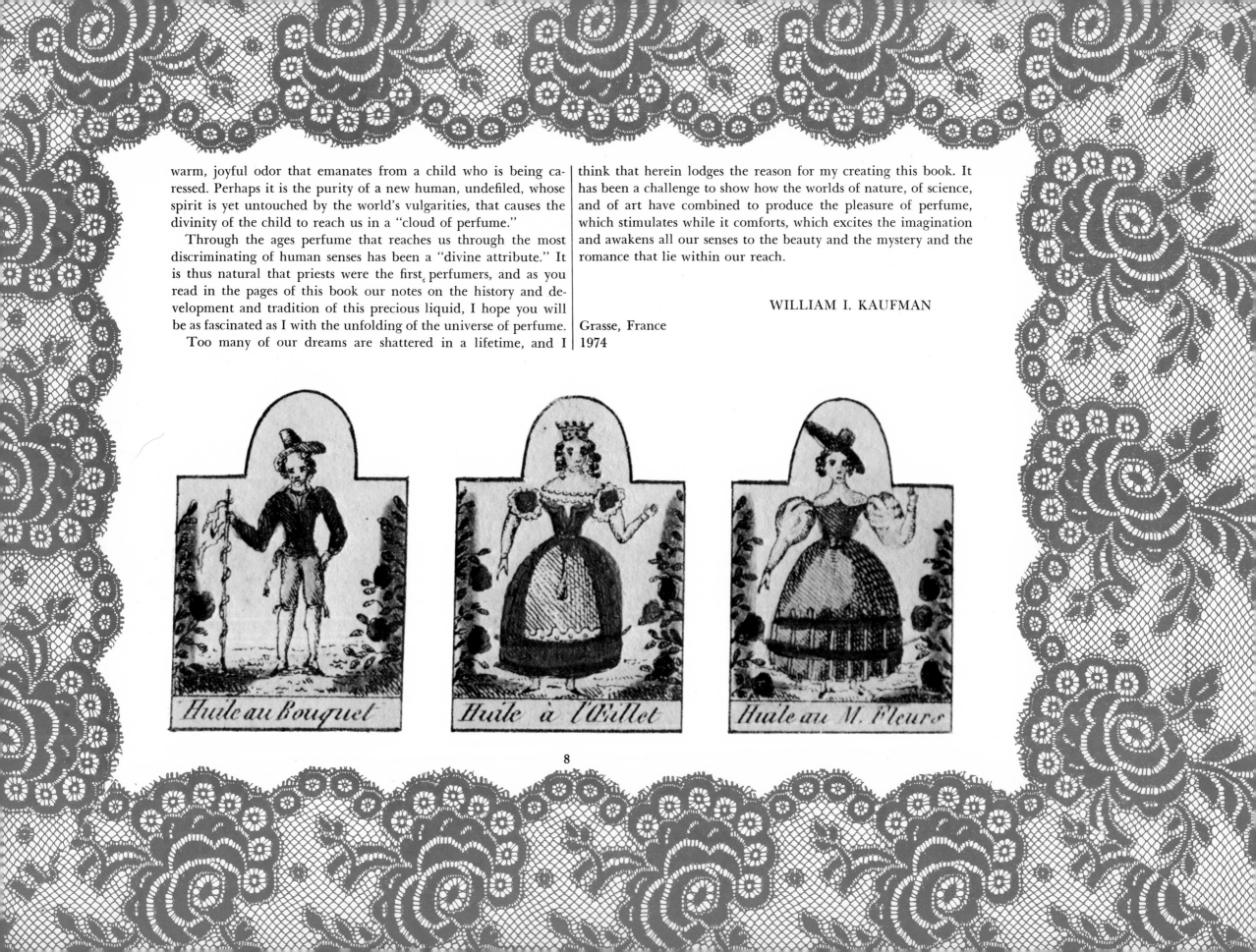

Huile au Bouquet    Huile à l'Œillet    Huile au M. Fleurs

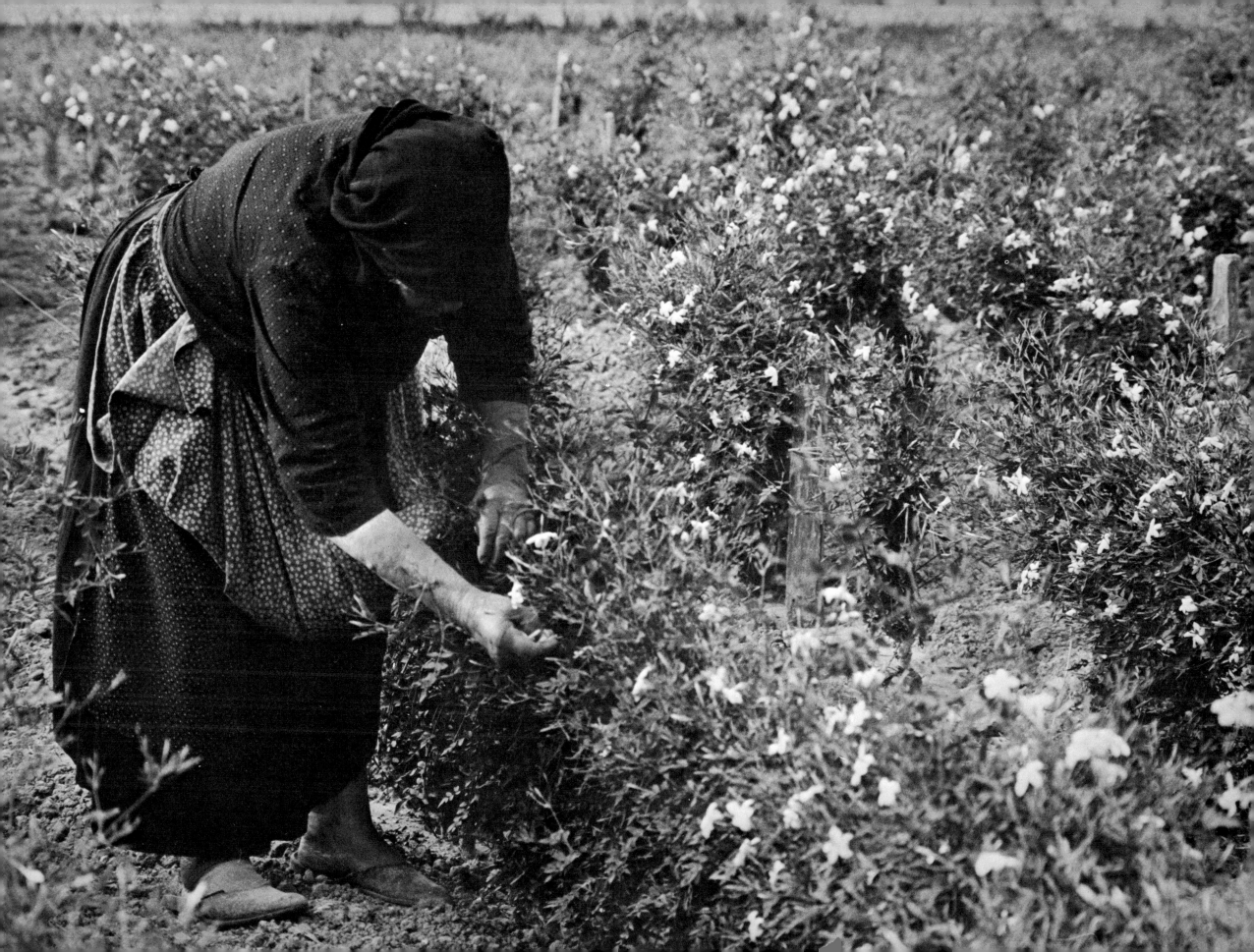

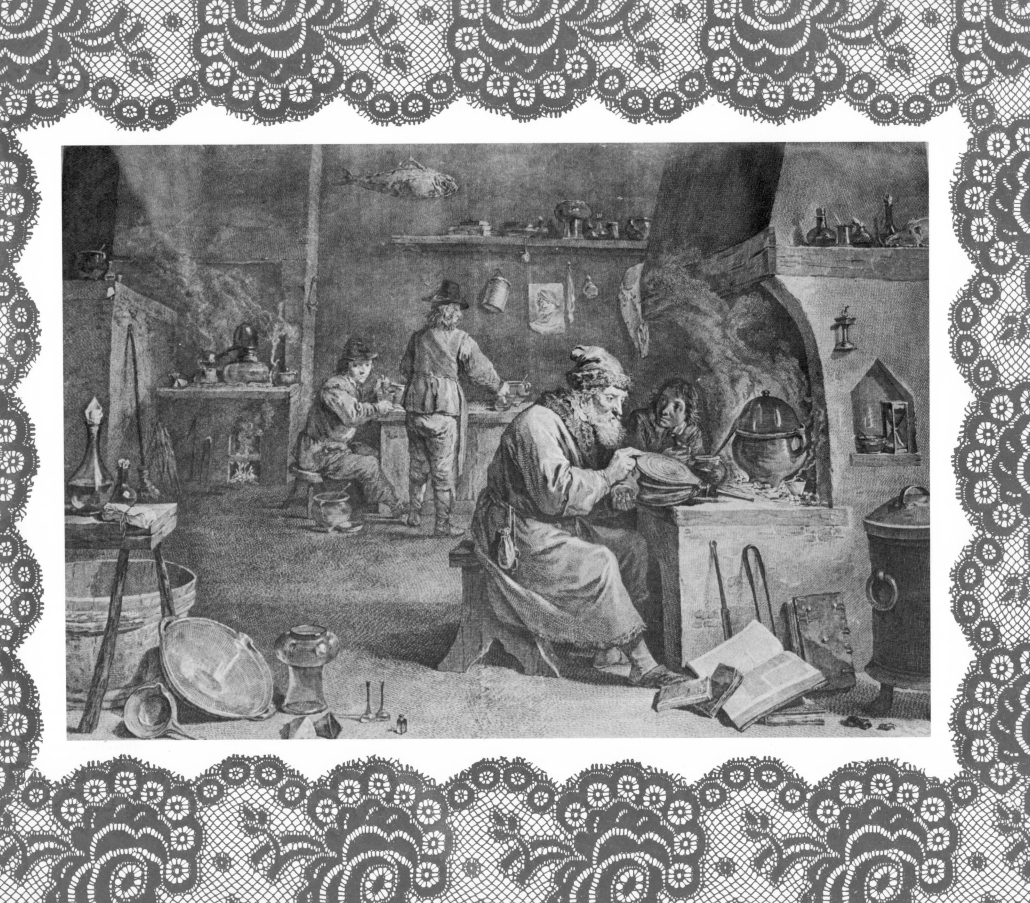

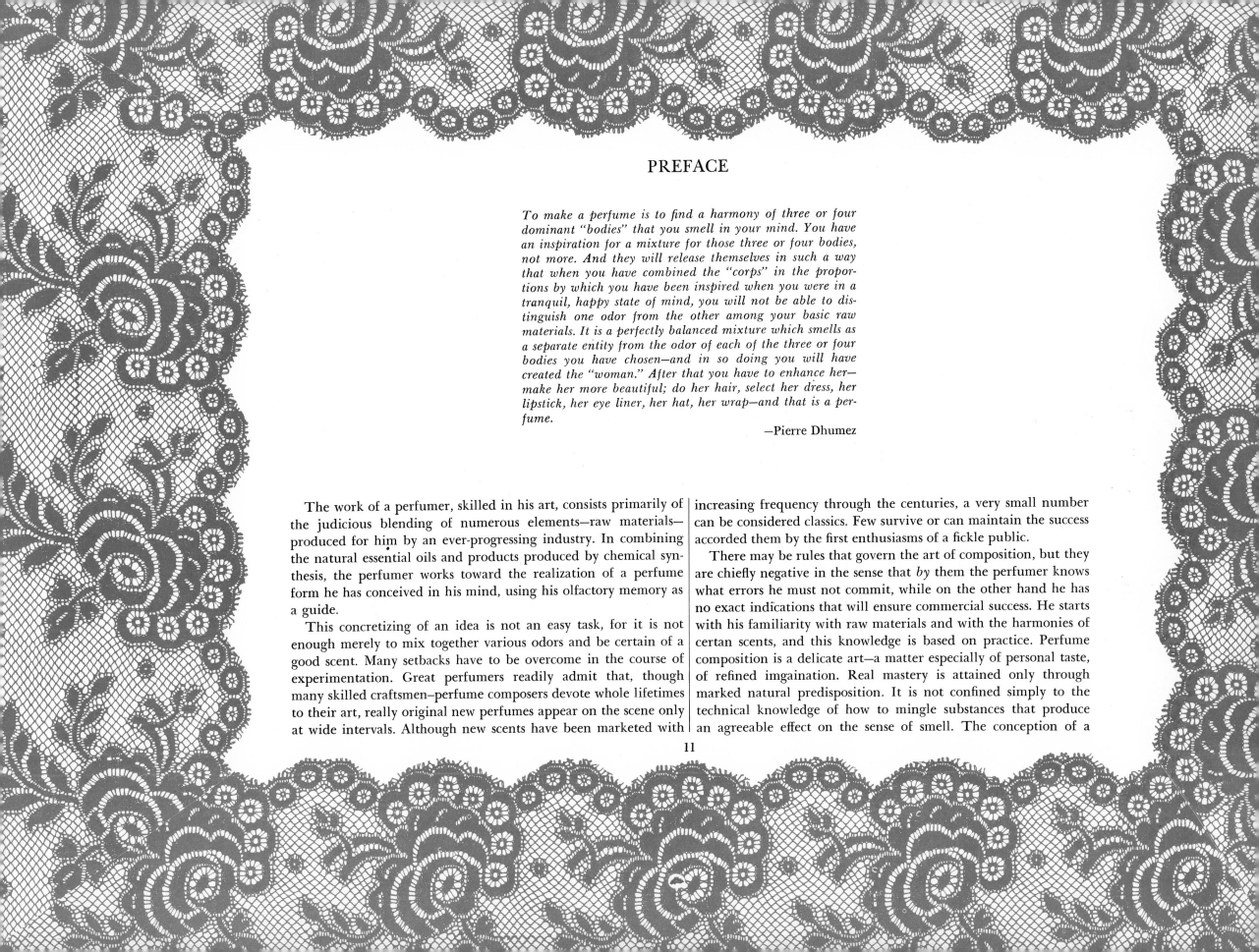

# PREFACE

*To make a perfume is to find a harmony of three or four dominant "bodies" that you smell in your mind. You have an inspiration for a mixture for those three or four bodies, not more. And they will release themselves in such a way that when you have combined the "corps" in the proportions by which you have been inspired when you were in a tranquil, happy state of mind, you will not be able to distinguish one odor from the other among your basic raw materials. It is a perfectly balanced mixture which smells as a separate entity from the odor of each of the three or four bodies you have chosen—and in so doing you will have created the "woman." After that you have to enhance her— make her more beautiful; do her hair, select her dress, her lipstick, her eye liner, her hat, her wrap—and that is a perfume.*

—Pierre Dhumez

The work of a perfumer, skilled in his art, consists primarily of the judicious blending of numerous elements—raw materials— produced for him by an ever-progressing industry. In combining the natural essential oils and products produced by chemical synthesis, the perfumer works toward the realization of a perfume form he has conceived in his mind, using his olfactory memory as a guide.

This concretizing of an idea is not an easy task, for it is not enough merely to mix together various odors and be certain of a good scent. Many setbacks have to be overcome in the course of experimentation. Great perfumers readily admit that, though many skilled craftsmen–perfume composers devote whole lifetimes to their art, really original new perfumes appear on the scene only at wide intervals. Although new scents have been marketed with increasing frequency through the centuries, a very small number can be considered classics. Few survive or can maintain the success accorded them by the first enthusiasms of a fickle public.

There may be rules that govern the art of composition, but they are chiefly negative in the sense that *by* them the perfumer knows what errors he must not commit, while on the other hand he has no exact indications that will ensure commercial success. He starts with his familiarity with raw materials and with the harmonies of certan scents, and this knowledge is based on practice. Perfume composition is a delicate art—a matter especially of personal taste, of refined imgaination. Real mastery is attained only through marked natural predisposition. It is not confined simply to the technical knowledge of how to mingle substances that produce an agreeable effect on the sense of smell. The conception of a

11

perfume form, the blending of elements, the imagination of the perfumer during his experiments, are the criteria of the art of perfume creation.

What are the early steps and thoughts of the perfumer as he composes? The idea is generally suggested to him by some material in nature or from the world of science that can help him develop a fragrance possessing the following features: (1) high stability under evaporation—that is to say, unvarying aroma; (2) tenacity, almost without volatility; (3) originality, which is the special attribute of the new scent that most frequently derives its values from a new harmony or balance of raw materials.

These elements must then possess features that differentiate them from the smell of those perfumes that are already known (no doubt a new perfume might result from the blending, in fresh proportions, of elements already known, but this is a rare occurrence and the result merely of happy chance). Thus the perfumer who has come upon a new basic substance with a particular odor that pleases him will endeavor to blend it with another equally pleasing and another and another until his perfume possesses all the necessary features mentioned above. He will continue his work methodically, guided by two principal ideas: association of odors —he will seek out scents harmonizing with the original base—and then he will look for a second category of harmonizing substances which, by contrast, will support and strengthen the earlier part of his work. Naturally he must avoid the effect of violent contrasts, modifying them by using suitable proportions from a perfect harvest of synthetic substances that have newly made their appearance as well as various natural fragrances known to the perfumer for centuries.

In this way, using his olfactory judgment, the perfumer obtains the substance of his scent. This being achieved, the most important part of his search has been accomplished. There remains the imparting of "character" and the perfecting of the composition. For this he has the aid of more precise rules, for he knows that to

give the flowery note he has the whole range of natural plants: jasmine for the note of sweetness up to the final moment of evaporation; rose for incomparable freshness; neroli for its velvety charm; jonquil for its penetrating sharpness; tuberose for a vaporous and disturbing note.

The initial impression should always be fresh and vigorous. If the scent does not suggest the actual presence of the flowers, fruits, herbs—all things of nature that titillate the sense of smell—it should at least be a reminder of them. It is necessary for the perfumer to combine all the components to stimulate a heightened awareness of his new odor. This is where infusions of animal matter come in. Amber, musk, civet, castorium, all impart a warm and living sensuous note. To fix the fragrances completely, orris root, benzoin, oak moss, and many, many other products aid the perfume composer.

Perfumes have varying degrees of volatility and are more or less rapidly diffused in the air. The scent must be vaporized and thoroughly criticized. The proportions of the ingredients may need to be revised, and if the perfumer's own sense of smell is not completely satisfied, he may wish to introduce new raw materials or remove some which displease him. The perfumer blends aromas as a painter blends his colors, as a musician chooses his chord progressions. Finally the perfume is left alone for a certain period of time so that the perfumer can allow the perfume form to mature and so that he can gain a fresh impression of his results before he returns to work at his "organ" of perfume materials.

This scent is a mixture of odorant substances selected and measured in proportionate degree in such a way as to create agreeable smelling sensations. But the appreciation of the scent is essentially a subjective thing. This subjective taste itself is prey to certain influences that qualify, modify, and sometimes transform it. The determining factor most frequently is fashion; the scent in vogue imposes itself on the public taste. Is it the perfume composer who creates this fashion, or is his part limited to expressing in scent a

## BÉLIER
...CAN : *du 21 au 31 Mars*
...LIPE – PHÉNIX – HOUX
...DÉCAN : *du 1er au 9 Avril*
...UL – TÊTE DE BÉLIER – PERSIL
...CAN : *du 10 au 20 Avril*
...UCINE – CAMÉE – GAZON

## TAUREAU
...CAN : *du 21 au 30 Avril*
...LAS – VIOLE – AUBÉPINE
...CAN : *du 1er au 9 Mai*
... – ROSSIGNOL – TAMARIS
...CAN : *du 10 au 20 Mai*
...RE – SCARABÉE – OLIVIER

## GÉMEAUX
...CAN : *du 21 au 31 Mai*
...ER – SPHINX – LE TRÉPIED
...CAN : *du 1er au 10 Juin*
...NNIA – MASQUE, MAIN
LES LOSANGES
...CAN : *du 11 au 21 Juin*
...ISSE – LICORNE – LAURIER

## CANCER
...CAN : *du 22 Juin au 1er Juillet*
...RIN – PÉLICAN – YUCCA
...CAN : *du 2 au 11 Juillet*
...M – CYGNE – LUNAIRE
...CAN : *du 12 au 22 Juillet*
...HAR – CRAPAUD – ROSEAU

## LION
...N : *du 23 Juillet au 1er Août*
...SOL – ABEILLE – PLATANE
...CAN : *du 2 au 11 Août*
...ROSA – AIGLE – PALMIER
...CAN : *du 12 au 22 Août*
...YLLIS – LION – ACANTHE

## VIERGE
... : *du 23 Août au 2 Septembre*
...RITE, CIGALE, VIGNE VIERGE
...CAN : *du 3 au 12 Septembre*
...NIUM – CORNE D'ABONDANCE
BLÉ
...CAN : *du 13 au 22 Septembre*

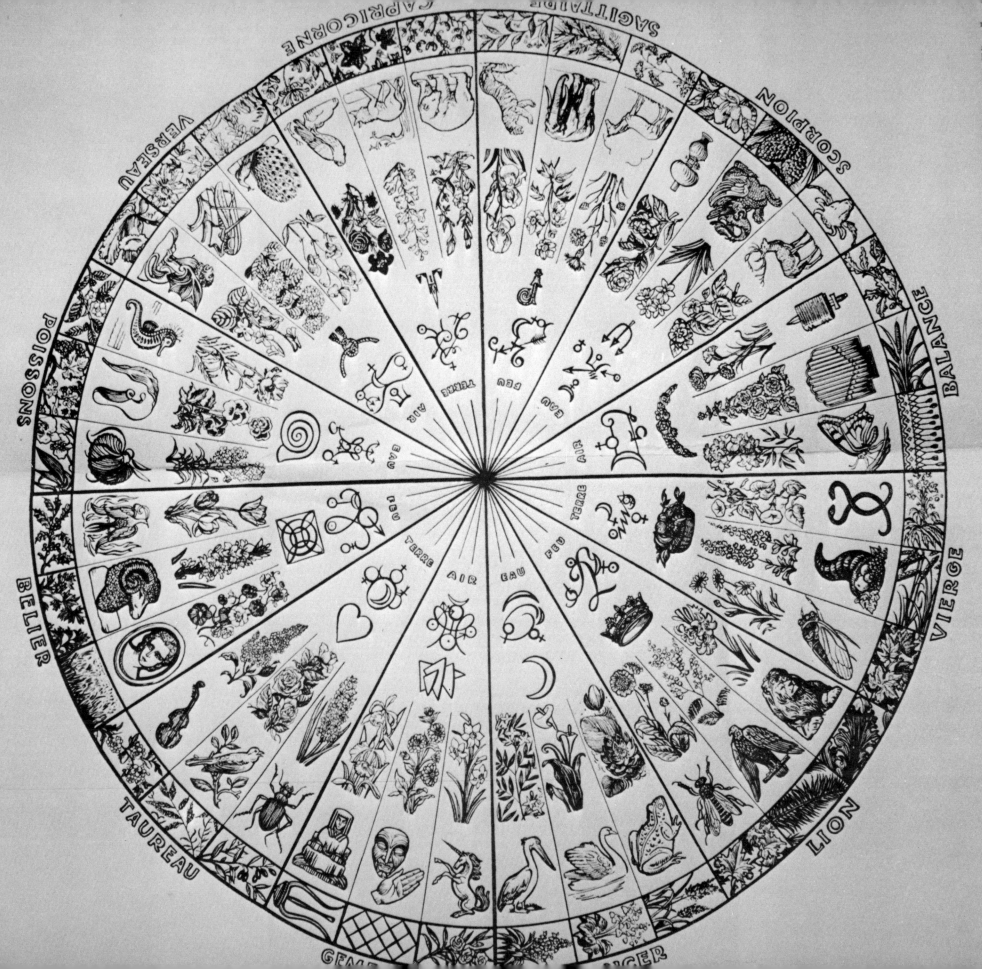

## SCORPIO(N)
1er DÉCAN : *du 23 Octob. au 2 No...*
BÉGONIA – CERF – TÊTE DE ...
2me DÉCAN : *du 3 au 12 No...*
ASPHODÈLE, DRAGON, POMMES D...
3me DÉCAN : *du 13 au 22 No...*
CAMÉLIA – LAMPE – MAGNO...

## SAGITTA(IRE)
1er DÉCAN : *du 22 Nov. au 1er D...*
BLEUET – CHEVAL – FÈ...
2me DÉCAN : *du 2 au 11 D...*
ANÉMONE – ÉLÉPHANT – C...
3me DÉCAN : *du 12 au 21 D...*
IRIS – TIGRE – FUSAI...

## CAPRICO(RNE)
1er DÉCAN : *du 22 au 31 ...*
GENTIANE – OURS – ...
2me DÉCAN : *du 1er au ...*
GUEULE DE LOUP – LOUP – ...
3me DÉCAN : *du 11 au 2...*
FLEURS NOIRES – EPER...
CHÈVREFEUILLE

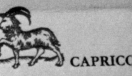

## VERS(EAU)
1er DÉCAN : *du 21 au ...*
POIS DE SENTEUR – PAON – ...
2me DÉCAN : *du 1er au ...*
HORTENSIA, SAUTERELLE ...
3me DÉCAN : *du 10 au 2...*
VIOLETTE – CHIMÈRE...

## POI(SSONS)
1er DÉCAN : *du 20 ...*
PAVOT – HIPPOCAM...
2me DÉCAN : *du 1er au ...*
PENSÉE – NÉPANTHE...
3me DÉCAN : *du 10 ...*
GIROFLÉE, NAUTILE...

preference for fragrance which he feels is more or less indicated, even dictated, by his customers? It must be admitted that there *is* a fashion in perfumery and that it is a perfumer's concern, if not to direct it, at least to reckon with it in his creations—a delicate and a subtle assignment which is not, despite careful stratagems, invariably crowned with success. Therefore, at the very start it is difficult to judge a scent—a difficulty that springs from the diversity of likes and dislikes in an age of constant evolution in consumer acceptance. Basically, the examination of a good scent produces a new pleasant sensation, while that of an ordinary scent gives nothing but the confused impression that results from an unsatisfactory mixture.

It has been said that "a new scent does more for the happiness of mankind than the discovery of a new star." The perfumer who has faith in his calling is never really satisfied; he never stops reaching for the star. The quest for perfumes is the subject of his intense personal application. Every day technical skill is producing new odors, materials of many kinds that furnish in and of themselves a pleasant odor; it is the task of the perfumer to employ them tastefully, to achieve beautiful results.

What is a synthetic in the world of perfume? It is a compound that is the complete and exact reproduction of a natural product in its nature and scent. It must not be confused with the word "artificial," by which is meant a compound that has a scent identical or close to a natural fragrance but which differs in constitution from that of the natural product. It must be acknowledged that, thanks to science, perfumes, which were formerly luxuries, have become available to all. Modern perfumery owes much to chemistry, but synthetic, artificial raw materials for perfume manufacture made by chemistry can never take the place of natural essences, nor are they intended to do so. Synthetic products are valuable auxiliaries by reason of the originality of their odor. It is necessary to use them in the creation of both luxury perfumes and more ordinary scents. Synthetics assist the perfumer to produce the most exquisite and renowned creations. One of the great men of perfumery described his industry best when he advanced the thought that it is a business of selling dreams and hope. Yes, dreams and hope. That is the end product. But it is the beginning, too.

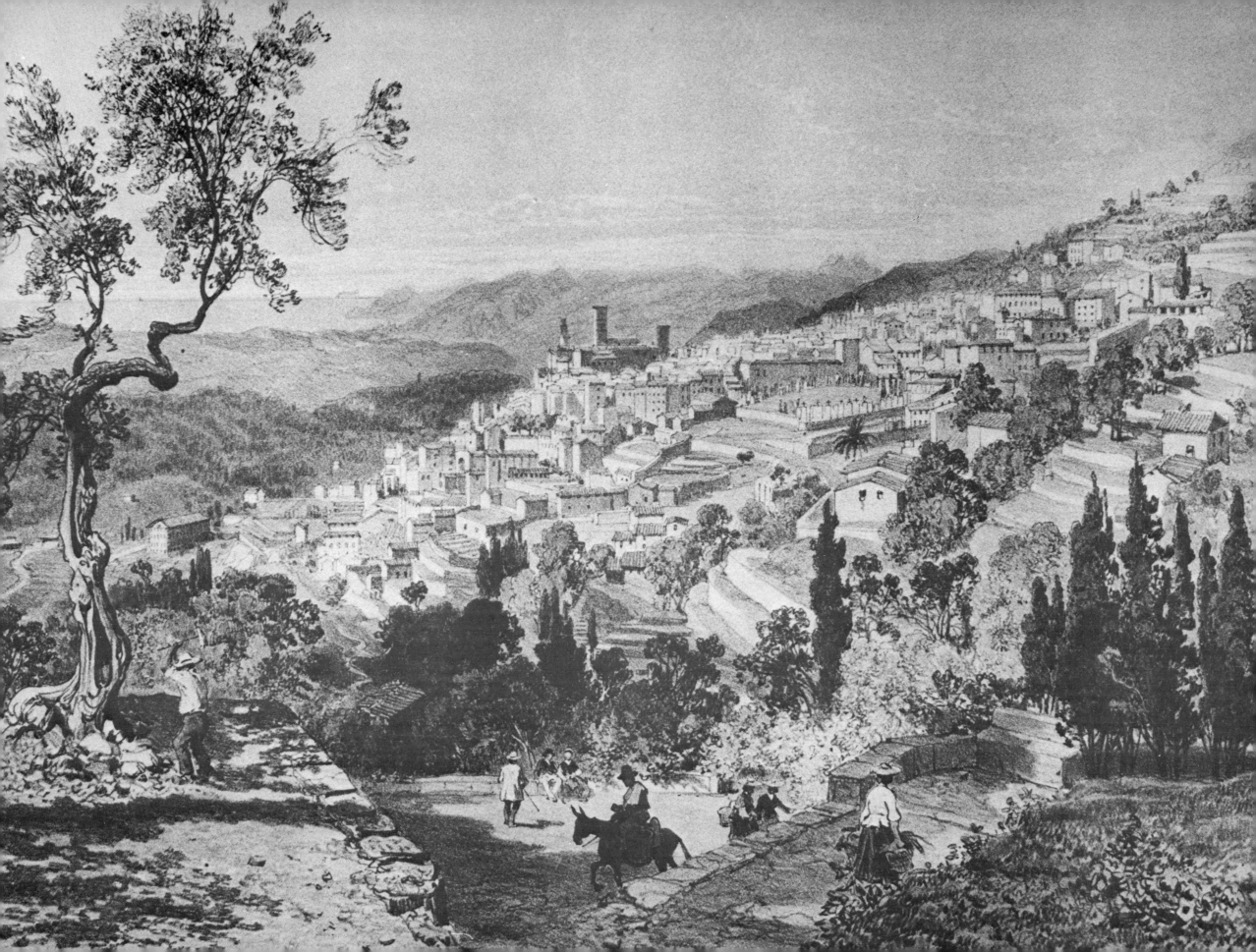

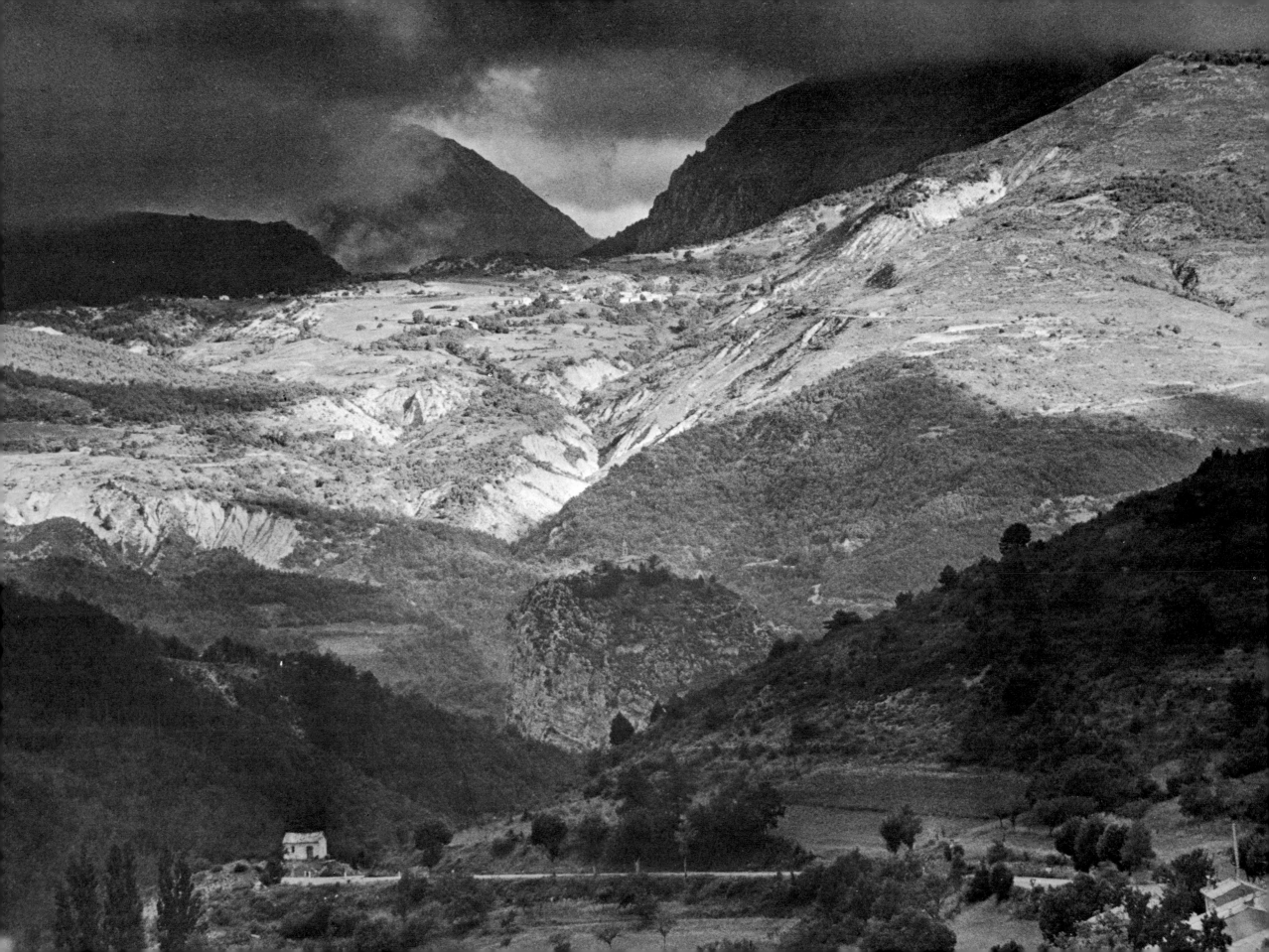

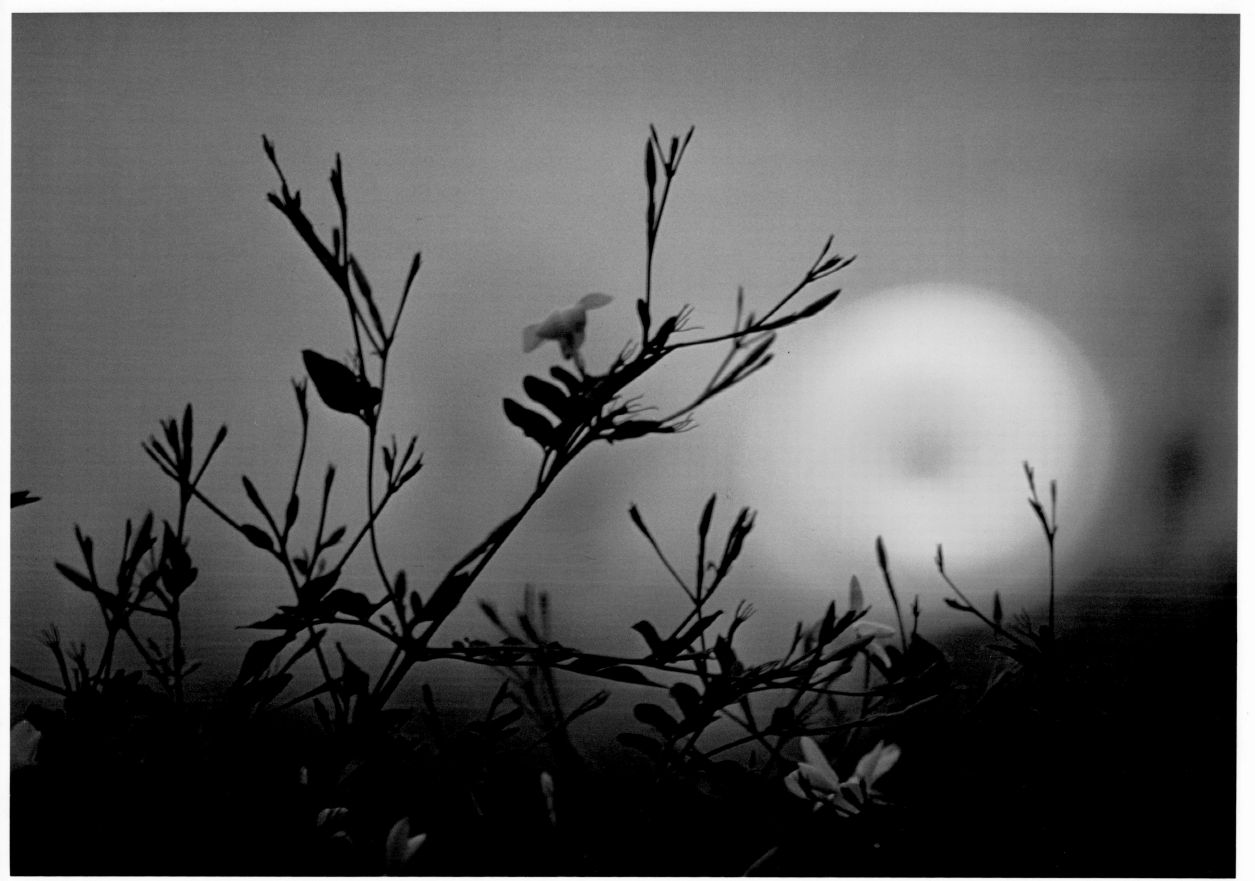

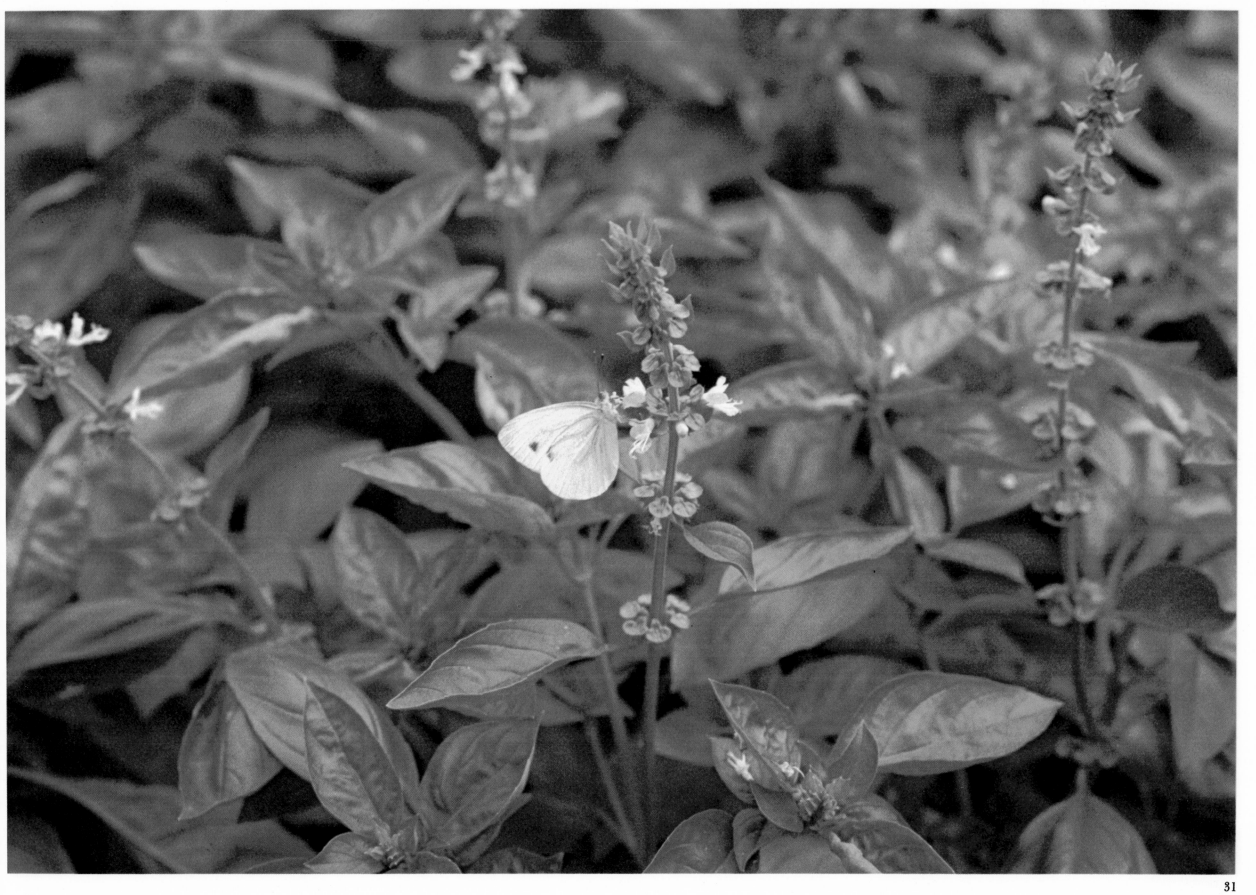

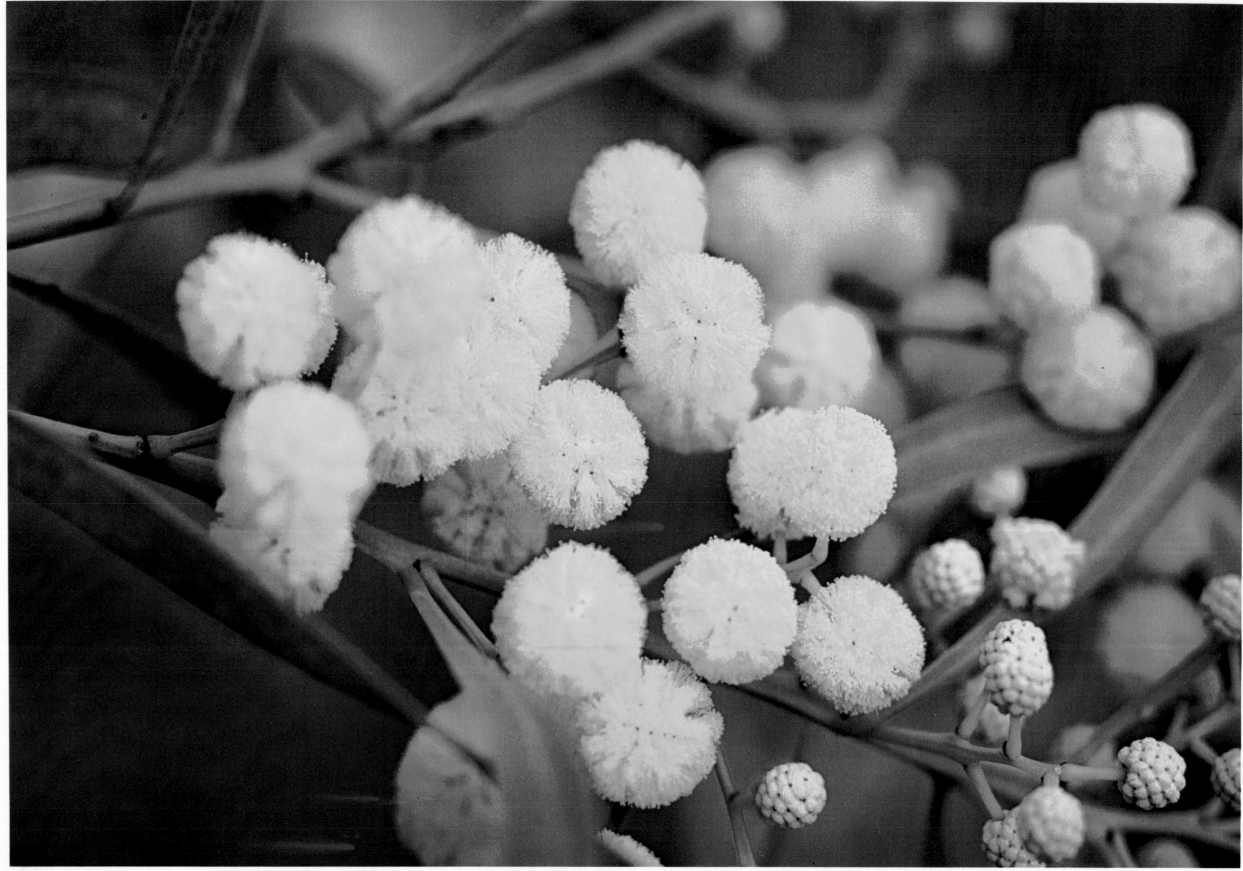

# PERFUME

## . . . and in the beginning

Perfume!!!!!

The very word fires the imagination with visions . . . the mystique of ancient religions, the eroticism of the Thousand and One Arabian Nights, the sultriness of the Dark Continent, the elusiveness of the Orient, the fragrance of the South of France.

> *And the Lord God planted a garden eastward in Eden. . . . And out of the ground made the Lord God to grow every tree that is pleasant to the sight . . . and every plant of the field before it grew, and every herb of the field before it grew.*
> —*Genesis 2*

The history of perfume parallels the history of mankind. From the time of Creation man has been conscious of the sweet smells and essences of flowers that have stimulated and pleased, and we think of Paradise as a place of fragrance.

Scholars place the Garden of Eden in the land of Mesopotamia lying between the Tigris and Euphrates. It is most beautifully envisioned by the poet Milton in *Paradise Lost:*

> *In this pleasant soil*
> *His far more pleasant garden God ordained.*
> *Out of the fertile ground he caused to grow*
> *All trees of noblest kind for sight, smell, taste. . . .*
> *Laurel and myrtle, and what higher grew*
> *Of firm and fragrant leaf: on either side*
> *Acanthus, and each odorous bushy shrub,*
> *Fenced up the verdant wall: each beauteous flower,*
> *Iris, all hues, roses and jasmine,*
> *Reared high their flourished heads between, and wrought*
> *Mosaic: underfoot the violet,*
> *Crocus, and hyacinth, with rich inlay*
> *Broidered the ground, more coloured than with stone*
> *Of costliest emblem*

The word "perfume" means "through smoke," and for primitive rites and in Biblical times perfume in the form of incense was used. "Perfume" consisted of various spices reduced to a fine powder and compounded for the purpose of honoring the deities, curing the sick, embalming the dead, and glorifying the human form.

Ancient doctors classified perfumes among medicines and prescribed them for many diseases, especially those affecting the nervous system.

Pliny in his *Natural History* mentions eighty-four remedies derived from rue, forty-one from mint, twenty-five from pennyroyal, forty-one from the iris, thirty-two from the rose, twenty-one from the lily, seventeen from the violet.

In the celebration of Egyptian religious festivals the burning of perfume ranked as the highest form of homage to their many gods. Originally ointments and fragrant oils utilized by the Egyptians were dispensed by the high priests, who might easily be called the world's first manufacturing perfumers.

Part of the embalming ritual in ancient Egypt consisted of filling the body with sawdust of fragrant woods and wrapping it in linen bands that had been dipped in essences. The skin was rubbed with cedar oil and myrrh.

Myrrh is probably the earliest aromatic gum of which we have a document; it is mentioned in several antique papyruses. One such, written about 2000 B.C. and housed in the Hermitage Museum in Leningrad, contains the following passage:

> *I will cause to be brought unto thee fine oils and choice perfumes, and the incense of the temples, whereby every god is gladdened. Of myrrh hast thou not much; all that thou hast is but common incense. Ashipu came and delivered me, and he gave me a shipload of myrrh, fine oil, divers perfumes, eye paint, and the tails of giraffes.*

Though perfumes were employed copiously for devotions, even greater quantities were used for cosmetic purposes. The Egyptians were extremely interested in hygiene and were the first to organize a system of baths, later to become the basis of the opulent thermal palaces constructed by the Greeks and the Romans. It was customary for the Egyptian to lubricate his body with scented oils and pomades after his ablutions. Myrrh, cinnamon, galbanum, as well as many other spices and substances, are mentioned in a papyrus from about 2000 B.C. that contains a recipe for making pastilles to perfume the breath.

Some Egyptian aromatics came from native soil, but the larger proportion of the essential ingredients used for perfume, such as myrrh and frankincense, came from Arabia. They were preserved and transported in bottles and vases of alabaster, onyx, glass, and other hard substances. The Egyptians made wood and ivory boxes, carved with fish and birds, to hold their cosmetics. Compartmented for the diverse preparations, they differed only slightly from those used by today's women.

To beautify themselves, the women of Egypt painted their eyebrows and underlined their eyes. Different types of eye cosmetic were used according to the season of the year, but it was considered absolutely necessary to cover the eyelids entirely with an ointment at least once each day. Lips and cheeks were always rouged, and women of high station stained their fingernails, toenails, and the soles of their feet with a reddish-yellow henna juice.

The most important perfume used by the Egyptians was *kyphi*. Scholars claim that when the tomb of Tutankhamen was opened, it was this odor that issued forth. So great was the renown of this toiletry that its use was later adopted by the Greeks and Romans. It is mentioned in the writings of the ancients, Dioscorides, Democritus, and Galen. Plutarch lists sixteen ingredients of this product, among which were honey, wine, cypress, raisins, myrrh, aspalathus, seseli, sthoenanthus, saffron, dock, juniper, cardamom, and aromatic reeds. He is quoted as saying: "Its aromatic substances lull to sleep, allay anxieties, and brighten the dreams. It is made of things that delight most in the night and exhibit their virtues by night."

Other cosmetics, compounded by the high priests and distributed by them, were highly favored *psagdi*, a perfumed ointment; *mendesium*, composed of oil of ben, myrrh, and canella; and *metopium*, made from almonds, honey, wine resin, myrrh, and calamus. *Aegyptium*, a perfumed ointment for the hands and feet, was much in demand. *Cyprinum* was tinted green with the extract of henna flowers and strongly impregnated with the scent of cinnamon.

Egyptian enthusiasm for perfumes and cosmetics is said to have reached its zenith during the reign of Cleopatra. Shakespeare pictures her excesses in this fashion:

> *The barge she sat in, like a burnished throne,*
> *Burn'd on the water; the poop was beaten gold,*
> *Purple the sails, and so perfumed that*
> *The winds were love-sick . . .*
> —*Antony and Cleopatra*

Released from captivity in Egypt, the Hebrews brought to their homeland the many skills they had acquired as slaves. One of these techniques was the art of perfumery. Directions for making the holy anointing oil are found in the Old Testament:

> *Take thou also unto thee principal spices, of pure myrrh five hundred shekels, and of sweet cinnamon half so much, even two hundred and fifty shekels, and of sweet calamus two hundred and fifty shekels.*
> *And of cassia five hundred shekels, after the shekel of the sanctuary, and of oil olive an hin.*
> *And thou shalt make it an oil of holy ointment, an ointment compounded after the art of the apothecary; it shall be an holy anointing oil.*
> —*Exodus 30: 23–25*

(A shekel was about half an ounce; a hin a little more than a gallon . . . in some translations the word "perfumer" occurs instead of "apothecary," for in those times both professions were combined in one.)

This oil served to make holy the tabernacle, the ark of the covenant, the altar of burnt offerings, the altar of incense, the candlesticks, and all the sacred vessels. It was also used to consecrate Aaron and his sons, conferring upon them perpetual priesthood from generation to generation.

As ordained by Hebrew Law, purification of women required the use of perfumes in great profusion. The first six months of the year this ritual was accomplished with oil of myrrh and the latter six months with other sweet odors.

Esther, desiring the freedom of her people, underwent this purification rite prior to appearing before King Ahasuerus, oppressor of the Jews, and perfumes were employed by Judith when she went forth to seduce Holofernes in his tent.

> *She pulled off the sackcloth which she had on, and put off the garments of her widowhood, and washed her body all over with water, and anointed herself with precious ointment, and braided the hair of her head and put a tie upon it, and put on her garment of gladness, wherewith she was clad during the life of Manasses, her husband.*
> *And she took sandals upon her feet, and put about her bracelets, her chains and rings, and her earrings and all her ornaments, and decked herself bravely, to allure the eye of all men that should see her.*
> —*Judith 10:3, 4*

The most complete description of the aromatics in use by the Hebrews is to be found in The Song of Solomon. It is true that symbolic meaning has been ascribed to this great poem, but even if taken in the figurative sense, the frequent mention of perfumes indicates that they must have been well-known and much appreciated at the Hebrew court.

The most luxurious and costly perfumes were reserved for use on the couches. In Proverbs 7:17 we read, "I have perfumed my bed with myrrh, aloes, and cinnamon." Nature was very kind to the land of Judea, and all about the prairies aromatic plants and shrubs abounded.

Traditionally the Hebrews anointed the heads of their guests to honor them. Undoubtedly one of the most familiar instances of this practice is the description of Jesus of Nazareth sitting at the table in Bethany in the house of Simon the leper:

> . . . As he sat at meat, there came a woman having an alabaster box of ointment of spikenard very precious; and she brake the box, and poured it on his head.
>
> —St. Mark 14:3

Not content with their natural personal attractions, Jewish women enhanced themselves, as did their Egyptian counterparts, with various cosmetics, particularly kohl for lining the eyes. A recipe for this kohl, which has been in use since the time of the ancient Egyptians, has come down to us in the following formula:

> Remove the inside of a lemon, fill it up with plumbago and burnt copper. Place it on the fire until it becomes carbonized. Then pound it in a mortar with coral, sandalwood, pearls, ambergris, the wing of a bat, and part of the body of a chameleon which has been previously burned to a cinder and moistened with rose water while hot.

Whether or not the Hebrews composed their eye cosmetics with this instruction, we do not know, but ancient writings tell us that Jezebel resorted to the seductive powers of kohl when she awaited Jehu.

Kings of Assyria offered incense and libations of wine before the altar of the sacred Tree of Life. Herodotus states that frankincense in the amount of a thousand talents' weight was used every year during the feast of the sun god Baal, in the rituals held on the great altar in the Temple of Babylon. Arabia alone furnished

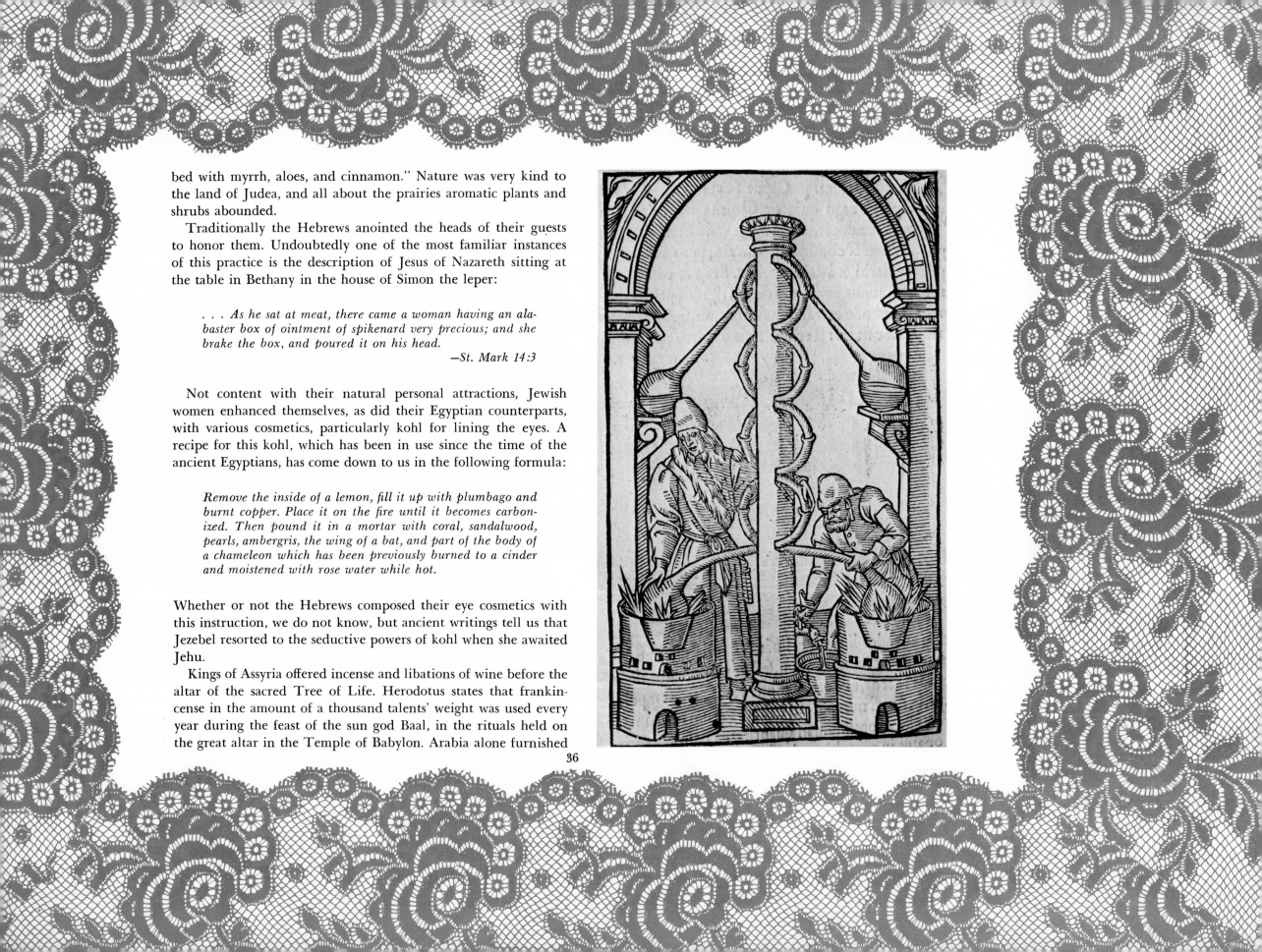

an annual tribute of a thousand talents of this precious perfume. Assyrians were strongly attracted to scent and used it so lavishly that, although the land was rich in aromatics needed as raw materials for the creation of fragrance, supplies of additional spices had to be imported each year from nearby territories.

Antiochus Epiphanes (175–163 B.C.), king of Syria, shared his love of fragrance with the populace. It is recorded that during the games at Daphne two hundred women were employed to sprinkle spectators with perfume from golden vessels during one of the royal processions. In a similar parade boys arrayed in purple tunics bore golden dishes of frankincense, myrrh, and saffron. They were followed by two incense burners, six cubits in height, made of ivy wood covered with gold and flanking a large square golden altar that stood in the center. Everyone who entered the arena was anointed with some perfume selected from one of the fifteen golden dishes, each filled with a different aromatic, such as cinnamon, spikenard, fenugreek, amarancas, lilies, and guests were coiffed with garlands of myrrh.

Hedonism appears to have reached new heights in the time of Assyrian King Ashurbanipal (669–626 B.C.), who not only painted his face with vermilion and made substantial use of cosmetics, but was known to affect feminine garb whenever possible.

According to Athenaeus, Alexander the Great (356–323 B.C.) rebelled at first at such excesses, but later on, having savored the fragrances of his enemies, he ordered the floors of his apartments to be sprinkled with perfumes. Myrrh and other sweet-smelling gums burned in his halls, and his tunics were soaked with scents.

Babylon was the world's principal market for the perfume trade. The Assyrians were skilled in the art of glassmaking and kept their essences in flacons or alabaster vases. They perfumed their bodies and burned sweet-smelling woods in their homes, and their Babylonian rivals quickly surpassed the art of their teachers.

Medes were as skilled as Babylonians in the art of making perfumes and cosmetics. The Greek historian Xenophon (c.430 B.C.–

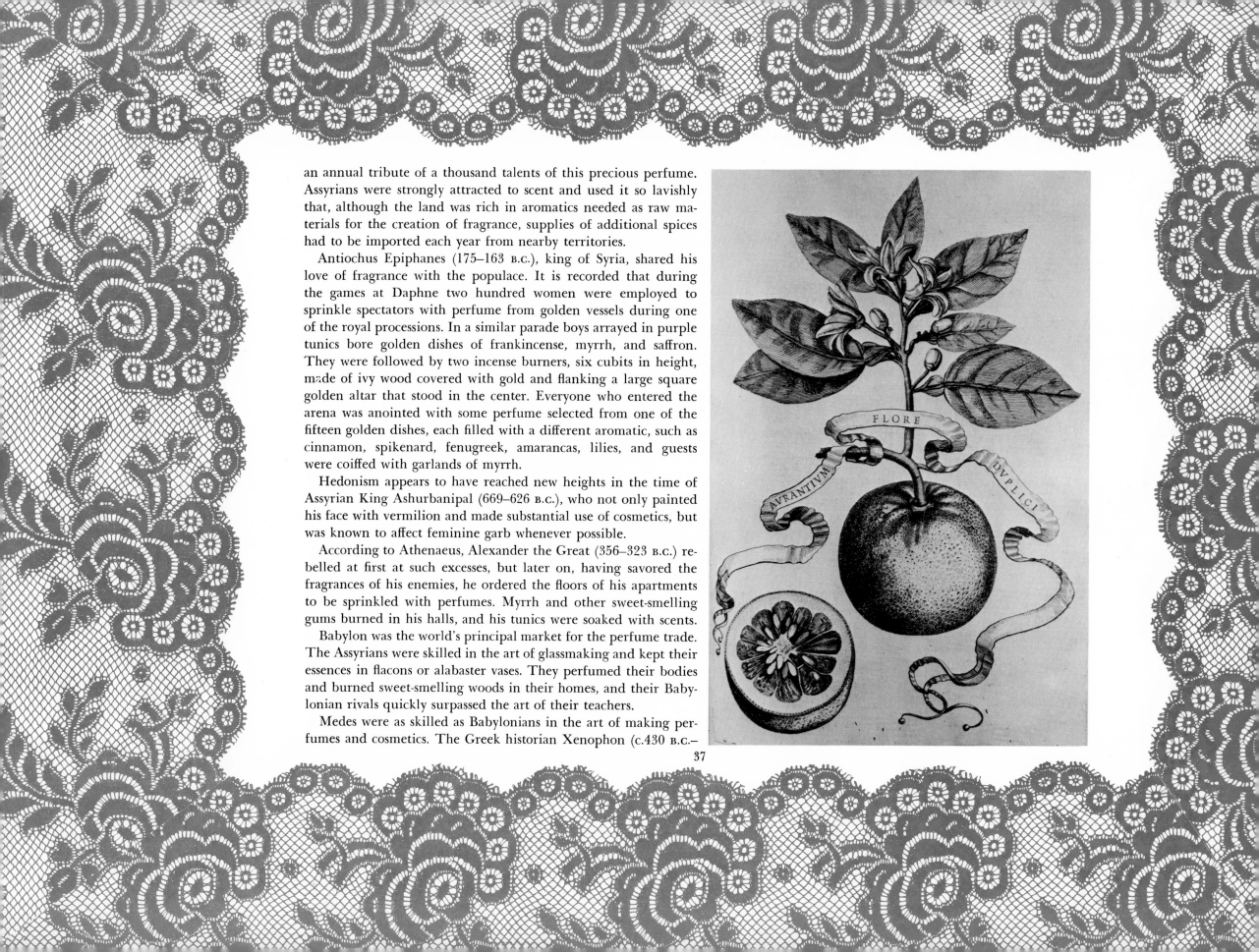

37

c.355 B.C.) in his work *Cyropaedia* tells that Cyrus, at the age of twelve, went with his mother to visit Astyages, the king. He saw his grandfather adorned with painted eyes, color on his face, coiffed in a luxuriant wig of flowering ringlets. The boy, believing all to be real, turned to his parent in utter admiration. "Oh, Mother, how handsome my grandfather is!"

In chainlike sequence Persians borrowed from the Medes their taste for perfume and cosmetics in their sacred and secular life. They were conscious of fragrance in its every phase. Their kings spent the sultry summers at Ecbatana but in winter resided at a palace named Susa, after the beautiful lily, "souson." Persians habitually wore crowns made of myrrh entwined with a sweet-smelling plant called labyzus.

Very early in their history they took special delight in the rose (*gul*). It was not uncommon at great feasts to have rose petals spread over the carpets and on the reclining couches. One of the most famous pieces of Persian literature chants a hymn of praise to this much-loved flower.

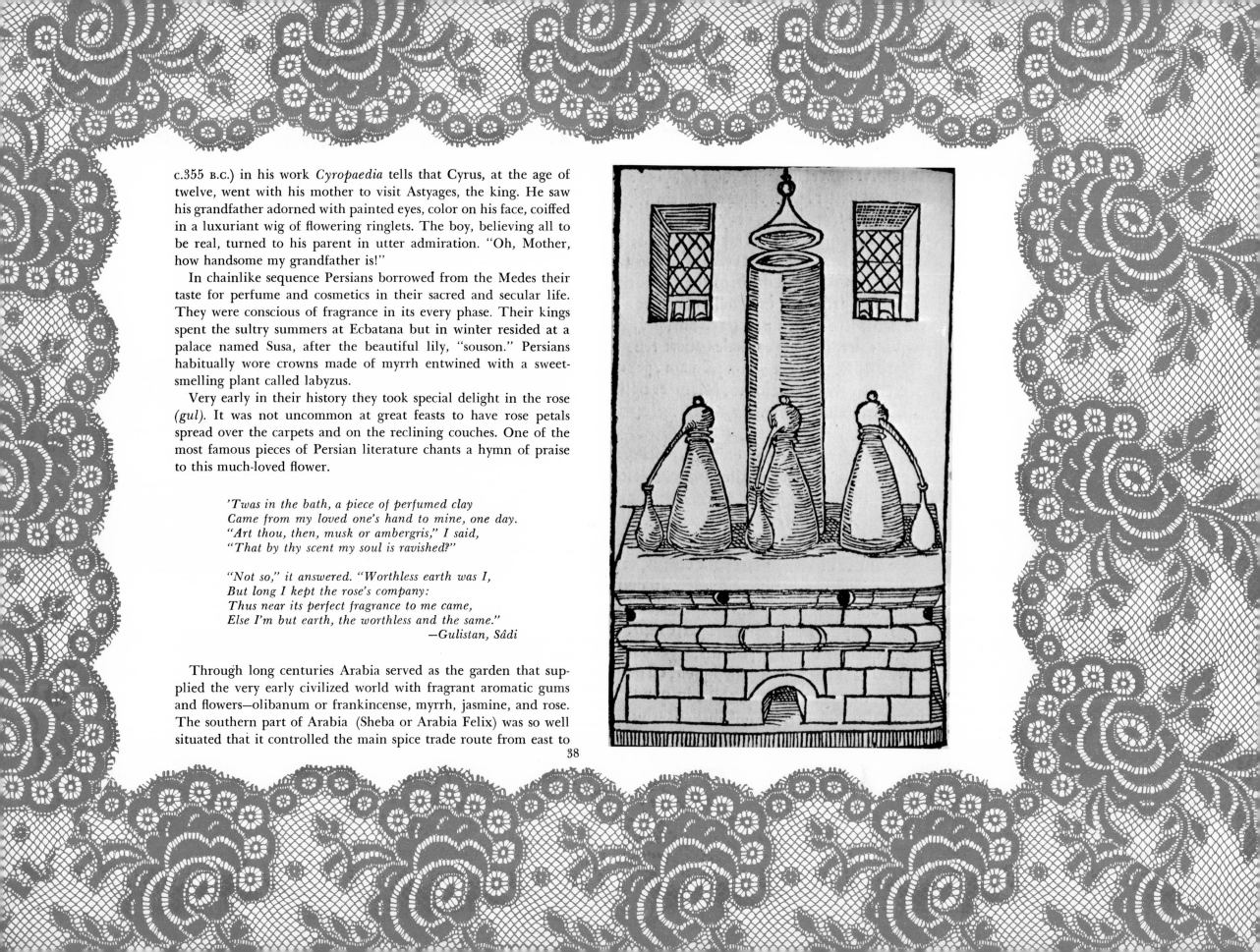

> *'Twas in the bath, a piece of perfumed clay*
> *Came from my loved one's hand to mine, one day.*
> *"Art thou, then, musk or ambergris," I said,*
> *"That by thy scent my soul is ravished?"*
>
> *"Not so," it answered. "Worthless earth was I,*
> *But long I kept the rose's company:*
> *Thus near its perfect fragrance to me came,*
> *Else I'm but earth, the worthless and the same."*
> —Gulistan, Sâdi

Through long centuries Arabia served as the garden that supplied the very early civilized world with fragrant aromatic gums and flowers—olibanum or frankincense, myrrh, jasmine, and rose. The southern part of Arabia (Sheba or Arabia Felix) was so well situated that it controlled the main spice trade route from east to

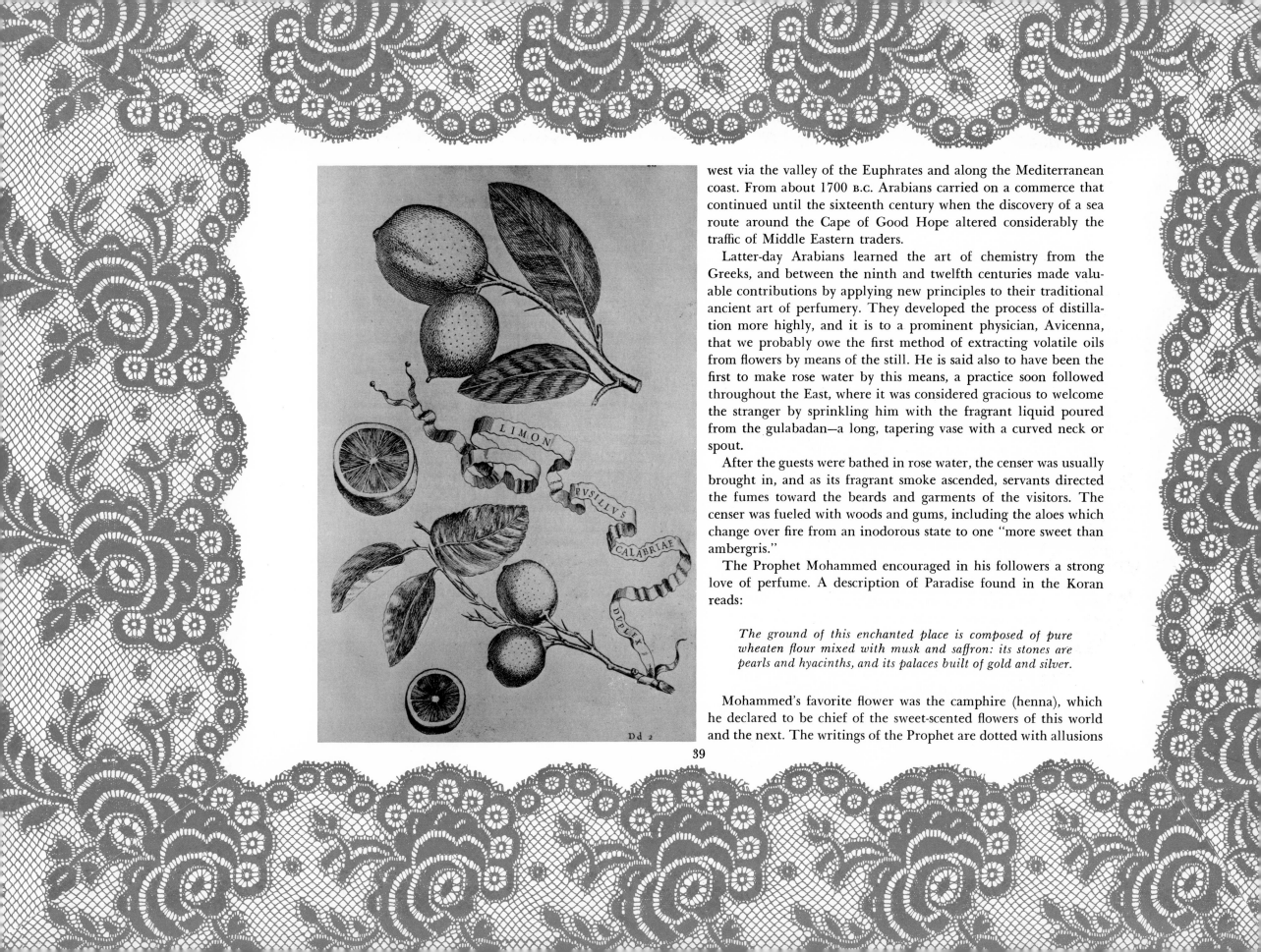

west via the valley of the Euphrates and along the Mediterranean coast. From about 1700 B.C. Arabians carried on a commerce that continued until the sixteenth century when the discovery of a sea route around the Cape of Good Hope altered considerably the traffic of Middle Eastern traders.

Latter-day Arabians learned the art of chemistry from the Greeks, and between the ninth and twelfth centuries made valuable contributions by applying new principles to their traditional ancient art of perfumery. They developed the process of distillation more highly, and it is to a prominent physician, Avicenna, that we probably owe the first method of extracting volatile oils from flowers by means of the still. He is said also to have been the first to make rose water by this means, a practice soon followed throughout the East, where it was considered gracious to welcome the stranger by sprinkling him with the fragrant liquid poured from the gulabadan—a long, tapering vase with a curved neck or spout.

After the guests were bathed in rose water, the censer was usually brought in, and as its fragrant smoke ascended, servants directed the fumes toward the beards and garments of the visitors. The censer was fueled with woods and gums, including the aloes which change over fire from an inodorous state to one "more sweet than ambergris."

The Prophet Mohammed encouraged in his followers a strong love of perfume. A description of Paradise found in the Koran reads:

> *The ground of this enchanted place is composed of pure wheaten flour mixed with musk and saffron: its stones are pearls and hyacinths, and its palaces built of gold and silver.*

Mohammed's favorite flower was the camphire (henna), which he declared to be chief of the sweet-scented flowers of this world and the next. The writings of the Prophet are dotted with allusions

39

to blossoms. He commented on the origin of the rose, and referring to the violet, he says:

*The excellence of the extract of the violets, above all other extracts, is as the excellence of me above all the rest of creation: it is cold in summer and hot in winter. The excellence of violet is as the excellence of El Islam above all other religions.*

Rival of the violet is myrtle, and again according to the Prophet:

*Adam fell down from Paradise with three things: the myrtle, the chief of sweet scented flowers in this world; an ear of wheat, which is the chief of all kinds of foods in this world; and pressed dates, which are the chief of the fruits of this world.*

Arabian women selected their cosmetics from a large number of preparations. There was *hemsia,* an almond unguent used as a cleansing cream or pressed into the navel to avoid dryness and unpleasant odors. There was a tooth powder called *souek,* made from the bark of the walnut tree. They employed *termentina,* a thick paste depilatory containing turpentine, and set much store by a face cream, a *schnouda,* composed of jasmine pomade and benzoin. They created *kourss,* a pastille made from musk and ambergris paste, which they burned in a censer to perfume the boudoir. Often ladies of the harem would roll the pastilles in their hands, fashion them into beads, string them, and wear them around the neck or ankles.

Divine origin was attributed to perfume by the imaginative Greeks. Their deities revitalized themselves with ambrosia and nectar—food unknown to mortals. Special perfumes were reserved for the exclusive use of these deities. Homer conveys to us his conception of Juno at her toilette:

*Here first she bathes, and round her body pours
Soft oils of fragrance, and ambrosial showers.
The winds, perfumed, the balmy gale convoys
Through heaven, through earth and all the aerial ways.
Spirit Divine! whose exhalation greets
The sense of gods with more than mortal sweets.*
—Iliad, *Chapter XIV*

In Greek literature women were depicted as magicians—persons most skilled in the preparation of perfumes. They were thought to possess mystic powers, and thus we have Circe detaining Ulysses on her isle by casting spells of sweet smokes—fumigations that intoxicated his senses; we have Medea boiling old Eson in an aromatic bath and transforming him into a perfect juvenile.

According to myth, it was the nymph Oenone who revealed to Paris some of the secrets of Venus's beauty, and it was by means of these "heavenly cosmetics" that Helen of Troy acquired the radiance that eventually proved so fatal to the Greeks.

An interesting poem by Antiphanes reflects the fact that special perfumes were used for special parts of the body, a practice particularly common to Greek athletes.

*He really bathes
In a large gilded tub, and steeps his feet
And legs in rich Egyptian unguents;
His jaws and breasts he rubs with thick palm oil,
And both his arms with extract sweet of mint:
His eyebrows and his hair with marjoram,
His knees and neck with essence of ground thyme.*

Homer alludes to the custom of offering dinner guests a bath after which they were rubbed with sweet ointments and conducted to the banquet hall. During the feasts perfume was brought in alabaster or gold bottles, and there were garlands of flowers to crown those present, as in the days of Babylonian luxury.

Socrates strongly disapproved of all this excessive love of perfume manifested by the men of his country. He wrote:

> No man is ever anointed with perfume for the sake of men, and as to women, how can they want perfume in their husbands when they themselves are redolent of it? If a slave and a free man be anointed with perfume, they both smell alike in a moment, but those smells which are derived from free labors require both virtuous habits and a good deal of time, if they are to be agreeable and in character with a free man.

Socrates' objection no doubt was based on the fact that perfume was often used to "disguise" unhygienic habits.

One of the earliest instructions on the manner in which perfume should be worn and applied appears in the works of Appolonius of Herophil, who wrote a treatise on the origins of perfume and the materials used in its composition.

> Perfumes appear sweetest when the scent comes from the wrist, so that perfumers apply scent to this part. Heat changes or destroys the character of a scent, and the effect on the sense of smell is immediately perceived when perfumes are brought into close contact with the skin.

Grecian women used cosmetics in the same manner as the Egyptian, Hebrew, Babylonian, Medean, and Persian women before them. They painted their faces with white lead and applied vermilion to their cheeks and lips with a small brush. They used kohl for darkening the eyebrows and eyelids. Hair dyes were as popular among the men as among the women.

An ancient Greek story tells how Lais, as celebrated for her wit as for her beauty, once repulsed Miron, the sculptor, who, at the age of seventy, fell desperately in love with her. The rejected suitor attributed his being cast aside to the fact that his hair was white. He therefore dyed his hair a splendid black and returned the following day, hoping for a better reception. He was doomed to disappointment. Glancing at him briefly, Lais laughed and asked, "How can I grant thee today what I refused thy father yesterday?"

Perfumers' shops of Athens served as meeting places for all classes of society. Often frequented by philosophers, statesmen, artists, and writers who came to discuss affairs of state, they attracted also those who would spread gossip, create scandal, and keep abreast of the latest changes in the world of fashion.

Proper protocol of the toilette was considered to be so vital in Athens that a tribunal was established to arbitrate on all matters of dress. A woman whose mantle was cut incorrectly, whose coiffure was neglected, or whose application of cosmetics was vulgar was liable to a fine. However, Grecian women did not truly need law enforcement to motivate them to maintain the elegant personal appearance of which they were so proud. They were extremely coquettish, and standards of beauty, as revealed in classical art, demonstrate that Grecians clothed themselves with great taste and gave particular attention to the manner of dressing their hair.

Romans, before they came under the influence of their Grecian captives, cared little for the refinements of civilization. The only perfume in which they indulged came from clusters of verbena and fragrant plants which they plucked from the fields and hung over the doorposts of their homes to ward off the evil eye. But as Roman conquest extended to the provinces of Magna Graecia, the southern part of Italy colonized by the Greeks, the centurions adopted the manner of the vanquished to a sickening degree.

The drolleries of the rich Roman matron were depicted by the satirist Juvenal sometime during the years A.D. 100–128:

> She hurries all her handmaids to the task;
> Her head alone will twenty dressers task:
> Psecas, the chief, with neck and shoulders bare,
> Trembling, considers every sacred hair.
> If a straggler from his rank be found,

41

*A pinch must for the mortal sin compound.*
*Psecas is not in fault; but, in the glass,*
*The dame's offended at her own ill face;*
*The maid is banished, and another girl,*
*More dexterous, manages to comb and curl:*
*The rest are summoned on a point so nice,*
*The first the grave old woman gives advice:*
*The next is called, and so the turn goes round,*
*As each for age or wisdom is renowned.*
*Such council, such deliberate care they take,*
*As if her life and honor lay at stake.*
*With curls on curls they build her head before,*
*And mount it with a formidable tower;*
*A giantess she seems, but look behind,*
*And then she dwindles to the pigmy-kind.*

Three kinds of perfumes were favored by the Romans: liquids (stymmata); unguents in the form of ointments or oils (hedysmata); and powders (diapasmata). As in Athens, perfumes were named for ingredients, some for the place in which they were originally produced, and others for the particular circumstance in which they were made. Like today's perfumes, each scent attracted its own enthusiasts. There was *rhodium,* made from roses; *melinum* from quince blossoms; *metopium* from bitter almonds; *narcissinum* from narcissus flowers; and many others. Most renowned of the perfume ointments was *susinum,* compounded of lilies, oil of ben, calamus, honey, cinnamon, saffron, and myrrh. Another famous unguent was *nardinum,* a mixture of oil of ben, sweet rush, costus, spikenard, amomum, myrrh, and balm.

These perfumes were applied to the entire body—the face, the hair, even the soles of the feet. All were poured in the bath and on clothing. They perfumed the Roman couches and the walls of the rooms. Even military banners were impregnated with sweet odors.

Perfumers were an important part of the commercial and social life of Rome, and Marcellus often mentioned the celebrated apothecary Cosmus.

In the city of Capua perfume venders occupied an entire street called Seplasia. They extracted some of their essences from flowers grown in Italy, but most of their raw materials were imported from Egypt and Arabia. Some were so costly that slaves who worked in the laboratories were stripped and searched before they were permitted to return home for the night.

The custom of spraying perfumes in the reception and dining halls was transmitted from the Greeks to the Romans, who also concocted a great number of compounds for the improvement and preservation of the complexion.

Ovid wrote a tome on cosmetics, of which only certain small fragments remain. Among them:

*Learn from me the art of imparting to your complexion a dazzling whiteness, when your delicate limbs shake off the trammels of sleep. Divest from its husk the barley brought by our vessels from the Libyan fields. Take two pounds of this barley with an equal quantity of bean flower and mix them with ten eggs. When these ingredients have been dried in the air, have them ground and add the sixth part of a pound of harkshorn of that which falls in the spring. When the whole has been reduced to a fine flour, pass it through a sieve and complete the preparations with twelve narcissus bulbs pounded in a mortar, two ounces of gum, as much of Tuscan seed, and eighteen ounces of honey. Every woman who spreads this paste on her face will render it smoother and more brilliant than her mirror.*

Romans also used *psilotrum,* a kind of depilatory for the face; *fucus,* a rouge for the cheeks; kohl, for underlining the eyes; barley flour kneaded with fresh butter to cure pimples; calcined pumice stone to whiten the teeth, and an assortment of hair dyes. False hair was much in fashion, and its use bordered on the ridiculous when the marble bust of Julia Semiamira, mother of the

Emperor Heliogabalus (c. 204–222), was outfitted with several different colored marble wigs which could be interchanged according to the whim of the decorator.

The infamous Nero squandered the Roman treasury on aromatic gums and perfumes. He had the roofs of his dining halls painted to represent the firmament, and as the banqueters gathered, fragrances showered down on them from silver pipes. He gave his wife, Poppaea, a lavish funeral at which more incense was burned than all of Arabia could produce in ten years.

Common to all Middle Eastern and Oriental countries was the use of incense both for religious and personal purposes. In fact, in Chinese the word "perfume" *means* incense. The same word, "*heang*," is applied to any and all fragrances. The Chinese classified their incense into six basic types: Tranquil, Recluse, Luxurious, Beautiful, Refined, and Noble, the use of each of which was supposed to induce the mood bearing its designation. Incense was selected to harmonize with the flowers that decorated the room in which it was to be burned.

It is thought that ceremonial burning of incense may have come to China from the south by the end of the third century; some scholars postulate that it came much sooner. The ritual use of incense was practiced in the home and also at shrines for the worship of Buddha.

Made from a combination of powdered sandalwood, dried patchouli leaves, and olibanum, this incense often was fabricated in stick form. Sometimes these joss sticks were more simply made from fragrant tinder wood mixed with water and clay, which was dried. Chinese women continued to use sticks of incense to scent their bed linens and personal things up to very recent times.

Sandalwood was highly prized as long as 2500 years ago. It was so lavishly used later on in paying homage to Buddha and to the philosopher Confucius that the great forests of the East were threatened with depletion. Today government preserves this commodity—one of the finest raw materials necessary to perfumery.

Aside from its use in religious worship, sandalwood incense was burned by mandarins in paying obeisance to their emperor. In the absence of the ruler the ceremony took place before an empty chair.

In the Chinese funeral rite the body was washed, perfumed, and dressed in fine raiment while incense burned continuously under the portrait of the deceased.

More than from historians, we learn about the uses of fragrance and cosmetics in China from the reading of the works of Li Po (701–760), great poet of the T'ang Dynasty.

> *Shake not your crown, if perfumed;*
> *Nor flap your garment, if spiced with lan!*
> *It is better to hide the chaste soul's radiance,*
> *The world hates a thing too pure.*
> —*"To the Fisherman"*

> *Fair one, when you were here, I filled the house with flowers.*
> *Fair one, now you are gone—only an empty couch is left.*
> *On the couch the embroidered quilt is rolled up; I cannot sleep.*
> *It is three years since you went. The perfume you left behind haunts me still.*

> *The perfume strays about me forever, but where are you, Beloved?*
> *I sigh—the yellow leaves fall from the branch,*
> *I weep—the dew twinkles white on the green mosses.*
> —*"The Long-departed Lover"*

In Cochin fishermen, about to set forth in their boats, insured a safe and successful trip by burning aromatic and consecrated woods on crude stone altars.

Musk was in great demand, as well as sandalwood, and was also prized for its medicinal properties. Considered a cure-all, its long-lasting odor has been savored through the centuries by all peoples.

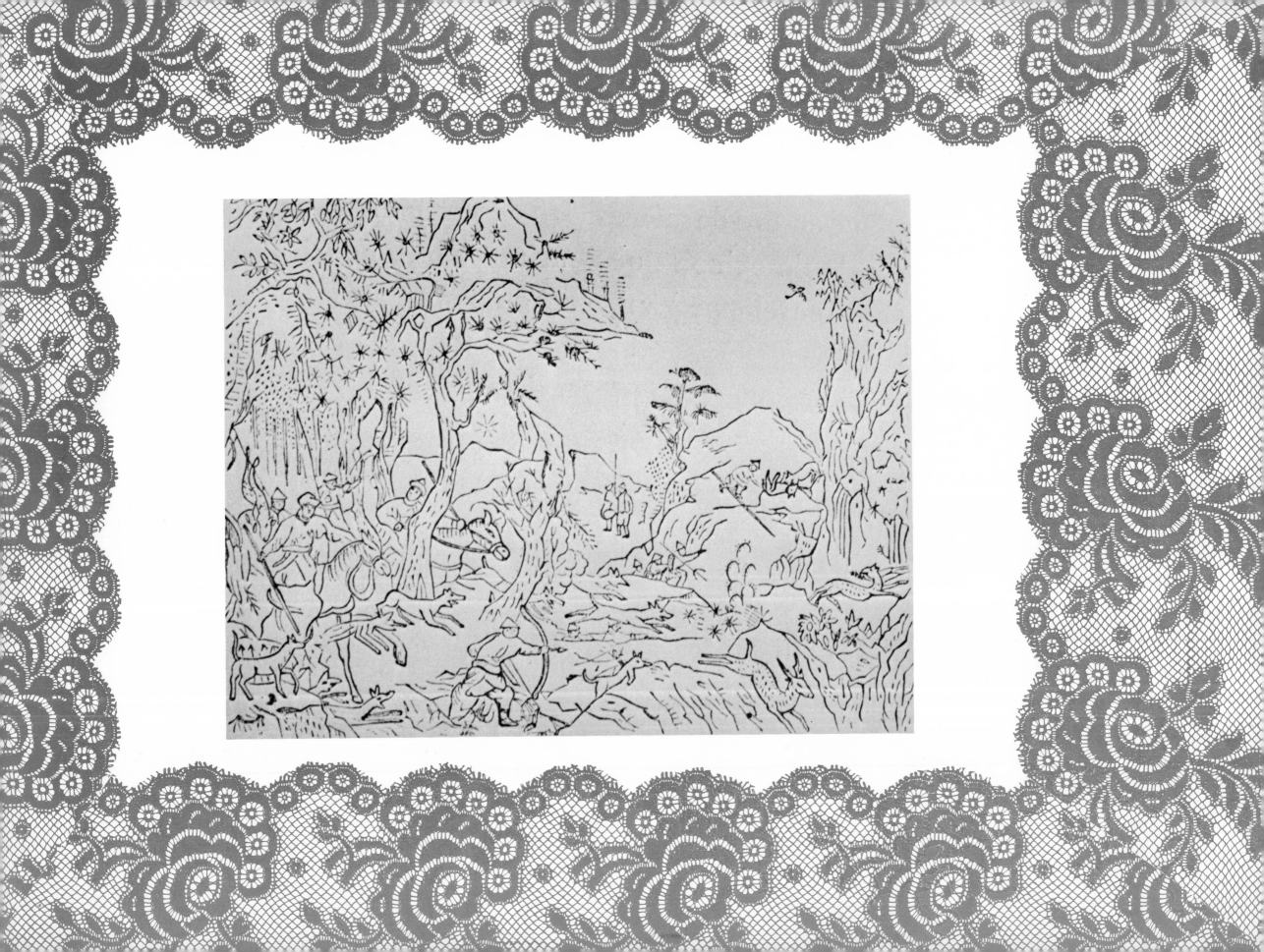

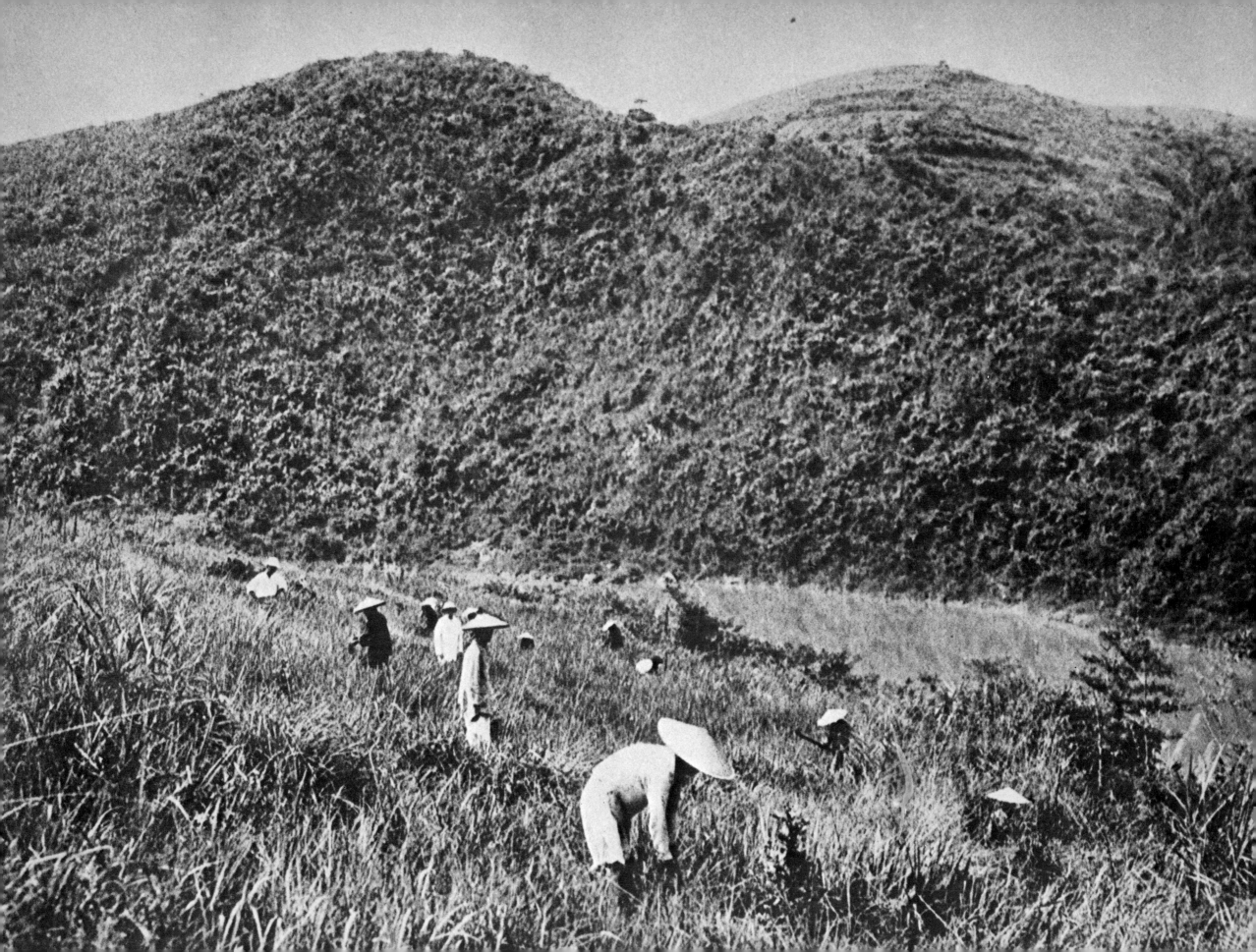

We read that seventy jugs of musk were mixed with the mortar for a certain mosque to keep the holy place forever fragrant. Almost from the beginning, musk has been considered invaluable as a fixative for perfumes, and in consequence, like sandalwood, the source of this commodity—the musk deer of the high Himalayas—has been threatened with extinction.

The fragrances of China are more notable for being strong than for being pleasing. Outside of their prevailing use of incense throughout the centuries, the Chinese have developed only a few oils and essences for perfume. This is surprising since several fine species of odoriferous woods grow in China and as botanists the Chinese have achieved worldwide recognition, having developed many varieties of flowers renowned for their beauty.

Tibet is another country with a strong tradition in the use of incense. Sometimes placed in a censer, Tibetan incense was more often burned in a gigantic altar with an aperture at the top.

The twenty-third chapter of the Saddharma Pudarika Sutra taught that the sacrifice of one's own person outranks all other sacrifices—that even burning one's finger as a sacrifice is superior to rescuing all the people of a state. The hero of this chapter, therefore, "perfumed his whole body, anointed it with fragrant oil, soaked all his clothing in oil" before offering himself to his God.

Another interesting practice was carried out in ancient Java, where a ceremony was performed prior to any dangerous hunting expedition. The participants made an animal sacrifice, said prayers, anointed themselves with sweet-smelling oils, and burned gum benzoin at the entrance of the caverns where they planned to hunt.

The perfume past of the Japanese begins when incense was introduced to them, about A.D. 500 by the Chinese. It has played a prominent part in Japanese life ever since. Special schools were established which taught the art of burning incense and selecting the proper type of burners to be used. Dances were created to be performed during incense-burning rituals. Special poetry was recited to induce beautiful, imaginative, aesthetic thoughts.

Related in the *Nihon Shoki*, most valuable annal of ancient Nippon, is the legend of the pieces of agar wood found on the shores of the island of Awaji in A.D. 595. When the agar was burned in the fireplace along with other woods, everyone was so moved by the marvelous fumes it gave off that they reserved its use to worship of the emperor. Until the fourteenth century agar was imported from India in large quantities, but the supply of this natural resource dwindled rapidly and with it the Japanese Kodo ceremony. Kodo, the art of perfumery, is still practiced today, but only by a very small tradition-observing minority.

With the diffusion of Buddhism during the Nara Era (710–784), the use of scent increased. In the temple of Todaiji there were magnificent incense burners made of white copper, red copper, and red sandalwood. They are now preserved in the Shosoin Treasure House. Innumerable other incense burners made of gold or silver were fashioned at this same period, along with certain masterpieces of Japanese ornamental art shaped after chimera or flowers.

Aromatic materials placed in these burners included the following: (1) resinoids: styrax and olibanum; (2) woods: agar wood, sandalwood, borneol, camphire; (3) barks: cinnamon; (4) roots: costus, angelica; (5) buds: cloves; (6) animal materials: musk, ambergris. All were imported into Japan from southern China, Indochina, Malaysia, Sumatra, India, and Africa.

The Nara Period and the Kamakura Period (785–1084) mark the moment when the use of fragrances, previously confined to Buddhist ceremonies, began to infiltrate into the customs of everyday life. Perfumes appeared both in sachet and paste forms for the scenting of rooms and clothing. The paste was composed of several powdered materials mixed well with honey, plum pulp, seaweed, charcoal, and salt. It was stored in a cool, dark place to maintain moisture. The principles used in its making form the

46

basis for similar pastes composed in Europe during the sixteenth and seventeenth centuries.

In the Genjo classic we find the description of a game—a sort of aristocratic pastime—in which the players try to guess the correct odor of perfumes. There were only six compounds, each named for one of the seasons: spring, summer, late summer, early autumn, late autumn, and winter.

Nature was further explored for the treasures it might contribute to fragrance during the Muromachi Period (1392–1499). Ingredients commonly used were clove, sandalwood, musk, styrax, benzoin, borneol, nutmeg, fennel oil, and of course the most prized of all, agar wood, the very texture and aroma of which were considered to be the highest expressions of beauty.

The guessing game reported in the Genjo story was rendered more challenging as the number of ingredients for scents increased during the Edo Period (1604–1853). Names of the various scents were inspired by poetry, songs, traditional legends, flowers, birds. The most notable perfume was Genji-ko, named for the twelfth century romance.

The art of Japanese perfumery became exquisite and elegant, and the history of Japanese perfume is rich in tradition. Just as traditional are the perfumes of India. The Hindus constructed their sacred temples of aromatic woods, the edifices themselves thus becoming permanently fragrant. The Hindus offered perfumed water to their God, Attar, whose body they washed with scented liquids. During wedding ceremonies a sacred fire was fed with perfumed oils and aromatic wood, so that the sweet-smelling fumes would please the senses of the bridal party and the guests.

Sandalwood and sandalwood oil, mentioned in Indian history as early as 500 B.C., were articles of barter between India and the Mediterranean nations many centuries ago. Sandalwood retains its sweet, penetrating scent for dozens of years and is pleasing when used for statuettes and necklaces. Like the Chinese and the Japanese, Indian sculptors favored this wood for the fashioning of graceful stands that supported their handsome porcelains and precious manuscripts.

Possessing types of climate and terrain for the cultivation of all possible vegetable species, India is a veritable riot of perfumery plants. Its perfume tradition dates back thousands of years, and Vedic legends mention this art. Historians and poets of bygone days vaunted the glories of India's profusion of plants and flowers, fruits and woods, roots and resins and grasses. It was the lure of these treasures that attracted the Portuguese and other European mariners to this vast country.

Records of these ancient navigators indicate how valuable they considered the spices and perfumes indigenous to the forests and fields of India. During the latter days of the Roman Empire, an account states, a matron kept a slave whose single duty it was to sprinkle the hair and clothing of her mistress with Indian perfumes. Young girls of that era preferred a single fragrant ointment such as pomade of rose, narcissus, or crocus, while the matrons' cosmetics contained a mixture of scents. A favorite of both men and women was the exquisite and still popular Indian tuberose.

Attar of roses was the first preference of the natives of India themselves. Next came jasmine, which Hindu poets call the "Moonlight of the Grove." Attar (otto) can be described as perfume concentrate. Rose and jasmine are of Indian origin, imported into Europe by the Crusaders. Aside from distillates of these two flowers, other specialties were keora and champac, two highly fragrant blossoms not found elsewhere in the world.

But there is so much more of Indian fragrance—musk, civet, ambergris, spikenard, patchouli, and khus-khus (vetiver). The Muslims of India particularly loved a scented powder called abeer which they rubbed on the face and body or sprinkled on clothing. It was composed of sandalwood, aloes, turmeric, roses, camphire, and civet. Among the Indians, perfume is reputed to give a "touch of joy" to life.

Patchouli, of the mint family, has a heavy, hypnotic, compelling odor characteristic of Far Eastern fragrances and is used to perfume Kashmir shawls—perhaps the oldest example of scenting a product to increase its market value. The oil of cinnamon, the spikenard and myrrh mentioned in The Song of Solomon in the Bible are all perfumes of India.

The use of agarbathies, incense sticks, dates back to the most ancient days. Made mostly in the south of India, produced in the millions, maybe even billions, they are burned like candles in temples, in private homes and in shops, as well as in front of the images of deities. They perfume all festive occasions today—weddings and the welcoming of the New Year, even the inauguration of business enterprises. In the centuries-old traditional manufacture of agarbathies, the ingredients are odoriferous roots, barks, seeds, leaves, flowers, wood, gums, moss, and lichen, in particular sandalwood, agar wood, deodar wood, khus-khus, costus, nut grass, spikenard, licorice and calamus roots, cinnamon, cascarilla, and kapur.

The long, long history of perfumes, including that of many countries, have laid the groundwork for the years immediately preceding our own era of new skills, new techniques, all the new aesthetic achievements of modern perfumery.

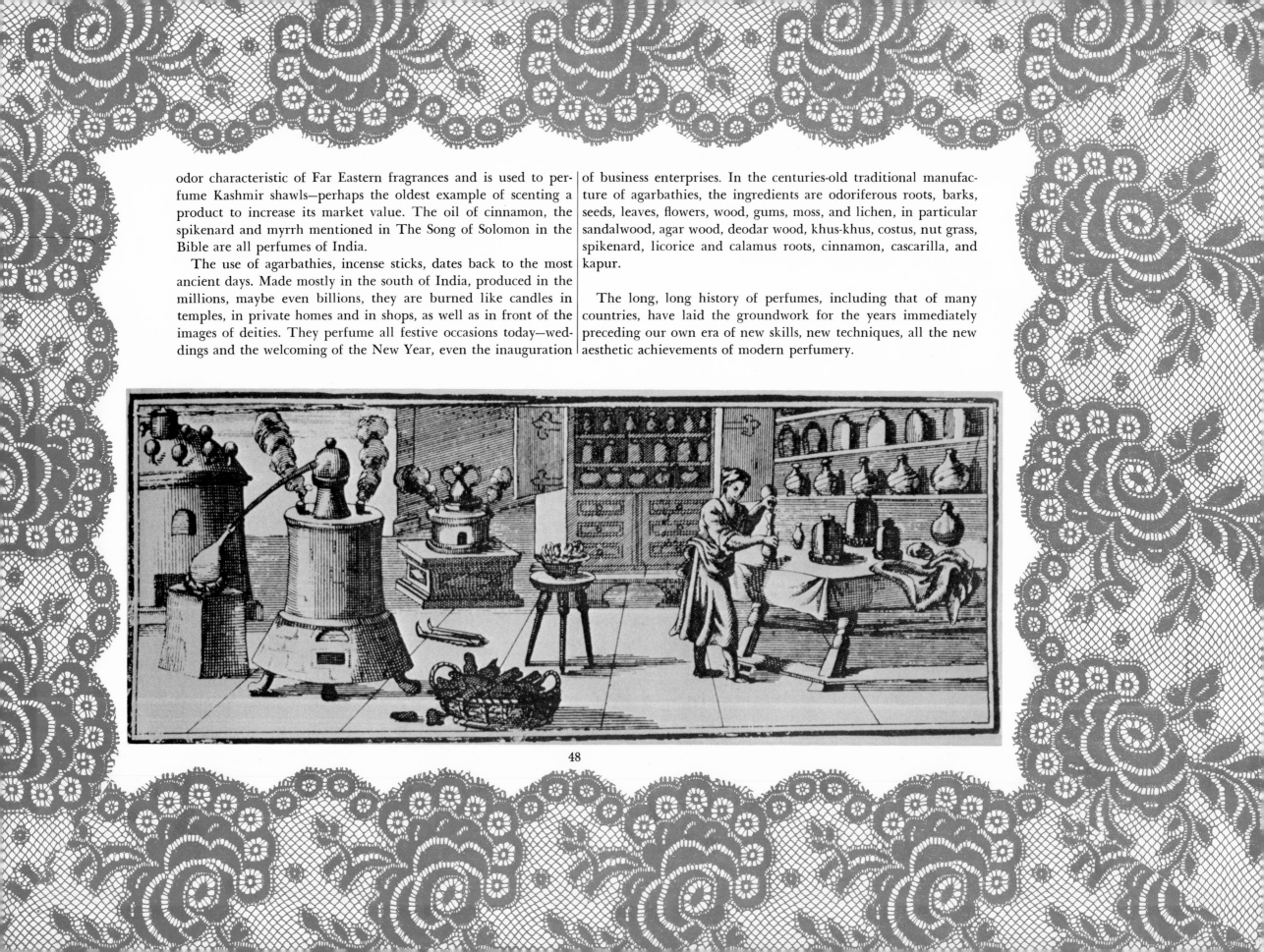

48

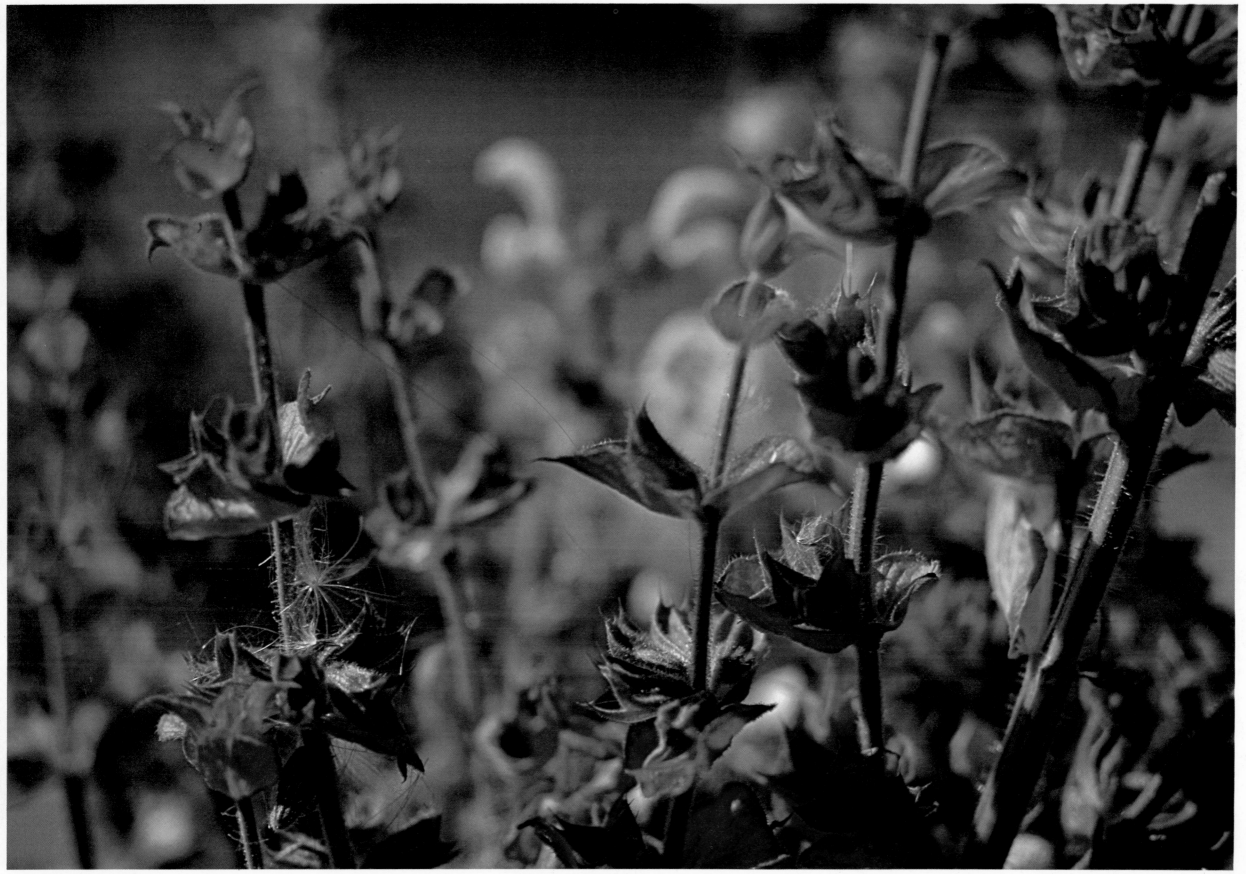

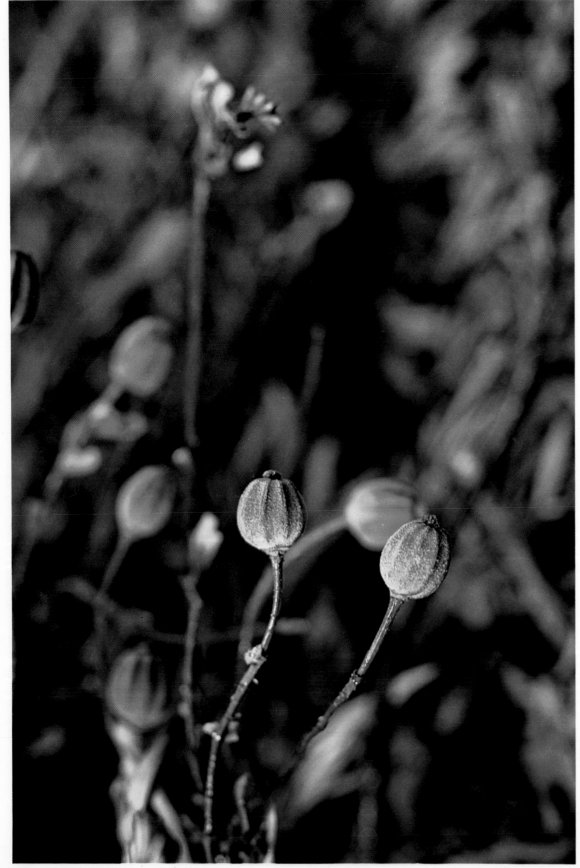

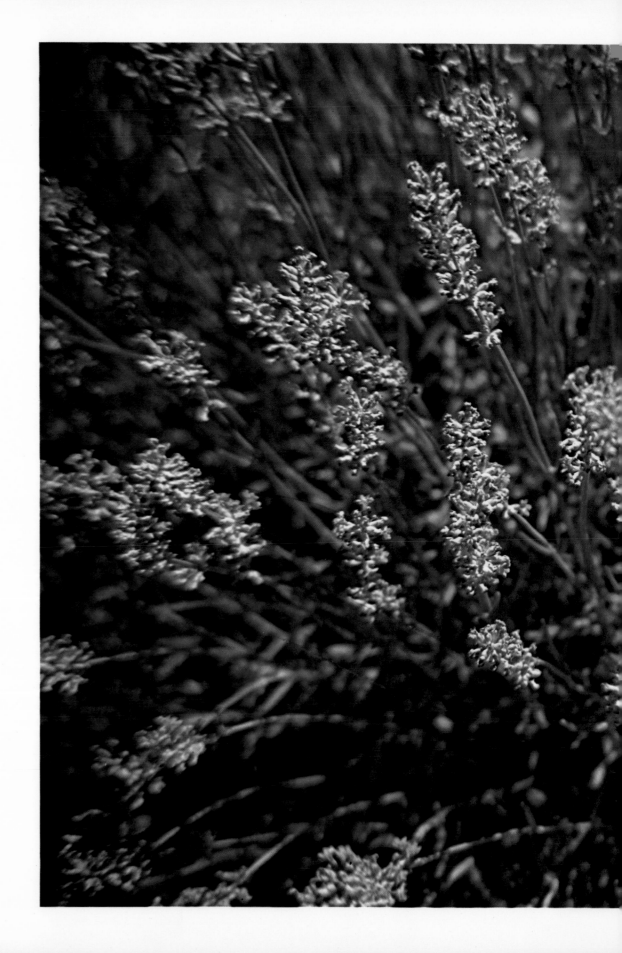

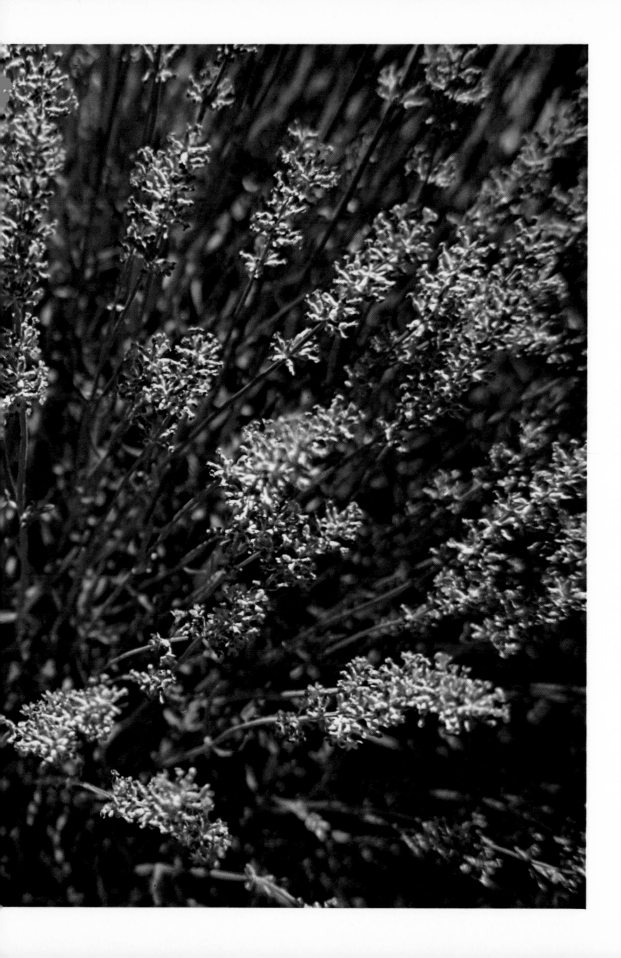

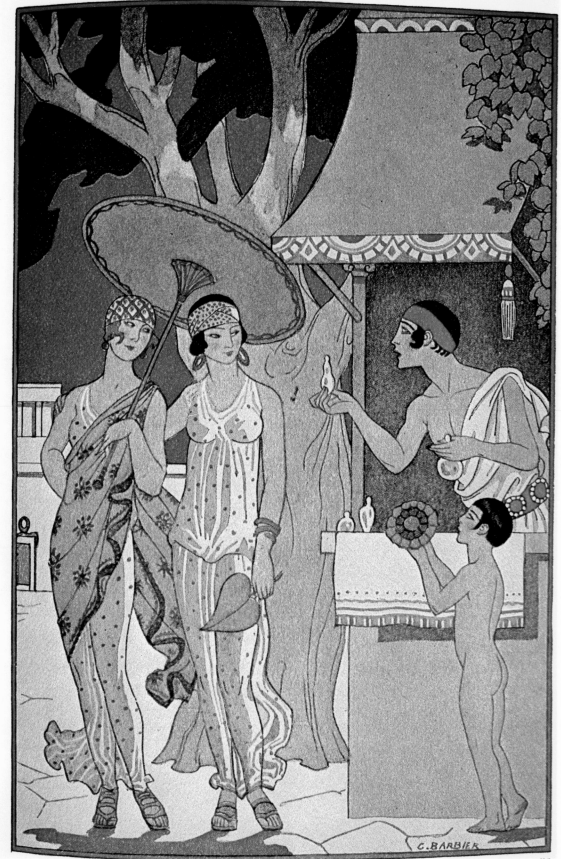

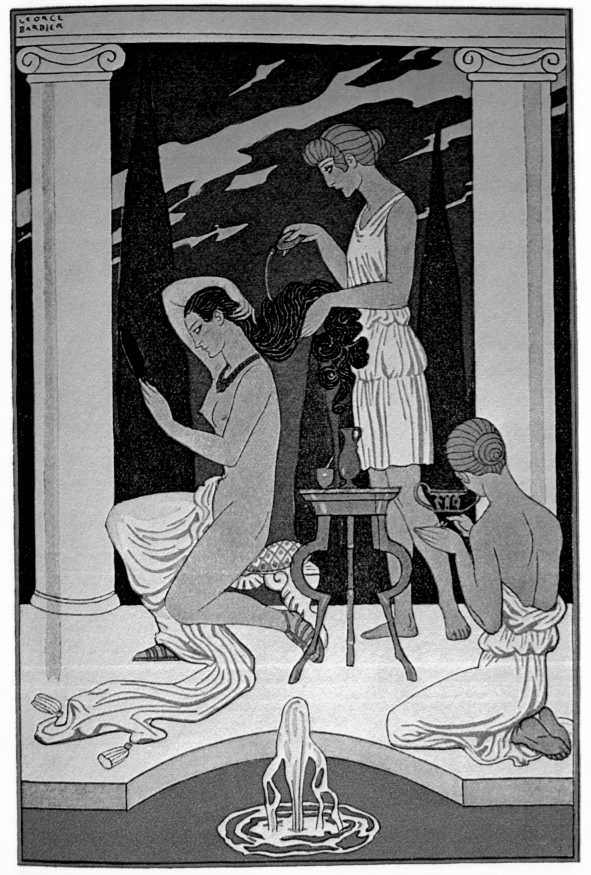

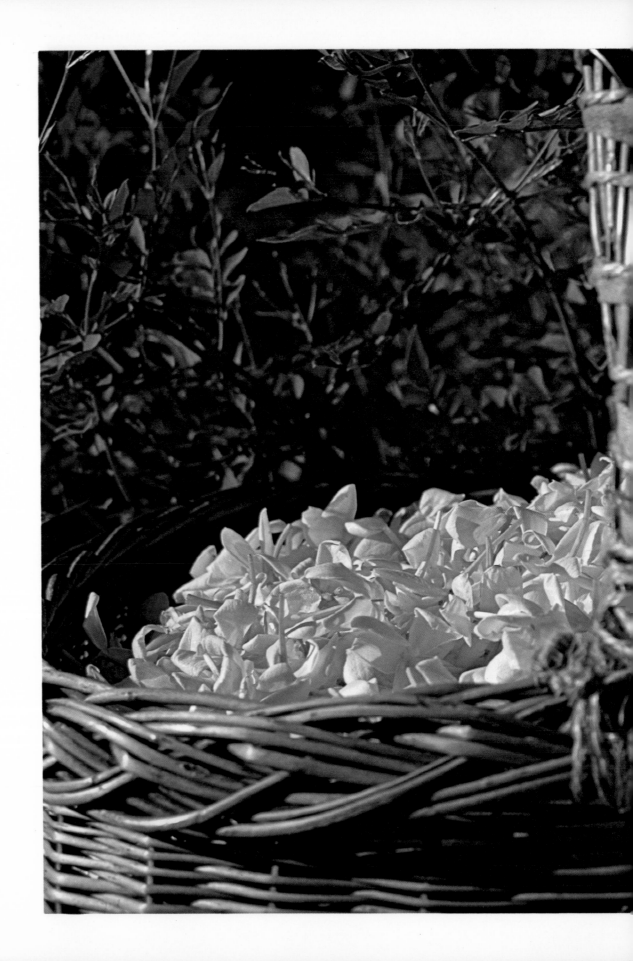

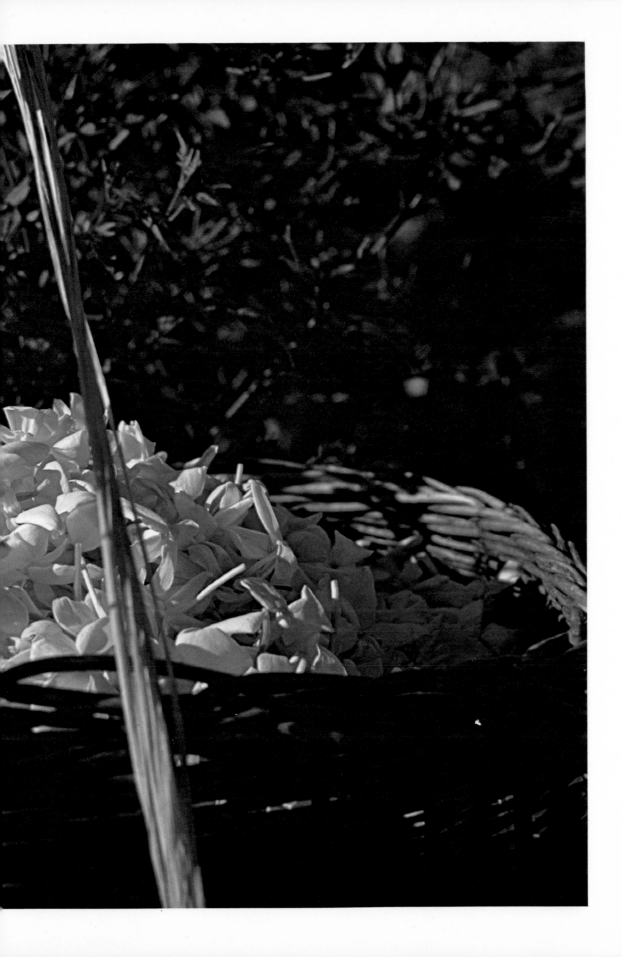

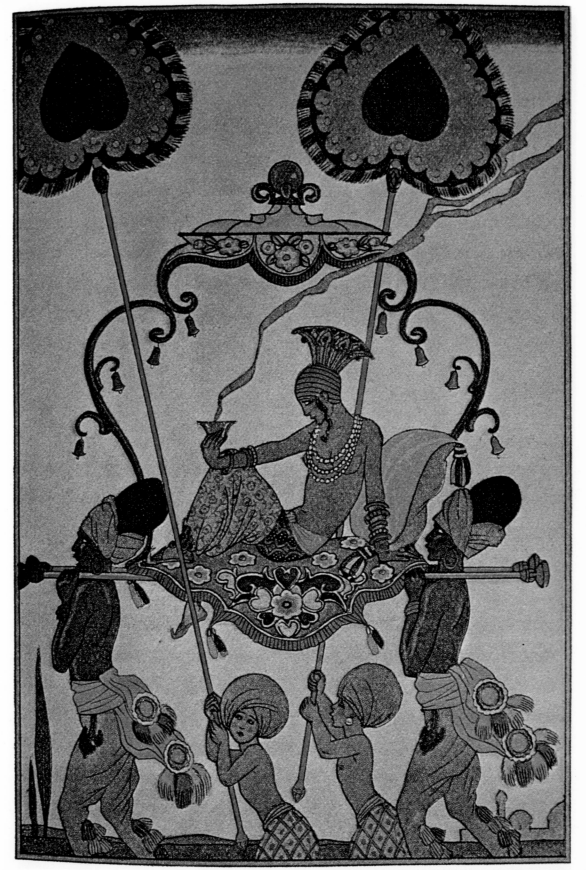

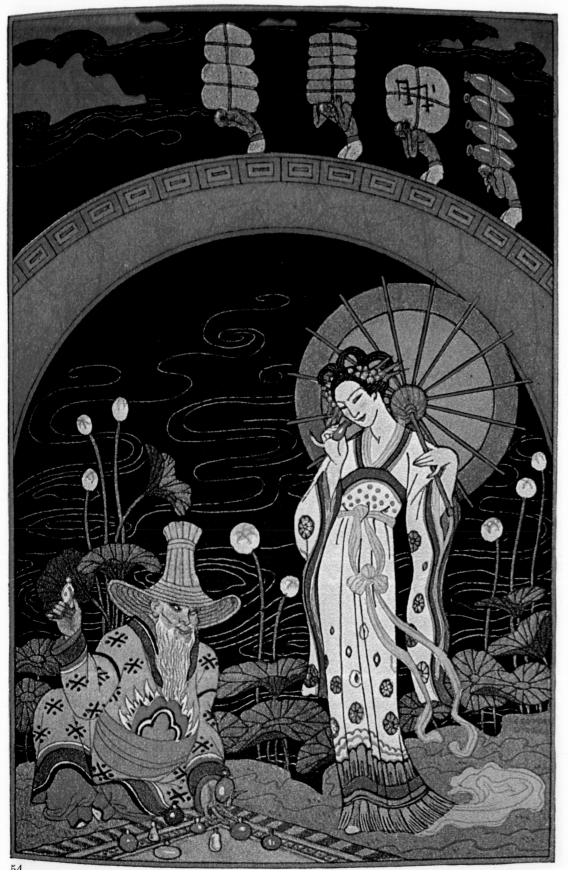

54

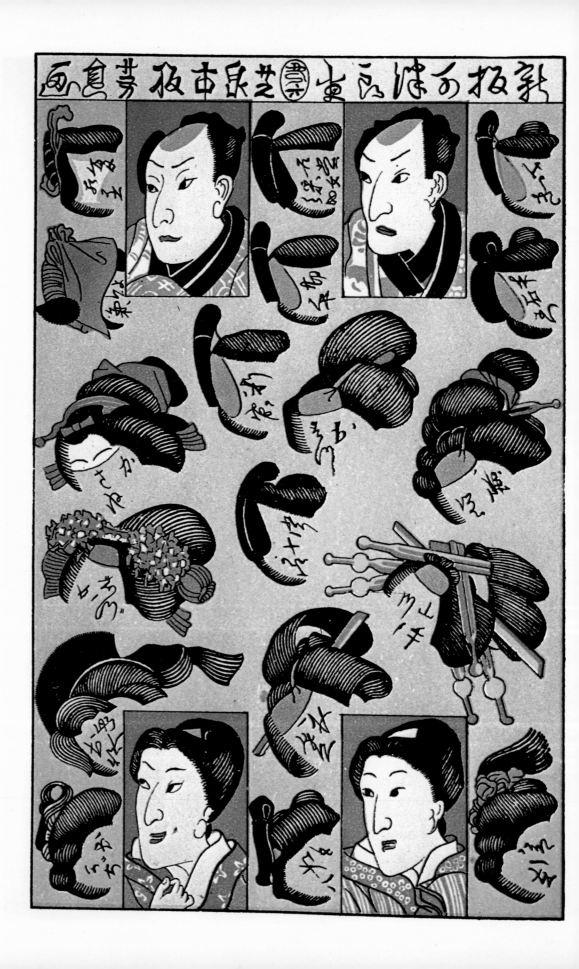

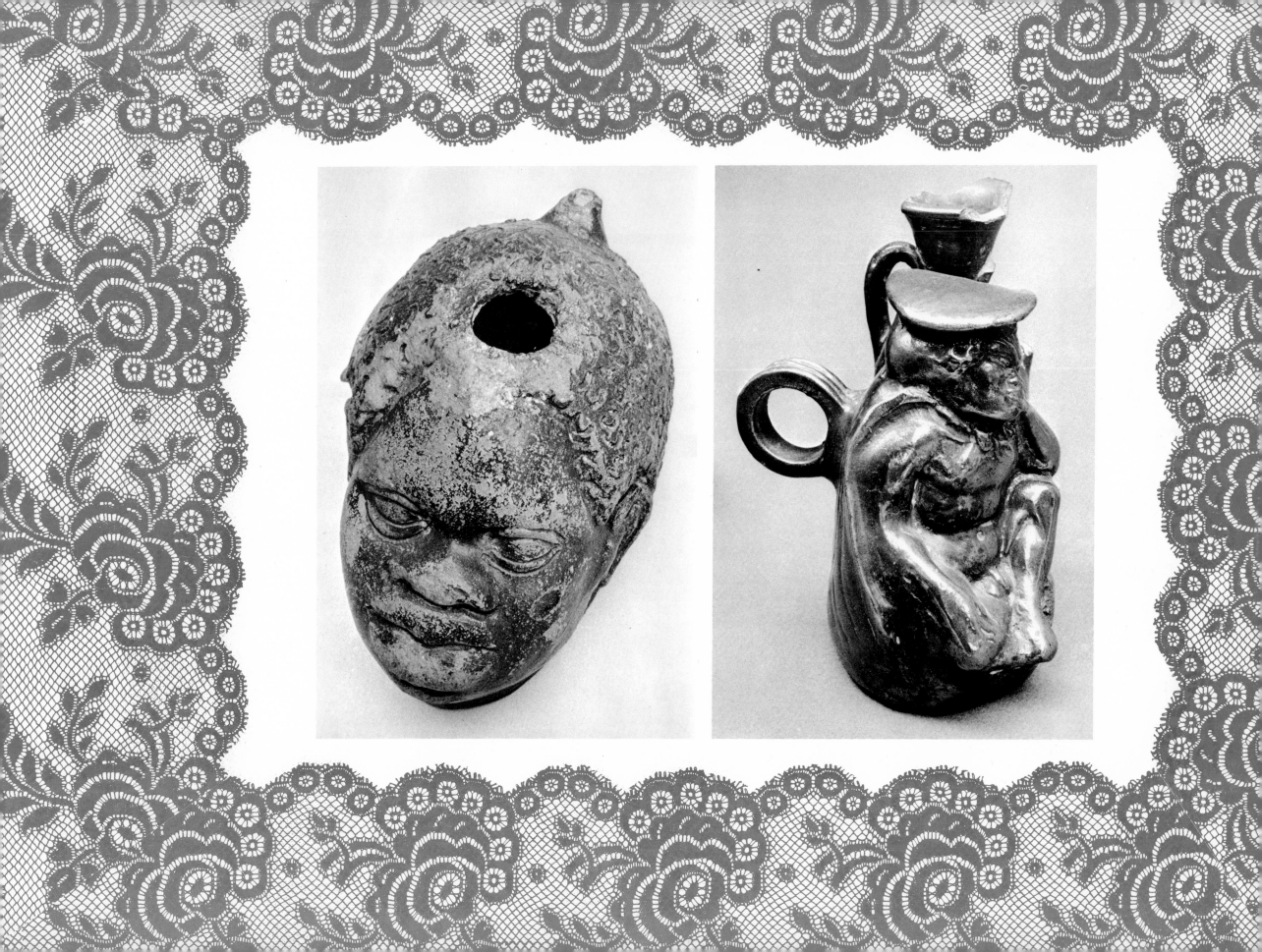

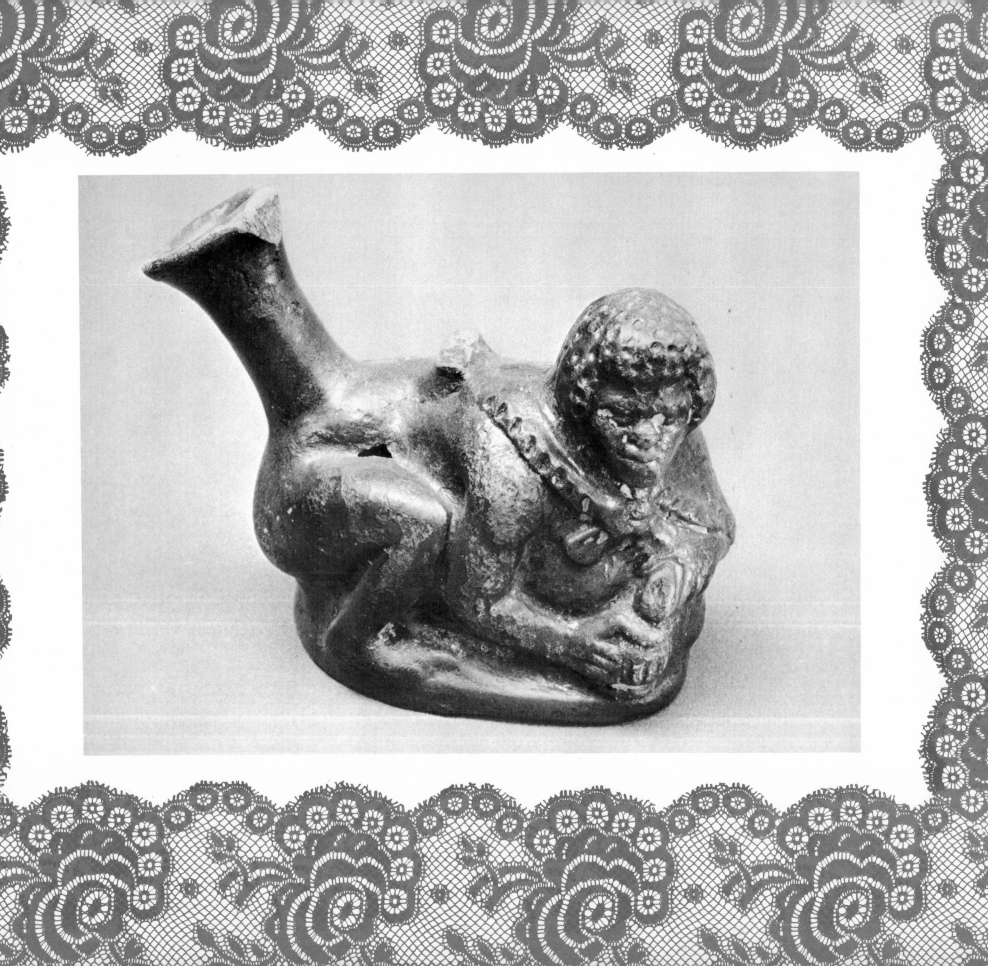

metrical layout of large blobs of glass of which Venice, some centuries later, was to make such effective use. Until the seventh century Italy retained a fairly important glass trade, especially to the Gauls. But the hedonism of Rome ceased with the coming of the Christian Era, and the art of glassmaking fell into obscurity for a number of decades.

The first Christians of Rome used small amphorae of glass for perfume and concentrated oils. These vessels were simple and generally coarse in quality. Infrequently, however, a consummate artist turned out one of the gilded vases later known as "Christian Glasses." A thin gold leaf on which were etched figures, symbols, or inscriptions was fixed with a thin layer of fused glass. This mode of decoration was noticeable not so much for its artistic value as for the novelty of the process. Apart from this very special example of the scent receptacle, we unfortunately are in almost total ignorance of glass of the first centuries of the Christian period.

Only the Arabians seemed to have done serious work as glassmakers during this epoch. Some rare specimens have come down to us, related very happily to perfumery. Antioch possessed great glassmakers, and Damascus also inherited the techniques of the artists of Sidon. Existing pieces from Damascus exhibit an art worthy of its Egyptian and Phoenician origins.

For a long time scholars suspected that Persia possessed an original art of glassmaking. They based their theories upon excavations that brought to light bottles ornamented with heraldic lines, noble medallions, red enamel on white enamel. Further research, however, has revealed that the Persians contented themselves with buying the glass from the manufacturers of Damascus.

The centuries passed. Little by little the barbarian invasions were repulsed. The Crusades followed, and the East, under pressure of the circumstances, reluctantly yielded the secrets of its sophisticated arts to a West in process of rebirth. The Crusaders carried home their fragrances in precious perfume containers. After a perilous journey to Palestine many knights brought their ladies the perfumes of the Orient, thus reviving their use and giving a new impulse to the pursuit of physical luxury. In the "Song of Roland" we find a passage about such a gift:

> *In a cedar wood chest, protected by Oriental carpets, a great number of bottles of fine glass, ornamented with gold and silver with stoppers of silver gilt or precious stones, held enclosed in their many-colored wombs all the perfumes and all the sweet scents of Araby and the Blessed. Face paints of brilliant tones and perfume paste in enchanting pots of painted earthenware or faience with lids embossed and inlaid with enamel.*

Blue kohl for coloring the eyelids was encased in bowls of cut crystal with golden stoppers, and the spatulas of gold and painted glass that served for the application of this exotic cosmetic were scarcely less luxurious.

Following the knights came the troubadours and the trouvères, who sang of the beauties of perfume and spread the knowledge of fragrance in the course of their pilgrimages from castle to manor house. The royal damsels welcomed gifts of scent bottles and took joy in the figured boxes that contained many sweet-smelling unguents presented to them by their swains.

Through the Middle Ages and the Renaissance Venice, as well as certain other provinces of Italy, held supremacy in the manufacture of glass for perfumery. The Italian glass industry was regulated by a strict code. From 1318 on, glassmakers were classified into various categories, each with its own standards. As early as 1224, on the occasion of the election of the Doge Lorenzo Tiepolo, glassmakers of Murano presented the Oricanni, scent bottles of great beauty. The inhabitants of Murano had a golden book in which were inscribed the names of families native to that island; their daughters were eligible for marriage to the patrician nobles of Venice, and their descendants retained their royal titles even when they followed the Murano family tradition and became

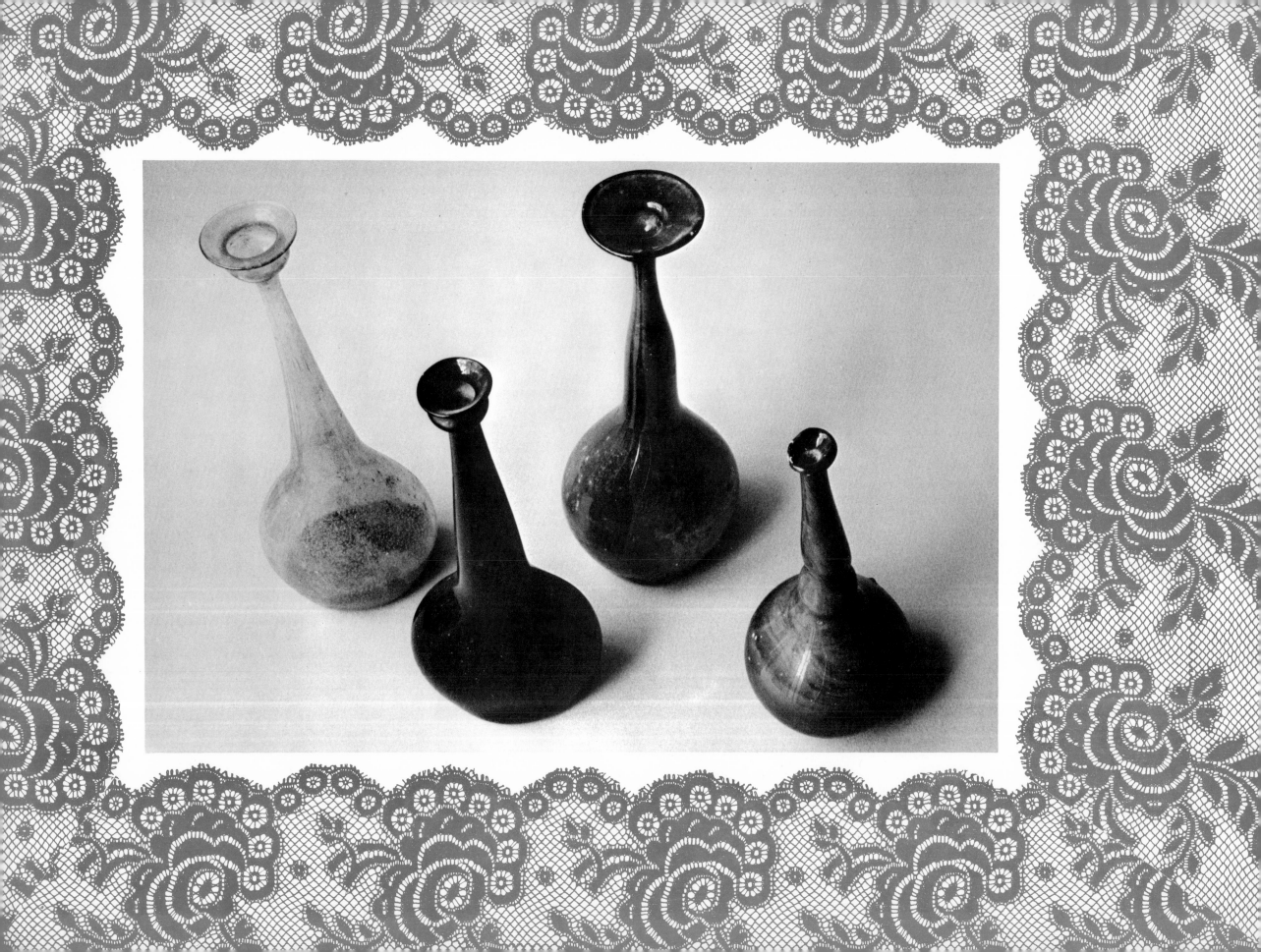

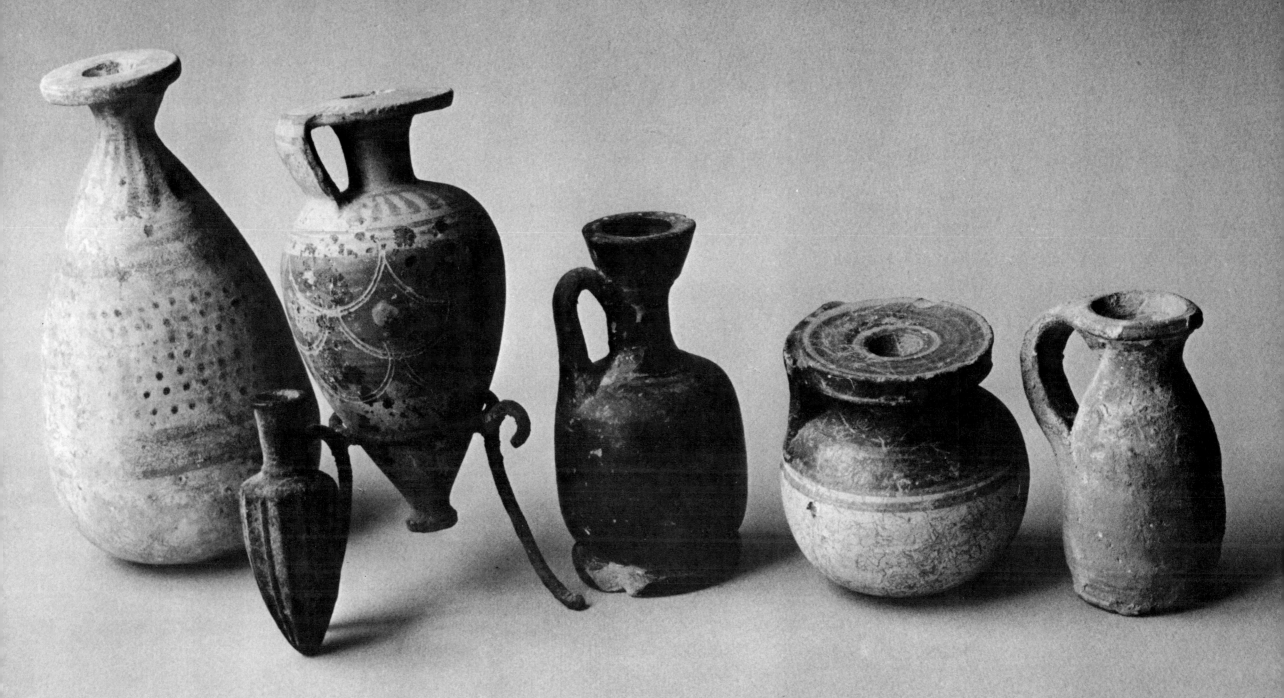

glassmakers. Work inside the factory was no less minutely regulated. So rigid was the control of the government that glassmakers were prevented from emigrating to Austria, France, Flanders, or England on pain of death. However, frequently laws cannot prevail against the promise of titles and wealth. Glass vessels put out by the Venice workshop were immediately acclaimed, and the creators of these flacons sought new fields to conquer. Proof of this fact is that in the year 1354 Vienna passed a regulation that reserved a special area in the marketplace for the sale of Venetian glass. An inventory of the property of the dukes of Burgundy in that same epoch mentions "a perfume pot in yellow Venetian glass, decorated with gold and with 20 pearls, also 3 vials in a glass of crystal fashion."

The craftsmen of Murano worked with equal success in all branches of glassmaking, and therein lies the secret of their great triumphs. They produced colorless glass of remarkable purity, both plain and crackled; glass tinted in the mass and glass sanded with gold, engraved, filigreed, or enameled. They made use of every combination of materials and techniques to embellish an object, to give it an original and a personal touch, irrespective of the purpose for which it was destined. While in Venice, in spite of the infinite variety of their models, we find a unique spirit developing, a single style of delicacy, an elegance—in a word, the art of Venetian glass.

Pieces decorated with paintings and enamels were set aside as objects of great luxury, a number of which still survive. One of the great enamelers was Biravino, famous in the history of Venetian glassmakers for having had his book of formulas stolen by one of his pupils, Giorgio, the hunchback. It was returned to him only in exchange for the hand of his daughter Marietta.

Another formula reserved for the making of perfume bottles was millefiori or "mosaic glass." The technique used to fabricate this beautiful product is almost as ancient as the glassmaker's art. Colored rods of glass were cut into small pieces, placed to form a design, and then carefully melted together. When the piece was fused adequately, it was ground and polished. Millefiori means one thousand flowers. The effect of this skillful blending was so stunning that scent bottles and other objects made from millefiori glass were in demand everywhere. (Unfortunately, the continued popularity of this work gave rise in the nineteenth century to numerous cheap reproductions that glutted the market and turned discriminating buyers away.)

In the course of the sixteenth century glassmakers redoubled their ingenuity to create a style of bottling worthy of a lotion called Golden Thread, a preparation that gave patrician ladies that warm blond tint so much in vogue and that was composed of black sulfur, alum, and honey.

To glasses and perfume bottles the artists of Murano added another astounding creation—glass pearls. They first appeared in 1528, born of the inspiration of Andrea Viadore, who made chaplets and necklaces of them. A perfumer of the time conceived the idea of piercing a small hole in the "pearl" through which he introduced a few drops of scent that evaporated on contact with the warm skin. Venetian ladies were intensely proud of them.

Gradually, as century succeeded century, Europeans constructed glassworks almost everywhere. Venice began to lose ground in the export trade. Her craftsmen confined their talents to manufacturing trinkets, pearls, and engraved mirrors.

Florence, on the other hand, produced in this period the exquisite perfume bottles ordered by the Medici (from the fourteenth to the seventeenth centuries) which were inspired by the works of Botticelli and Perugino. These powerful princes are said to have preferred cut crystal, and later Catherine de Médicis introduced these beautiful scent decanters to the courtiers of France with the aid of her perfumer, René the Florentine. Lucrezia Borgia used minute bottles of crystal and gold, carved in the figure of a heart or a skull. According to historians, they contained acqua toffana, which was mixed with a penetrating per-

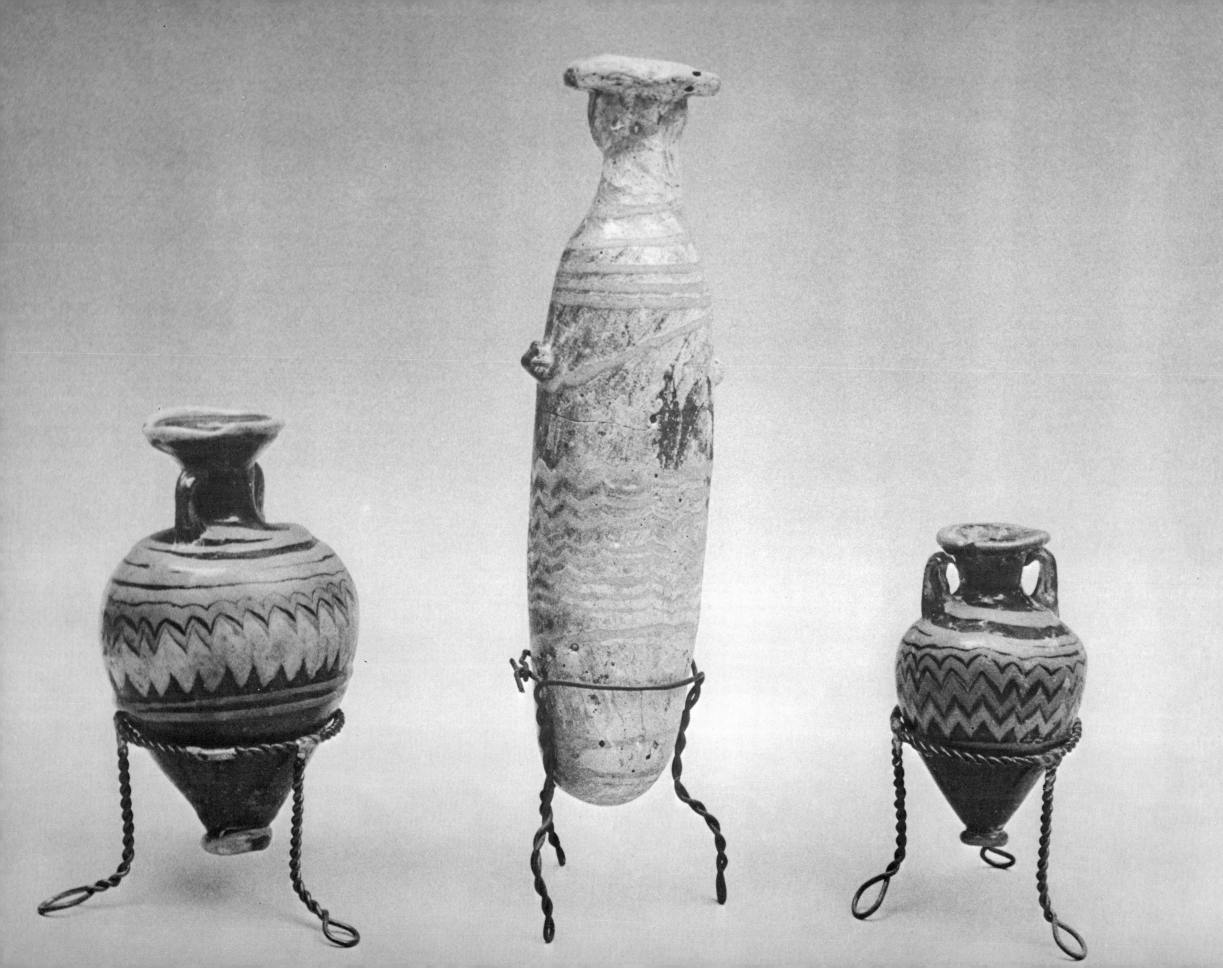

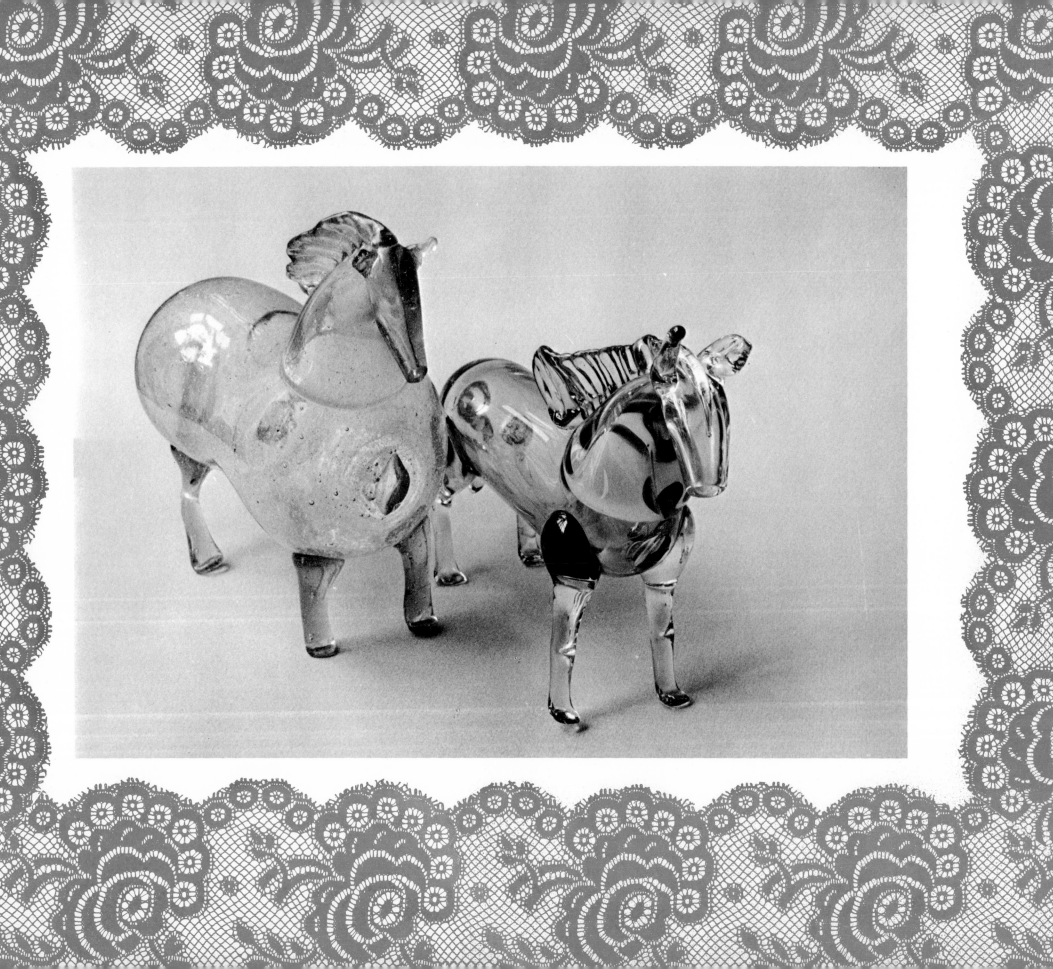

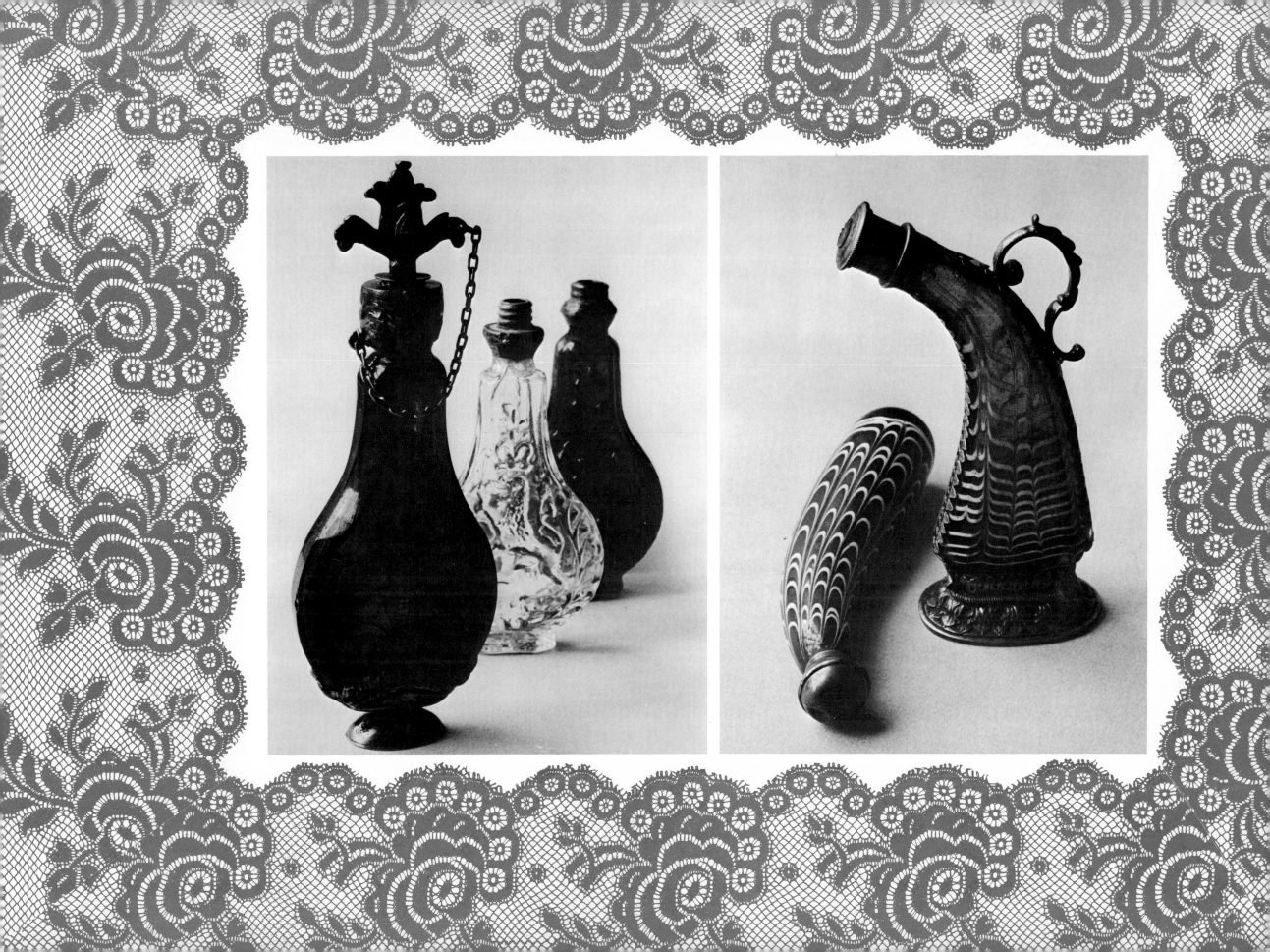

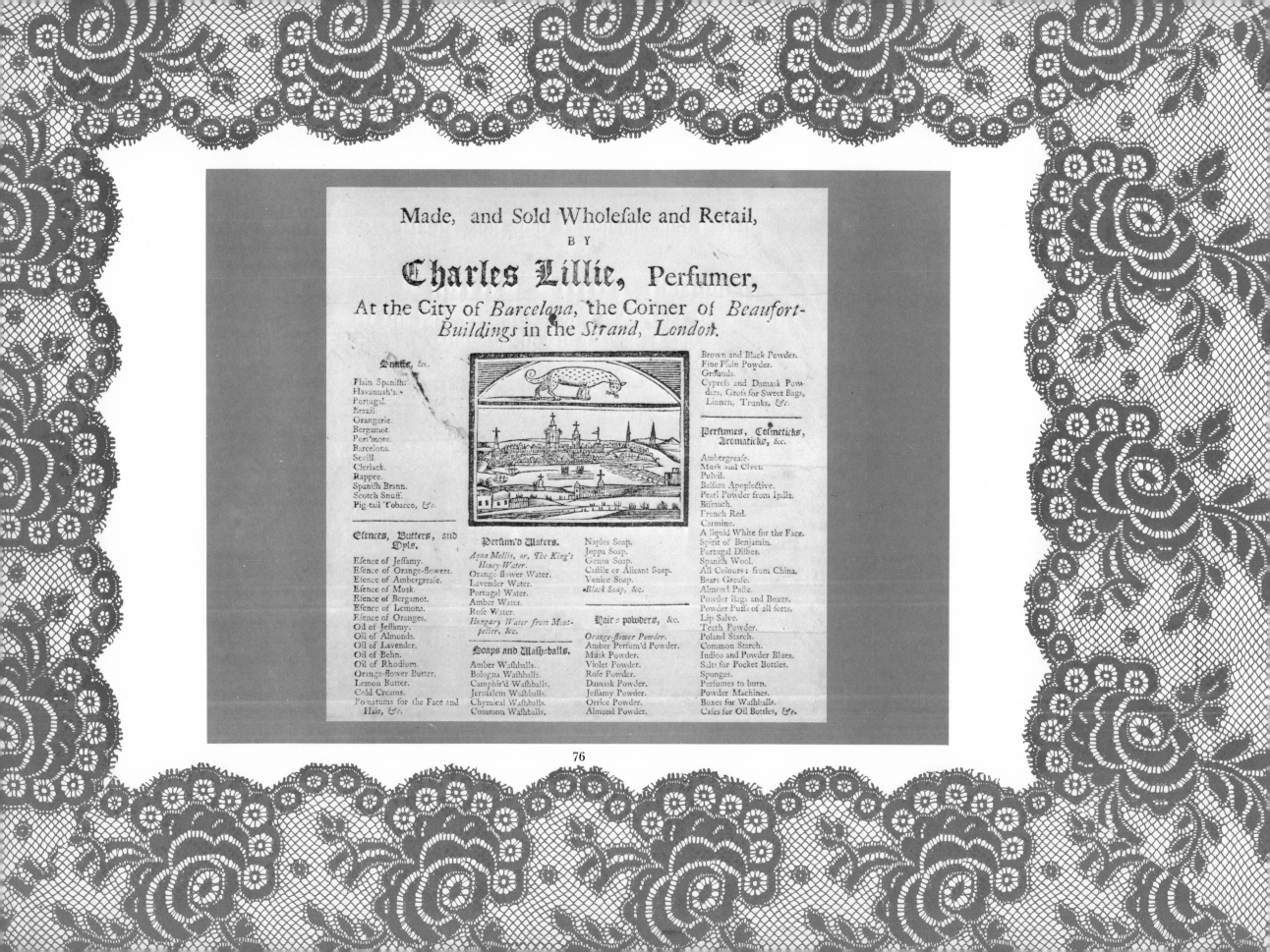

Made, and Sold Wholesale and Retail,

BY

# Charles Lillie, Perfumer,

At the City of *Barcelona*, the Corner of *Beaufort-Buildings* in the *Strand*, *London*.

**Snuffs, &c.**

Plain Spanish.
Havannah's.
Portugal.
Brazil.
Orangerie.
Bergamot.
Port'more.
Barcelona.
Sevill.
Cleriack.
Rappee.
Spanish Brann.
Scotch Snuff.
Pig-tail Tobacco, &c.

**Essences, Butters, and Oyls.**

Essence of Jessamy.
Essence of Orange-flowers.
Essence of Ambergrease.
Essence of Musk.
Essence of Bergamot.
Essence of Lemons.
Essence of Oranges.
Oil of Jessamy.
Oil of Almonds.
Oil of Lavender.
Oil of Behn.
Oil of Rhodium.
Orange-flower Butter.
Lemon Butter.
Cold Creams.
Pomatums for the Face and Hair, &c.

**Perfum'd Waters.**

*Aqua Mellis, or, The King's Honey-Water.*
Orange-flower Water.
Lavender Water.
Portugal Water.
Amber Water.
Rose Water.
*Hungary Water from Montpellier*, &c.

**Soaps and Wash-balls.**

Amber Washballs.
Bologna Washballs.
Camphir'd Washballs.
Jerusalem Washballs.
Chymical Washballs.
Common Washballs.

Naples Soap.
Jeppa Soap.
Genoa Soap.
Castile or Alicant Soap.
Venice Soap.
*Black Soap*, &c.

**Hair-powders, &c.**

*Orange-flower Powder.*
Amber Perfum'd Powder.
Musk Powder.
Violet Powder.
Rose Powder.
Damask Powder.
Jessamy Powder.
Orrice Powder.
Almond Powder.

Brown and Black Powder.
Fine Plain Powder.
Grounds.
Cyprefs and Damask Powders, Grofs for Sweet Bags, Linnen, Trunks, &c.

**Perfumes, Cosmeticks, Aromaticks, &c.**

Ambergrease.
Musk and Civet.
Pulvil.
Balsam Apopleftive.
Pearl Powder from India.
Bismuth.
French Red.
Carmine.
A liquid White for the Face.
Spirit of Benjamin.
Portugal Dishes.
Spanish Wool.
All Colours; from China.
Bears Grease.
Almond Paste.
Powder Bags and Boxes.
Powder Puffs of all sorts.
Lip Salve.
Teeth Powder.
Poland Starch.
Common Starch.
Indico and Powder Blues.
Salts for Pocket Bottles.
Sponges.
Perfumes to burn.
Powder Machines.
Boxes for Washballs.
Cases for Oil Bottles, &c.

fume formulated with musk, violet, and civet and which enabled her to eliminate persons who stood in her way.

In the Middle Ages the French imported much of their glassware, but Henry II (1519–1559) took an interest in glassmaking and even had a factory erected at Saint-Germain-en-Laye, to which he brought two Italian craftsmen. The first artistic pieces were offered to the beautiful Diane de Poitiers to contain, among other elixirs for the complexion, the famous lotion called "The Secret of Diane."

One of the most interesting facts of this period is that many of the artists of Murano migrated to Rouen, France, where they labored at making glass pearls. Early statutes dated about 1593 indicate that special favors were accorded these artists. These glass pearls replaced for citizens of modest means the elegant pomander or amber apples fashioned in gold or gems for the rich. Filled with perfume, they were to be held in the warmth of the hand so that the essences might be released. Queen Catherine de Médicis acquired lasting fame for her perfumed gloves, but she was no less fond of her small cut-glass bottles that came first from Italy and later from Rouen.

Henry III made excessive use of perfumes and beauty balms. His dressing table was furnished with several hundred bottles in all shapes and colors. He commanded the artists of Rouen to produce a glass mask for him under which he placed a paste designed to whiten his complexion.

Records show that a corporation of glassmakers was formed at Augsburg, Germany, in 1303, but it was not until the second half of the sixteenth century that the famous glass engraving for which Germany became renowned was perfected. Italian influence can be seen in this work. The Emperor Charles IV, thoroughly bored at Prague, sent for Italian artists to manage his factory for the cutting of rock crystal and gems. A German by the name of Lehmann learned his craft in that city and took to cutting glass by means of a lathe and a wheel of his own invention. He gained fame in his ever more exacting demands upon himself regarding the quality of the glass, and gradually he was able to imitate rock crystal closely. This engraved glass, with its typical heraldic ornaments and engraved phrases, was to meet with wide acclaim in the course of the following century. The city of Frankfurt am Main also had important glassworks that specialized, owing to the quality of the sand in the region, in the manufacture of utensils for the chemical, perfumery, and drug trades.

In England there was no national glass industry during the fourteenth century, but in the sixteenth century initial attempts were made to establish one, with no great success. Later on, however, Italians from Murano settled in London, attracted by all kinds of advantages, which unfortunately they lost with the passage of time. In 1567 Jean Quarre, a native of Holland, founded a glassworks at Savoy House; some men from the Vosges Mountains of France settled in the county of Sussex, and finally, at the end of the seventeenth century, thirty-three concerns were occupied in glass manufacture. Due to a lack of wood for fuel, they had problems, and for this reason Great Britain lagged behind Italy, France, and Germany in the manufacture of glass used for flacons of perfume.

Perfumers themselves enjoyed no great vogue in England until the reign of Henry VIII, and in the successive reigns of Mary and Elizabeth there was no big demand for perfume containers. Elizabeth I, however, perfumed not only her garments but also the reception rooms of her palaces, the hangings, the seats, even the animals she kept as pets. All the fragrances used for these purposes came from France or Italy in their original bottles. The rigorous austerity of Protestantism excluded the delights of perfume, thought to have a pernicious effect upon the soul, until the queen openly expressed her pleasure in fragrance and all London awoke to its luxury.

An increasing number of bottles, stumpy, square, or hexagonal, in flint glass, a glass made with silica sand, came into being. A purely English invention, these flasks stand as the forerunners of some of today's most sophisticated perfume containers.

The Spanish technique in glassmaking came to fruition very early in the sixteenth century because of the Arabian influence. Spanish glassware was very Oriental in design and form. Nevertheless, one should not confuse it with the actual Oriental products, for it showed a much more fanciful trend. Barcelona, in 1503, delivered 274 glass pieces to King Ferdinand, who gave them to Queen Isabella, and when the Venetian ambassador Navagoro visited Spain, he particularly noted a toilet set of eighty vials in which the glass, the gold and other metals, the enamels, and the paintings formed a very beautiful, exotically imaginative ensemble. Seville, Toledo, and other towns manufactured bottles for distilleries of flowers and fruits as well. Even those for common use retained a certain originality of form, while receptacles for costly aromatic liquids were embellished with green and yellow enamels, a specialty of the Iberian Peninsula during the Renaissance. Bizarre in form, they feature multiple handles, reminiscent of the many-limbed Hindu gods.

France advanced slowly in the art of the flacon for the glassmakers were too often at loggerheads with the sovereign authority in their attempts to define their position among the nobility. It could be said that a Frenchman was noble *although* he was a glassmaker, whereas a Venetian was noble *because* he was a glassmaker. So much time was spent claiming the privilege of French nobility that these discussions engendered a torpid spirit in the glassblowing workshops which was prejudicial to the progress of the art.

While from the beginning of the sixteenth century the Council of Venice exacted terrible penalities of glassmakers emigrating from Murano, nothing prevented the expatriation of Italian glassmakers. Several European countries profited greatly from their skill, to the detriment of the Venetian glassmaking industry. While other countries made inroads in the European markets, the Venetians in their turn tried to create products similar to those of their competitors. In Germany Venetian émigrés were creating perfume holders of streaked cream-white glass. This effect was achieved by sprinkling chips of colored glass onto the surface of the marver plate over which the lump of molten glass, attached to the gathering iron, was rolled before further blowing.

The handsome German red ruby glass made its appearance and was first described by Johann Kunckel (1630?–1703), chemist and glassmaker. It is doubtful that Kunckel actually invented the glass that has borne his name ever since, but certainly his famous work *Ars Vitraria* is responsible for our knowing about the method of its fabrication.

Ruby glass is made by adding gold chloride to the glass mixture, which is an odd grayish color and turns red only after it has been reheated. The Bohemians specialized in this glass, and a century later Fred Egermann (1777–1864) invented Lithyalin glass— a glass that looked like semiprecious stones. It was produced in shades of dark red, brown, gray-green, bluish-green, or solid color that was marked and veined. Egermann was soon imitated in his native country and abroad.

Also in Germany Henry Schwanhart, noting the change in the surface of the glass when he dropped a spot of hydrofluoric acid on his spectacles, came upon mat glass by accident. The discovery led him to create beautiful glassware with a mat surface decorated with designs in clear glass.

It was this kind of innovation that the Venetians tried to incorporate in their own traditional techniques. The great artist Diolarmi Nagagnati was encouraged to furnish the Italian perfumers with bottles of topaz and hyacinth glass, and toward the end of the eighteenth century the manufacture of bottles in the English style was authorized at Murano. All this imitation resulted only in the decline of Italian glassmaking, so much so that in 1797, during the French occupation of Venice, General Berthier could not find a single artist–glassmaker worthy to be sent to France, despite the fact that his government had commanded him to find one. Yet somehow, irrespective of all this, Venice retained a reputation so firmly established that every European country turned to her for manufacturing secrets.

In the seventeenth century France, due to the specialization of small glassworks, began to make considerable progress, though they were still under the spell of Venice. The kings took a keen interest in this new industry, several of them establishing new glassworks generally devoted to the manufacture of tableware and toilette services of great luxury.

The single most important factor in the evolution of French glassmaking during the seventeenth century was the refinement in the art of perfumery and the fact that the members of the court were obliged to smother themselves with scents to mask other odors, sometimes due to poor hygiene. During the reign of Louis XIV the great glassmaker Bernard Perrot expressed his genius in ornamenting his creations with cameos on which portraits were represented. The court of Louis XV was known as "The Perfumed Court," and Madame de Pompadour treated a perfumer with the same deference she gave to a great artist. Madame Du Barry launched the fashion of Eau de Cologne, which was to enjoy a greater and greater popularity as the centuries passed.

The eighteenth century saw the development of glassworks in Normandy and Lorraine. At Tourlaville Richard Lucas de Nehon received royal patronage for the creation of bottles and flasks, and the glassworks at Saint-Quirin produced numerous objects, the harmony and perfection of which have remained without equal. Typical perfume containers of the period of Louis XV are of enameled or ribbed glass or of crystal. They were embellished with chasing of gold and silver. Each bottle was different. Some were decorated with cameos, others with medallions; sometimes they were white, sometimes colored; always they were elegant.

Frequently they were part of a traveling case. In the reign of Louis XIV the perfume bottles in the *necessaire* were usually ribbed, squat and low, made of green or tinted glass and closed

with metal stoppers. But the flacons of the period of Louis XV were more decorative, varied in design. Some were made of metal and had stoppers of gold. The traveling cases were made of leather, wooden marquetry, tortoiseshell, sharkskin, or procelain and carried, in addition to the vials of perfume, boxes of face paints and hair pomades. Finally Marie Antoinette, patroness of both the perfume and glassmaking industries, was responsible for the establishment of the Queen's crystal and enamel factory at Saint-Cloud. She adored all perfumes, but especially rose and violet, which she adopted as her regular scents.

At this same time the royal glassworks of Sèvres was established. The output of this new factory, situated in the foothills of Meudon, was of the highest quality. But it had to contend with the heavy competition of Bohemian glass, the vogue of which was at its height.

Then came the Revolution and the Terror. In spite of the suppression of all luxuries, perfumes were still in demand, although in very small quantities. There was a "Guillotine" perfume and a "Sanson" perfume, but with the onset of the Directoire a veritable mania for luxury broke out. The Muscadins, the Incroyables, and the Merveilleux made use of the most astounding face paints, powders, creams, and perfumes. Bottling for perfumery made enormous progress. The glassmakers obtained letters patent confirming their privileges and special authorizations to make crystal or crystalline glass, formerly confined only to certain manufacturers.

In England, in this most important period of perfume history, wood firing was replaced by coal, making it necessary to work with closed crucibles instead of uncovered pots. Closed crucibles necessitated the presence of more fusible elements than open crucibles. A creative glassworker conceived of adding lead oxide to increase the fusibility of the mass and in so doing invented crystal, or glass having a lead base. It was, however, some years before this product came into general use. Aside from this, the English had to struggle from 1690 to 1785 against high taxes and government supervision.

79

Nevertheless, flint glass made amazing strides. French customers especially preferred English glassware to their own. The English crystal was superior in a certain aspect to rock crystal, for when cut in prisms, it reflected the light like a diamond. English bottles were cut with prominent facets, which appeared, especially at night, like so many gems, against which the transparency of the Italian and German glass could not compete. However, this cutting involved a thickness of glass which ruled out any fanciful shapes. The objects were heavy, solid and comfortable but without great delicacy. The glass stoppers lacked originality, and obviously there was no question of coloring the glass.

An important influence at this time was the fact that French artists expatriated themselves to London, tempted by the fine remunerations offered. Such are, in a few words, the profound reasons for a new orientation of the English glass industry. The banal round forms of the bottles gave place to some original polygonal forms. The artisans of the crystal industry sought increased beauty and increased depth of cut. So it is that, despite blockades and governmental supervision, English perfume bottles were purchased by all who could pay the fabulous prices, until 1848 when the craze for flint glass subsided.

The opulent, elegant eighteenth century undoubtedly gave us the greatest number and the greatest variety of perfume container designs. Porcelain came into its own and quickly ranked second to glass as a material for flacons. There had been many previous attempts to produce porcelain, but not until 1708 did experiments succeed in Dresden. Germany was in the vanguard with porcelain manufacture, but other European countries soon followed suit. In Meissen Johann Joaquim Kändler created an entire world of figurines which not only made charming ornaments but could also be used as pastille burners to scent the room or as containers for perfumes and cosmetics.

The Germans also perfected a method by which real lace could be dipped into the porcelain mixture. When fired, the actual lace was destroyed but the design remained. In England Chelsea porcelain was especially important. Artists were innovative with its material. This period in flacon making is familiar to all collectors. The style was much later imitated by the French, who also produced many beautiful pieces after the handiwork of the Chelsea craftsmen.

Chelsea scent bottles and similar ones were fabricated from separate molds for the different parts of the body so that variations could be made using a single figure as a basic theme. Clowns and harlequins were in great demand; other Chelsea pieces came in the form of girls, birds, animals, flowers. By the middle of the nineteenth century a very high value was placed on Chelsea porcelain.

In eighteenth-century Saxony beautiful porcelain scent bottles were encased in boxes that had the outward appearance of baskets or bouquets of roses, irises, and other flowers, all done in relief. Other materials, of course, were also used. There are beautiful examples of glass and gold perfume flacons in shapes not unlike those we have today, but the workmanship is extremely elaborate in every detail and exquisite in its delicacy.

In Spain, during this same century, the glassworks of La Granja gained distinction in the manufacture of chandeliers, services of engraved glassware, and perfume bottles. But the major contribution of this factory was the achievement of high-intensity coloring in the mass.

Holland, meanwhile, secured for itself a place in the history of glassmaking in the eighteenth century through the skill of its technicians in diamond engraving. Invented in Germany, this mode of decoration was perfected during the seventeenth century by Franz Grinvoot, an artist of Rotterdam, who substituted stippled work for parallel cutting.

In America a German immigrant, Caspar Wistar, opened a factory in Philadelphia for the making of buttons and glass. That was in the year 1740. Today experts estimate that only a few (possibly thirty) authentic pieces of precious Wistar glass are extant.

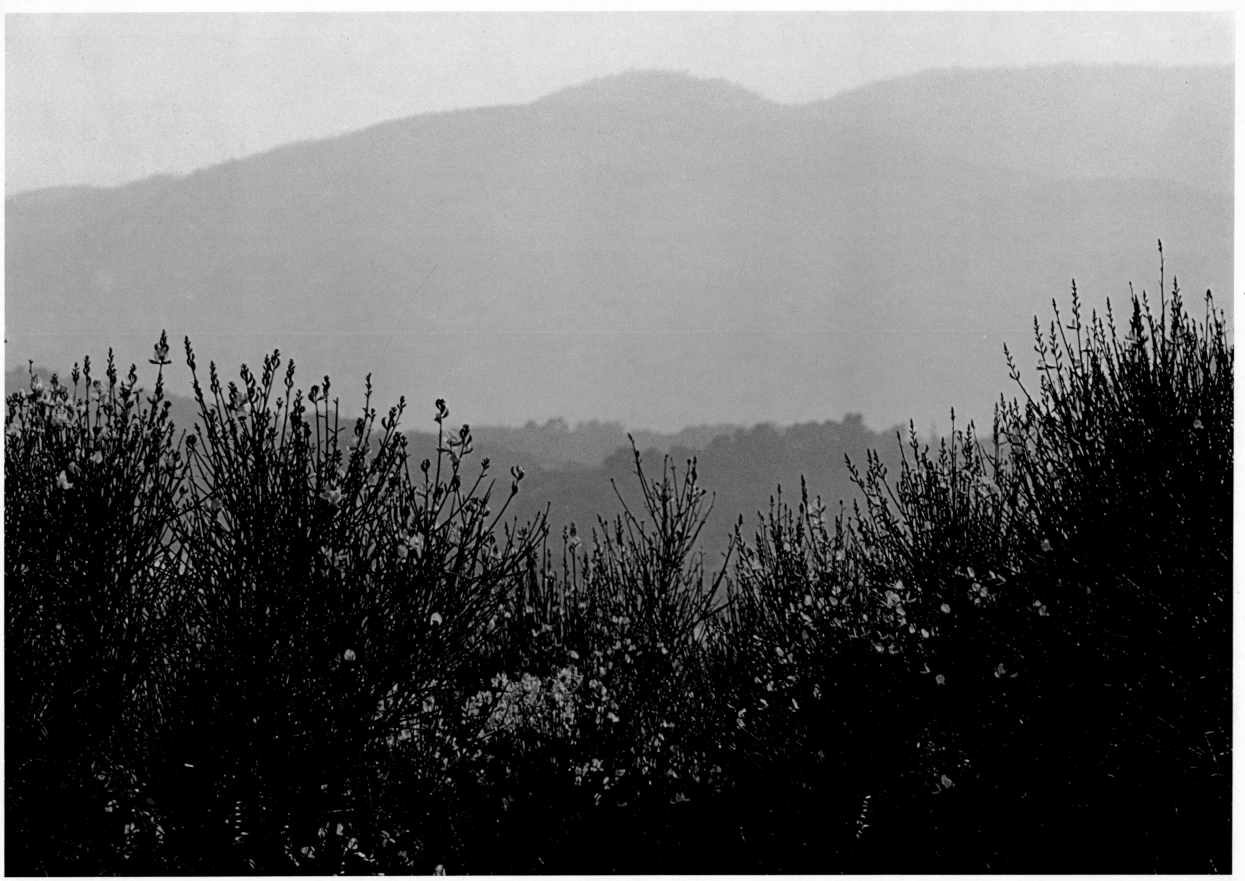

81

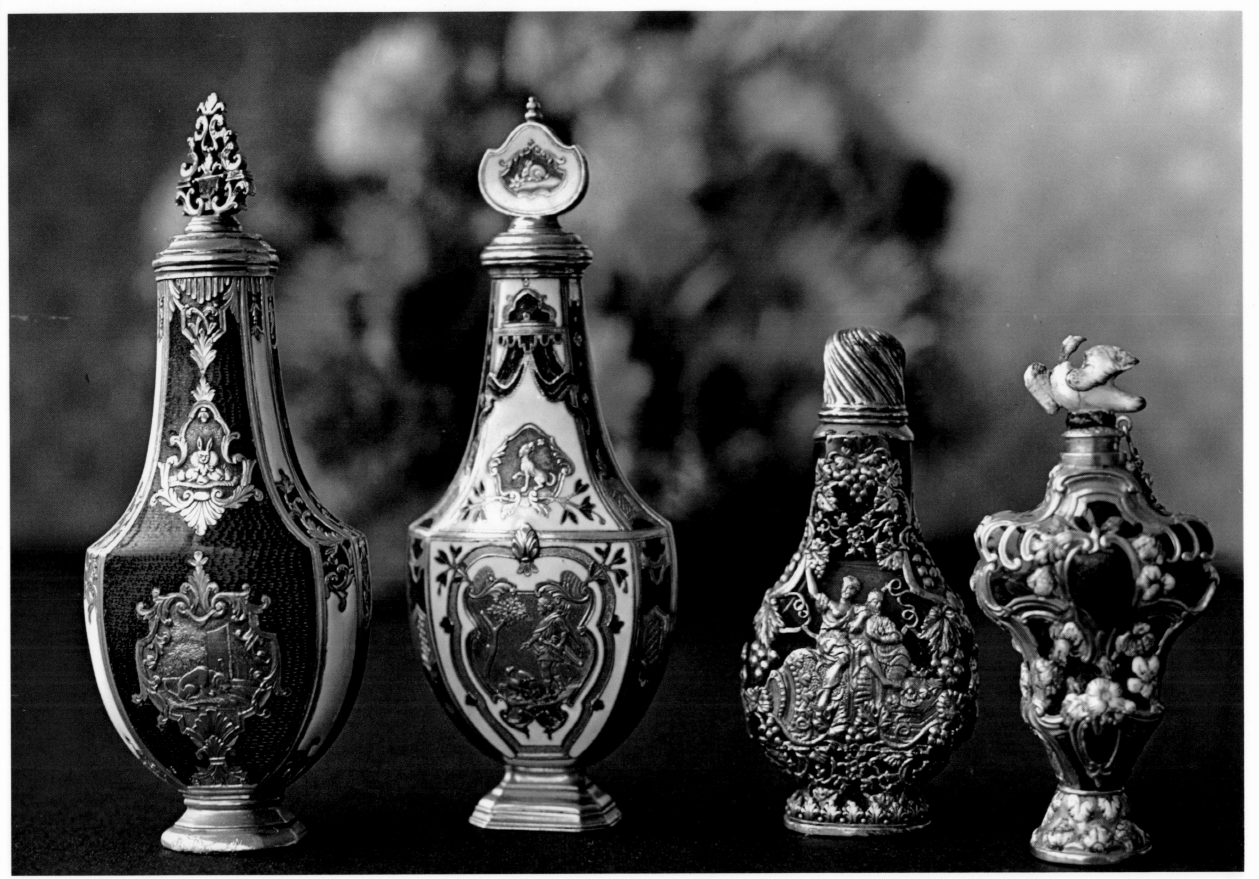

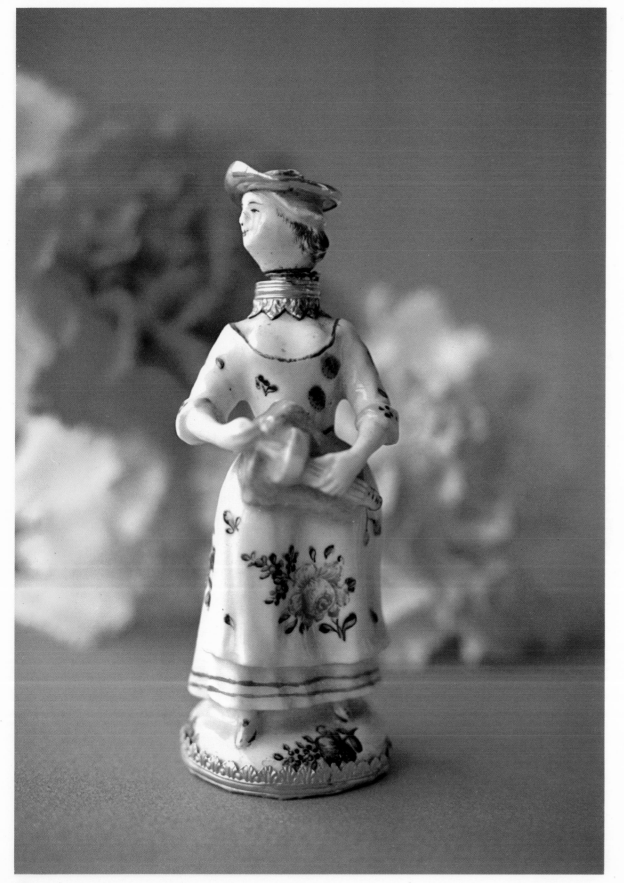

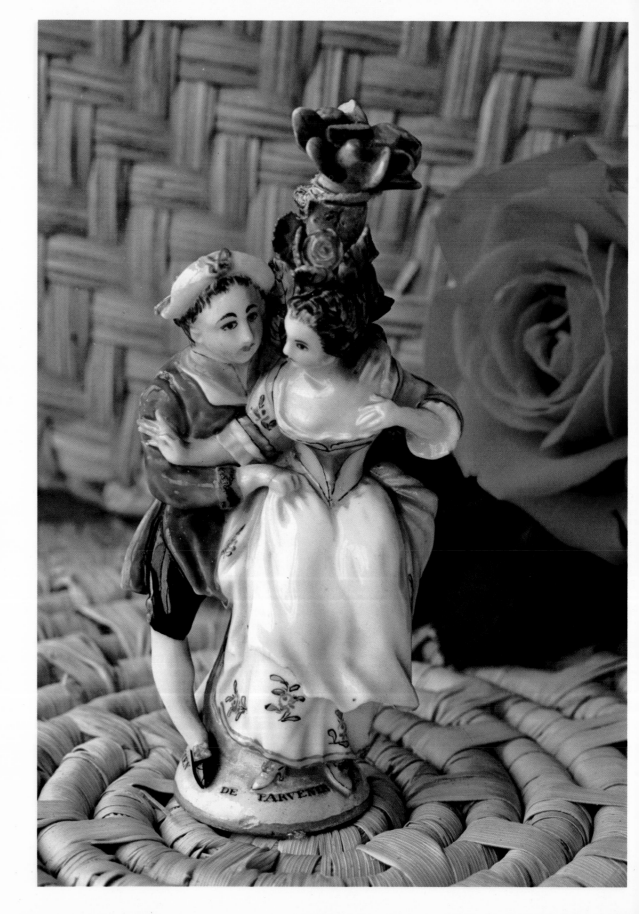

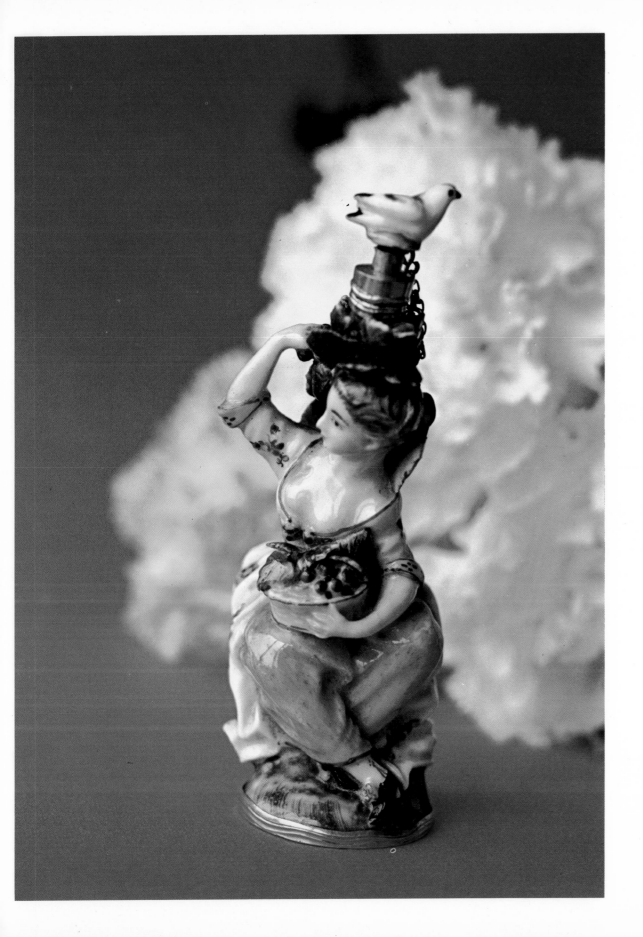
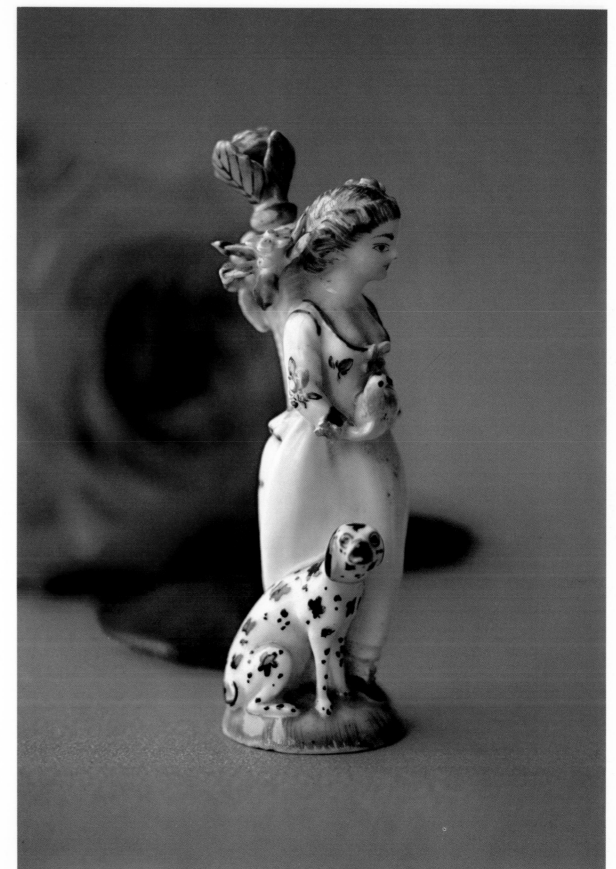

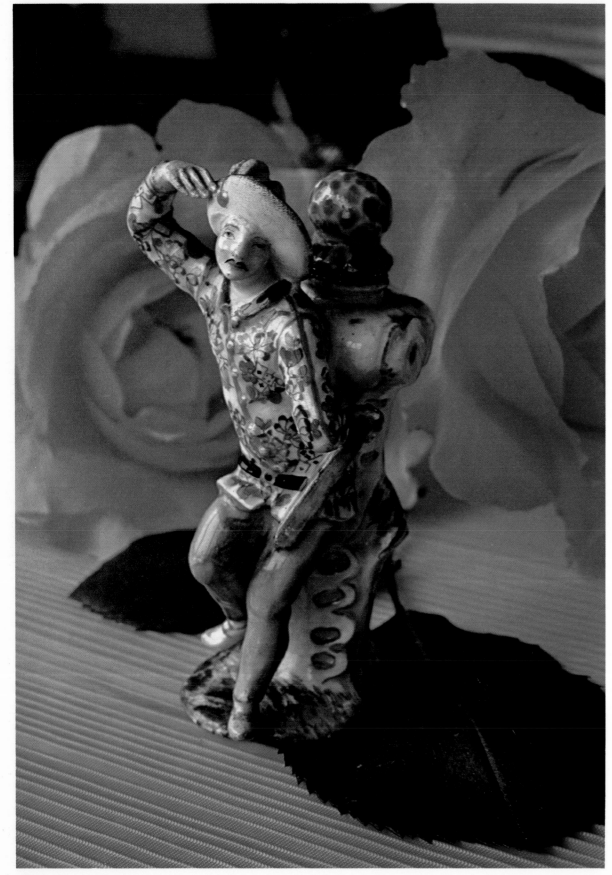

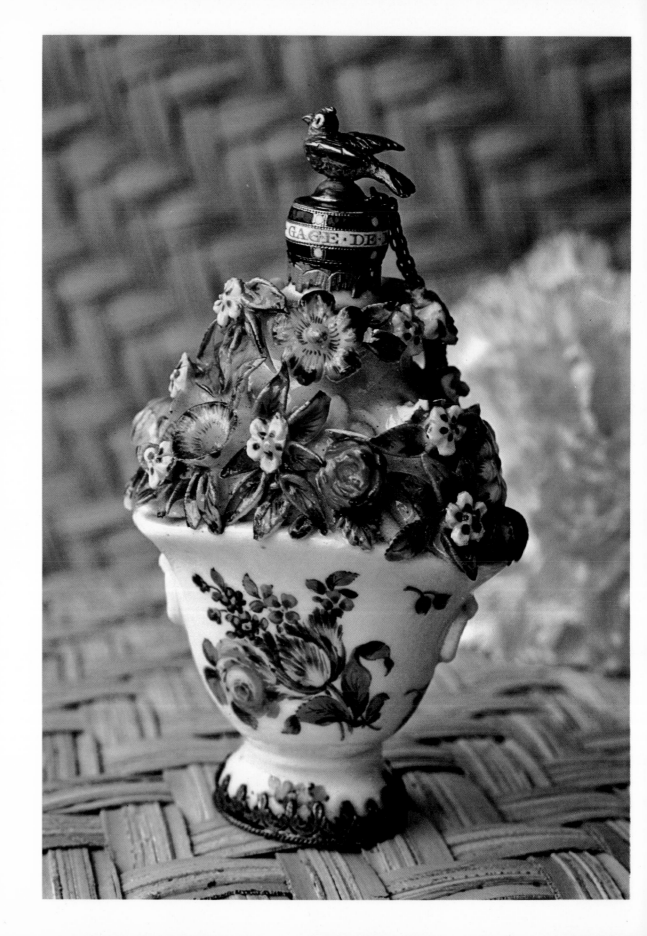

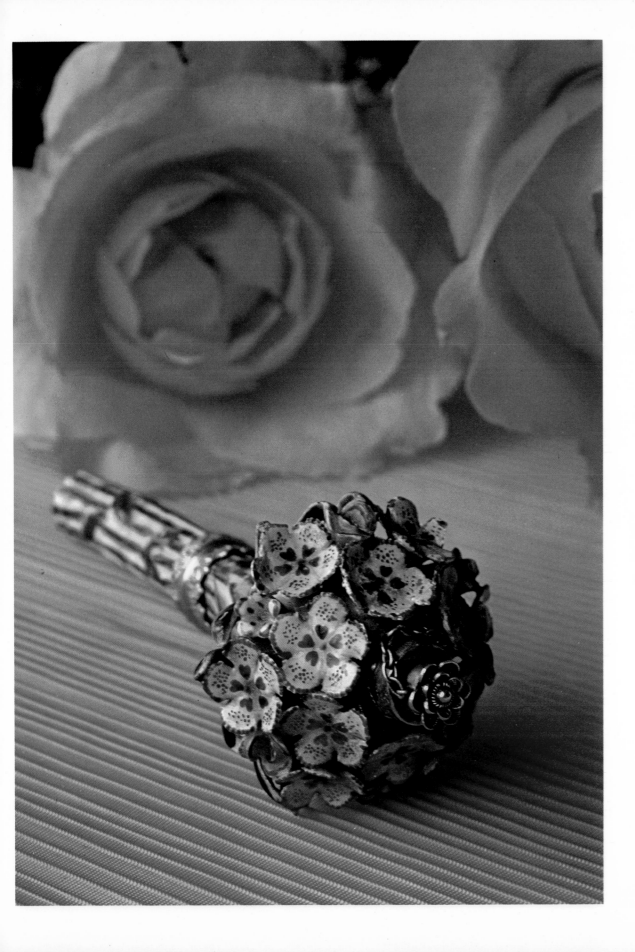

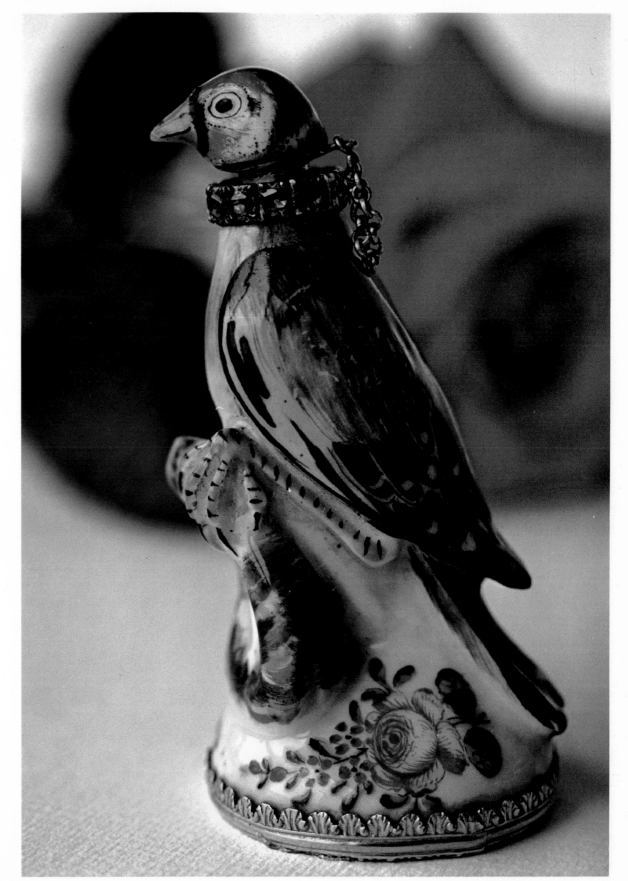

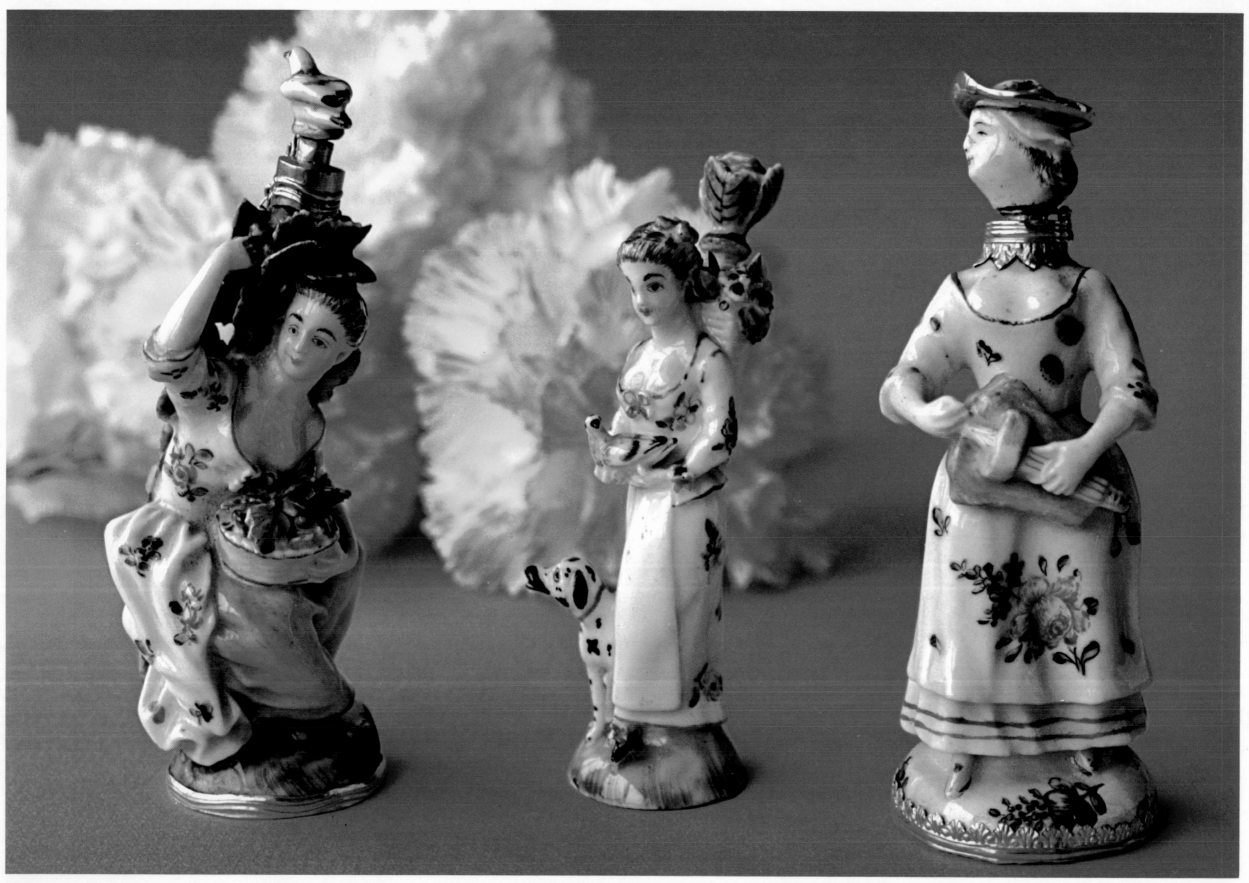

The really glamorous glassmaker of Colonial times was Henry William Stiegel, whose lavish style of living caused him to be called "Baron." He set up a feudal type of town complete with glass factory, homes for the workmen, a school, and a church, along with his own fantastic mansion, which boasted hand-carved woodwork, fabulous tapestries, and a bandstand on the roof. Stiegel rode in a coach-and-four, and as he approached his castle, canons were fired in salute. It was Baron Stiegel's ambition to match the quality of European glass in this country, and one would judge him successful by the respect in which his work is still held. Unfortunately, Stiegel suffered a financial crisis and was forced to sell everything, including his glass collection, which boasted fine enameled pieces and others of amber, amethyst, emerald green, and sapphire blue. Any authentic Stiegel glass that can be found today is worth a fortune.

The third important American glassmaker was Deming Jarves. Called the Paul Revere of New England glass, Jarves started a company at Sandwich on Cape Cod. His factory developed a pressing device which became the basis for a hundred-million-dollar business and is still called Sandwich glass. Unfortunately, due to a general glassmaker's strike in 1888, the factory at Sandwich was closed, never to reopen.

French perfumery began to develop along scientific lines at the beginning of the nineteenth century. The distillation process wrought changes that introduced the beginnings of industrial methods, and the ancient village of Grasse in the South of France began to emerge as a busy center of essential oils. Several firms founded in the earlier centuries expanded their marketing programs beyond the borders of France. After Waterloo the Emperor was altogether too disillusioned and skeptical to interest his people in luxury, and all fashion was restrained. The use of perfume was not. Eau des Belles, Eau de Sainte-Alliance, Parfum des Rois, and other fragrances created a furor.

In the reign of Charles X romanticism showed its influence in grooming as well as in literature. Perfumes in vogue had fresh, charming names which evoke pleasant memories: Le Parfum de Psyche, La Dame Blanche, Du Troubadour, Le Parfum aux Mille Fleurs.

The circumspect reign of Louis Philippe previewed French bourgeois domestic virtue and encouraged the smooth progress of a perfumery that utilized all the advantages of scientific chemistry without losing any of its traditional high quality. Men and women of fashion bathed themselves in a deluge of eau de toilette. The French sought surcease from the barricades of 1848 in a vibrant period of pleasure and prosperity. Floral perfumes enjoyed enormous success. Bottles of clear crystal with distinct lines were manufactured for the greatest perfumes. They were created to suit the taste of the important perfumers, real innovators in style and design.

At about this point, a Frenchman with the unlikely name of O'Reilly opened a glassworks in Paris, the products of which were beautiful enough to compete with the finest English flacons. His glass, no less elegant, was finely engraved and much better smoothed by grinding. He made bottles formed like amphorae, ornamented with classic figures of dancing girls. The design of the figures and the folds of the drapery attested to his tasteful, almost miraculous skills. Unfortunately, O'Reilly lived only until 1830.

Concurrently with him, Baccarat and Saint Louis made a strong bid for the perfume buyers' trade. Baccarat employed 1500 workers during the Empire in shops where crystal was made with wood fuel. Saint Louis, on the other hand, worked from the beginning with coal in open crucibles. This eliminated the negative action of the coal gases on the crystal. As a result of their combined artistry, perfumes were sold for the most part in bottles of high value and magnificent design. The faces were simple, plain, with cut sides. Encrustations were no longer considered desirable. Only crystal was used, and the beaded or point style of cut class was much in favor. Certain very costly perfumes were presented in

97

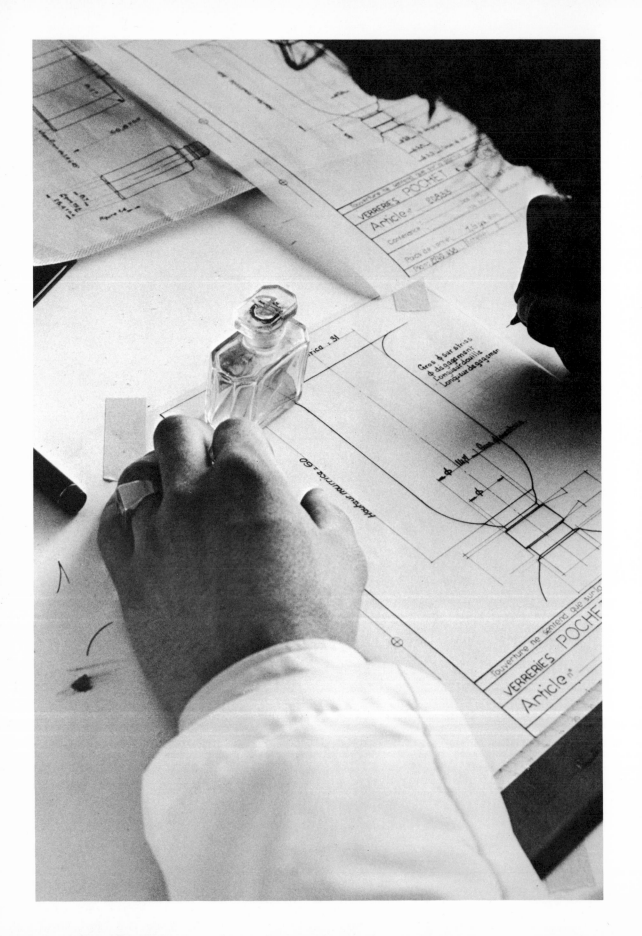

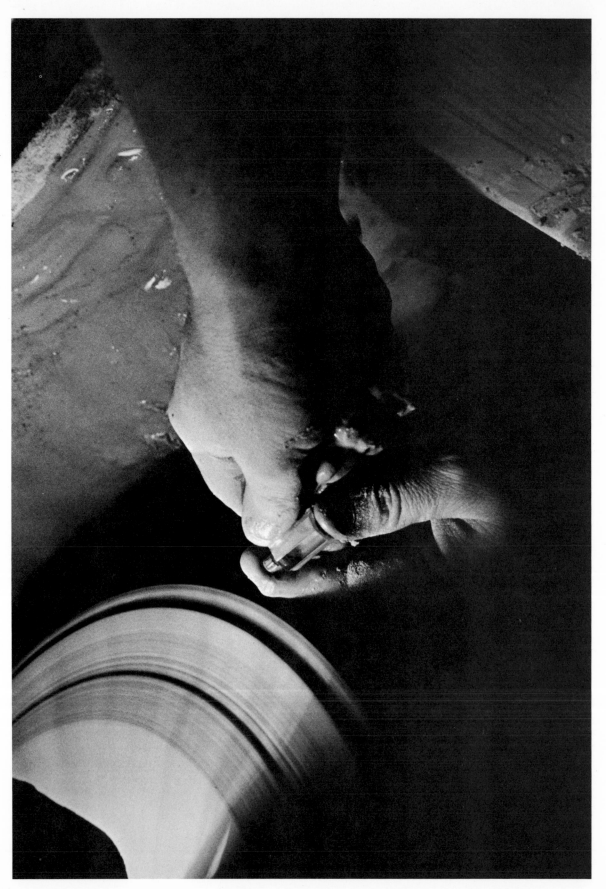

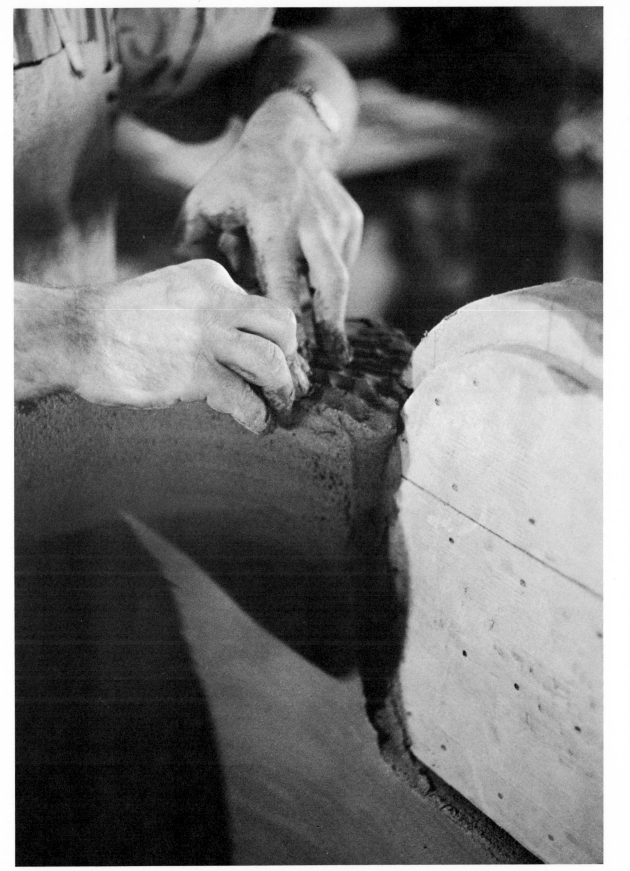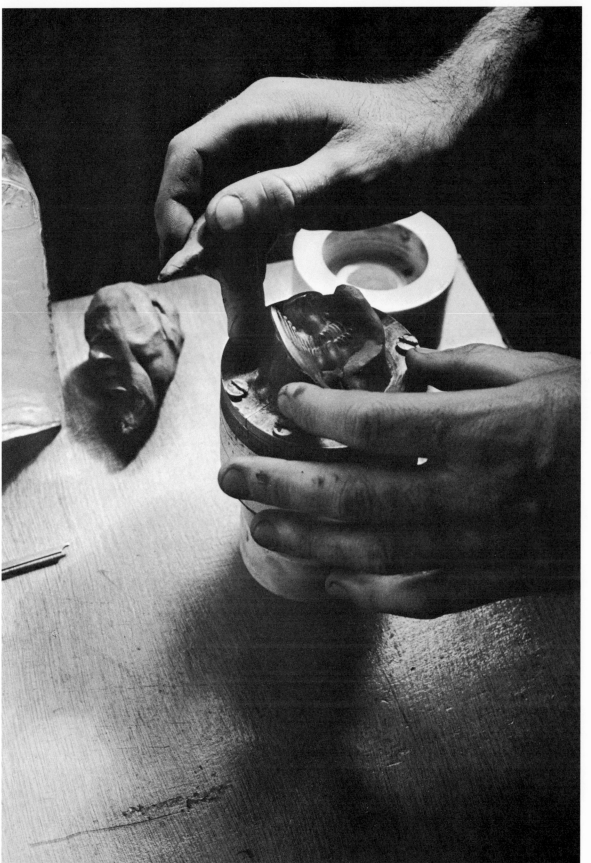

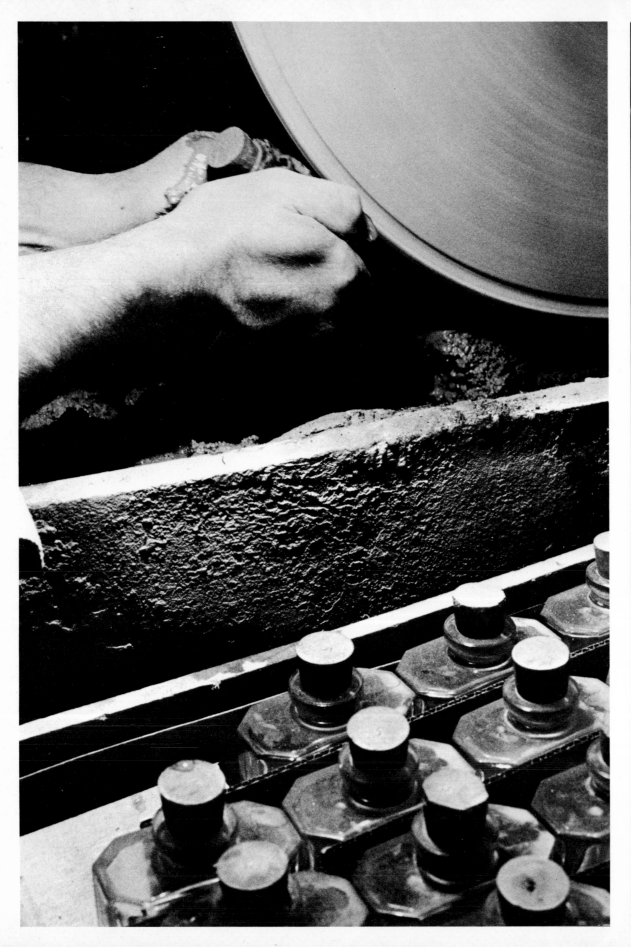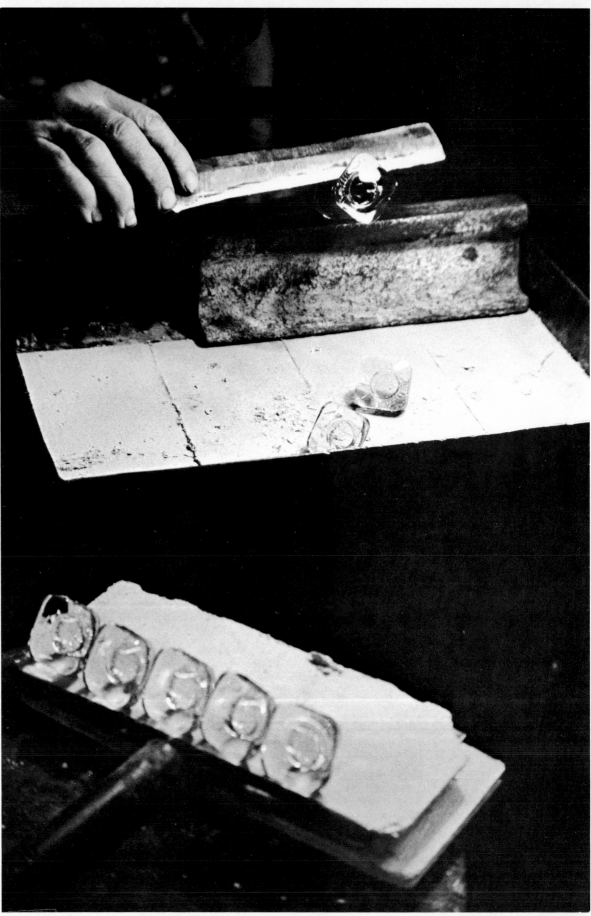

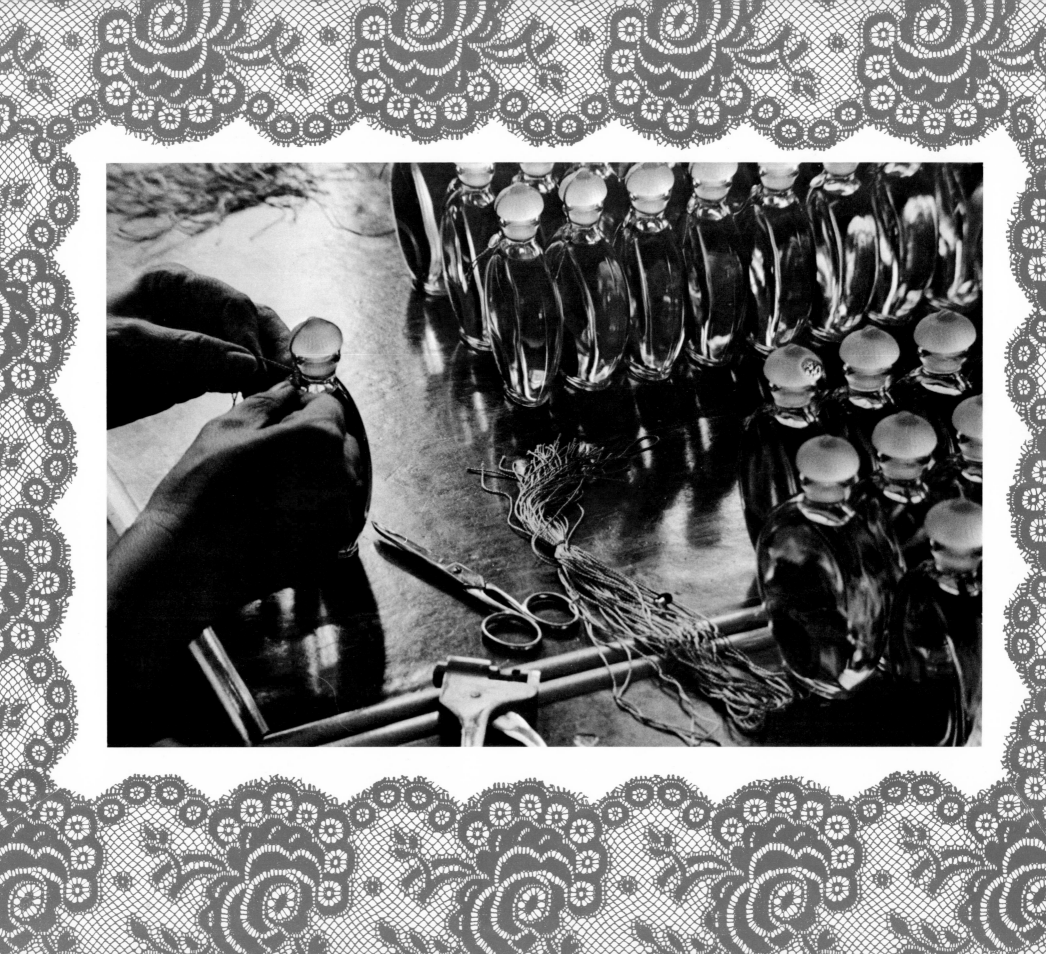

crystal bulbs, ornamented with a profusion of golden stars or bees. Stoppers were of precious metals. Less expensive scents were packaged in bottles of ordinary glass, gray or greenish in color, but the public was becoming more demanding, and the birth of advertising made people more conscious of the product. Perfume merchants therefore insisted that glassmakers create exclusive original or amusing forms for them.

Between 1815 and 1845 the mode of perfume presentation was entirely modified. Through advertising the label was made the important sales element, while the importance of the bottle became almost negligible. This situation was corrected, however, during the Second Empire when the marketing of perfume did a complete about-face. The fanciful and incessantly changing labels gave way to the trademark which stabilized the identification of the perfume with the perfume maker. Finally, advertising such as we know it today turned its efforts again to attracting the consumer through beautiful, exotic, elegant, bottling and packaging.

Frequently these perfume containers were sheathed in cases of precious wood, encrusted with medallions of gold, silver, or enamel, and lined with silk or velvet. The Rousseau factory in Paris created handsome perfume holders of two or three layers of glass, intensely colored and engraved on the wheel. The famous firm of Gallé, in Nancy, produced containers of perfect transparency or translucence. The artist glassmaker Lalique brought an even greater note of originality and harmony into the making of the perfume flacon. During this time all sorts of perfume gift items —pocket flasks, bulbs of scent, necklaces of hollowed-out and perfumed pearls, wings with hollow settings containing a perfume wax, made their reappearance. Perfumes were boxed and beribboned in every way imaginable.

Today the choice and quality of the materials cannot be compared with those of past centuries. Nevertheless, certain perfumers still seek to attain complete harmony between their perfume and the flacon in which it is presented.

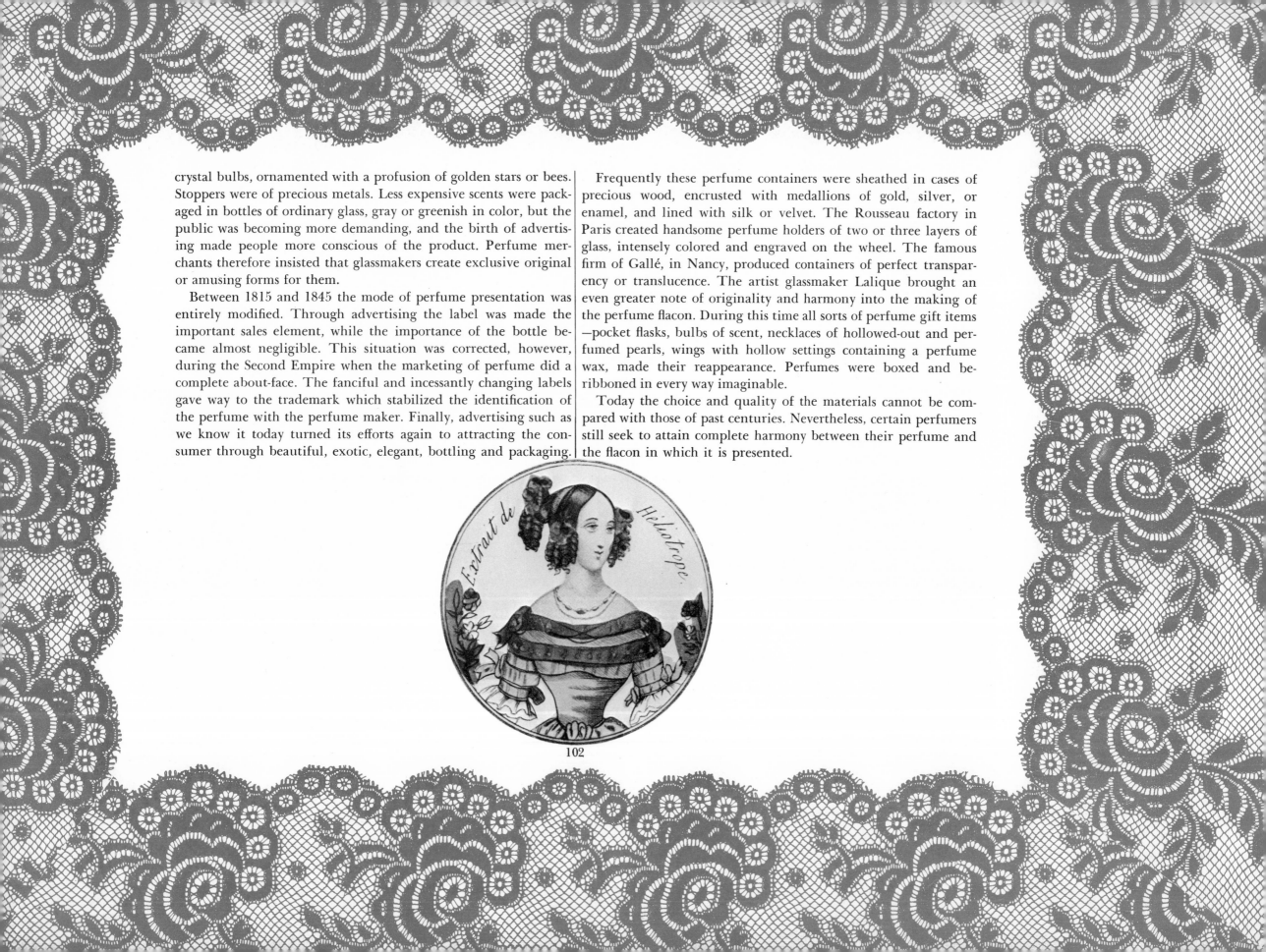

102

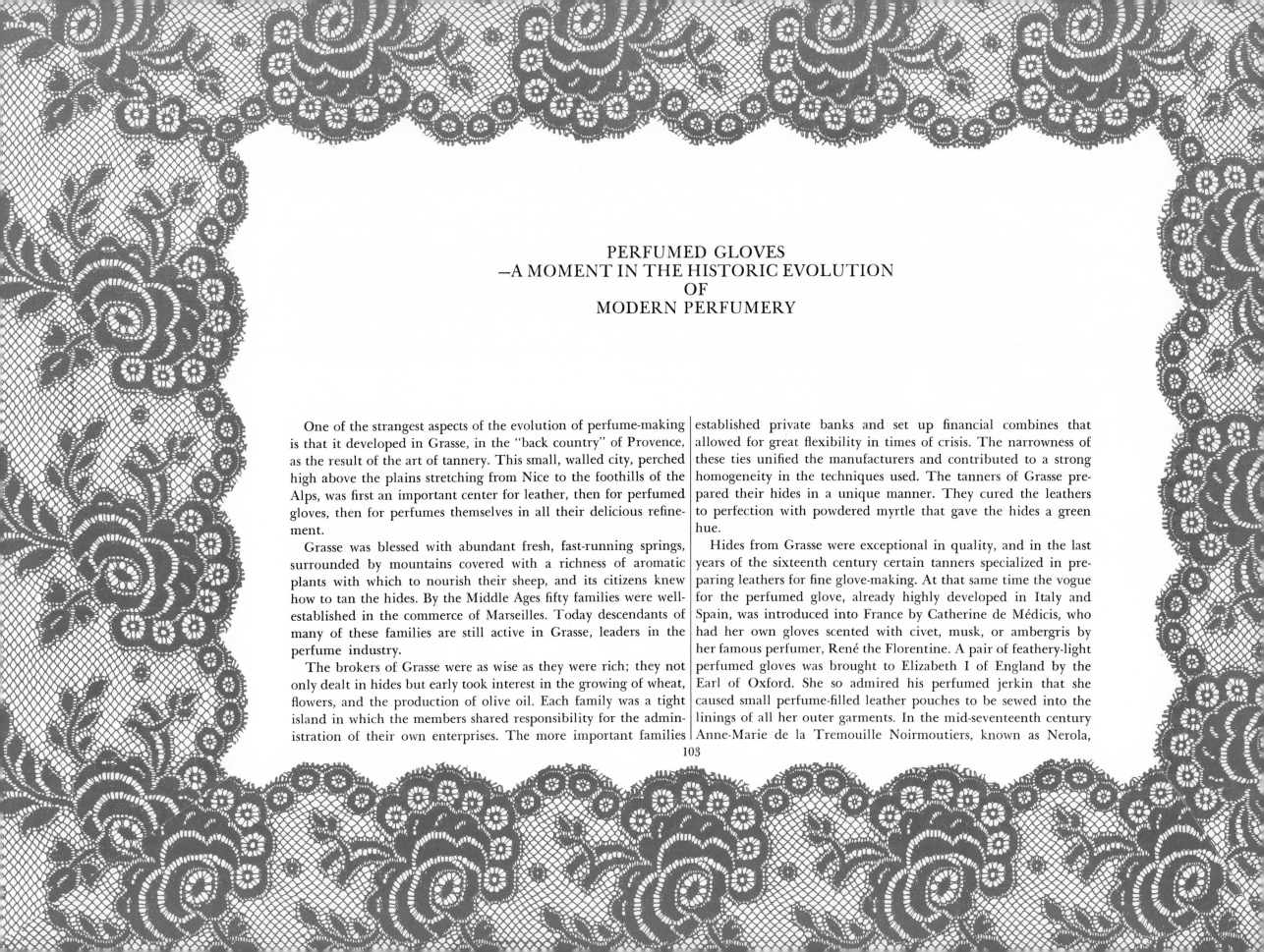

# PERFUMED GLOVES
## —A MOMENT IN THE HISTORIC EVOLUTION
## OF
## MODERN PERFUMERY

One of the strangest aspects of the evolution of perfume-making is that it developed in Grasse, in the "back country" of Provence, as the result of the art of tannery. This small, walled city, perched high above the plains stretching from Nice to the foothills of the Alps, was first an important center for leather, then for perfumed gloves, then for perfumes themselves in all their delicious refinement.

Grasse was blessed with abundant fresh, fast-running springs, surrounded by mountains covered with a richness of aromatic plants with which to nourish their sheep, and its citizens knew how to tan the hides. By the Middle Ages fifty families were well-established in the commerce of Marseilles. Today descendants of many of these families are still active in Grasse, leaders in the perfume industry.

The brokers of Grasse were as wise as they were rich; they not only dealt in hides but early took interest in the growing of wheat, flowers, and the production of olive oil. Each family was a tight island in which the members shared responsibility for the administration of their own enterprises. The more important families established private banks and set up financial combines that allowed for great flexibility in times of crisis. The narrowness of these ties unified the manufacturers and contributed to a strong homogeneity in the techniques used. The tanners of Grasse prepared their hides in a unique manner. They cured the leathers to perfection with powdered myrtle that gave the hides a green hue.

Hides from Grasse were exceptional in quality, and in the last years of the sixteenth century certain tanners specialized in preparing leathers for fine glove-making. At that same time the vogue for the perfumed glove, already highly developed in Italy and Spain, was introduced into France by Catherine de Médicis, who had her own gloves scented with civet, musk, or ambergris by her famous perfumer, René the Florentine. A pair of feathery-light perfumed gloves was brought to Elizabeth I of England by the Earl of Oxford. She so admired his perfumed jerkin that she caused small perfume-filled leather pouches to be sewed into the linings of all her outer garments. In the mid-seventeenth century Anne-Marie de la Tremouille Noirmoutiers, known as Nerola,

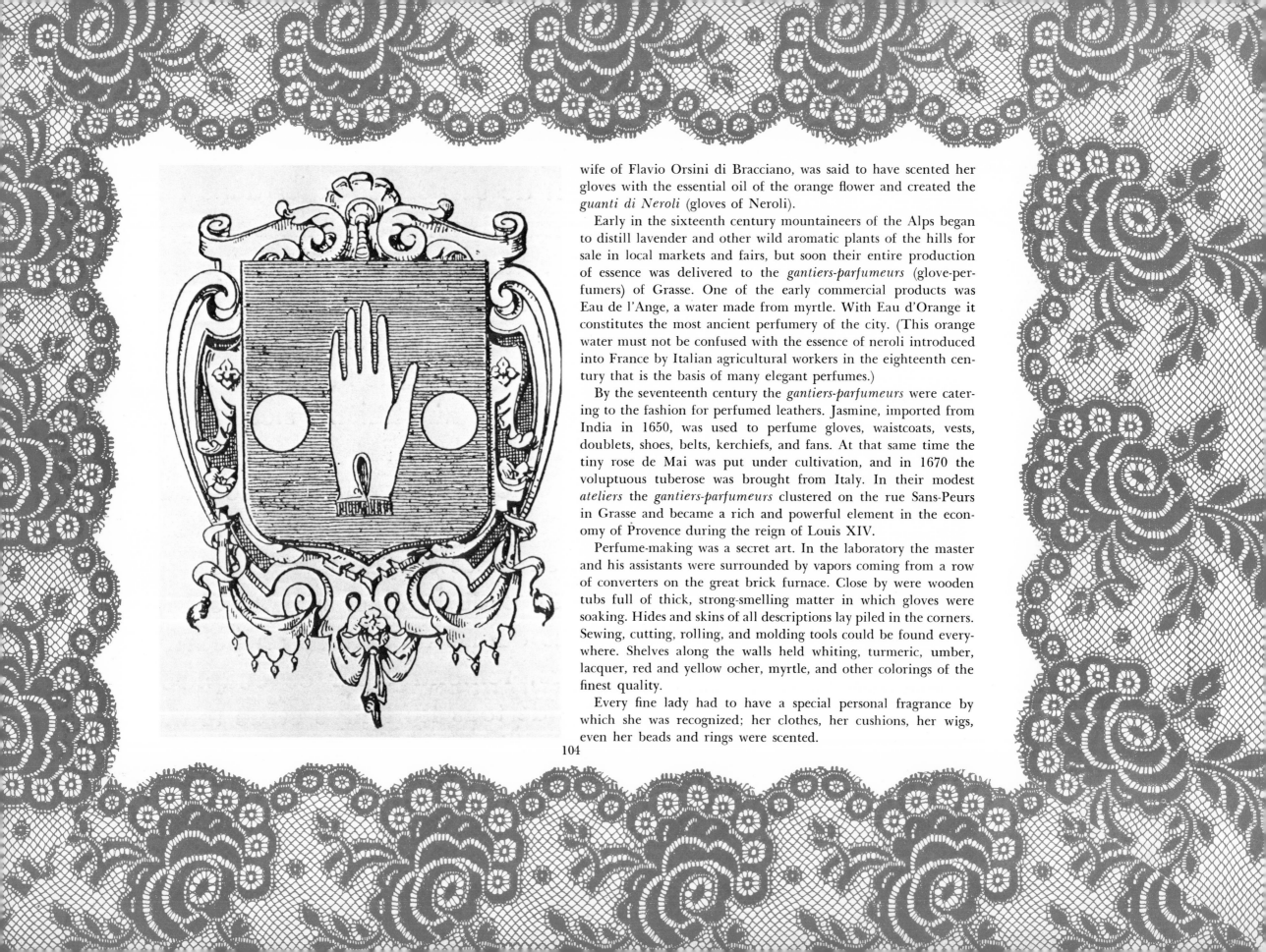

wife of Flavio Orsini di Bracciano, was said to have scented her gloves with the essential oil of the orange flower and created the *guanti di Neroli* (gloves of Neroli).

Early in the sixteenth century mountaineers of the Alps began to distill lavender and other wild aromatic plants of the hills for sale in local markets and fairs, but soon their entire production of essence was delivered to the *gantiers-parfumeurs* (glove-perfumers) of Grasse. One of the early commercial products was Eau de l'Ange, a water made from myrtle. With Eau d'Orange it constitutes the most ancient perfumery of the city. (This orange water must not be confused with the essence of neroli introduced into France by Italian agricultural workers in the eighteenth century that is the basis of many elegant perfumes.)

By the seventeenth century the *gantiers-parfumeurs* were catering to the fashion for perfumed leathers. Jasmine, imported from India in 1650, was used to perfume gloves, waistcoats, vests, doublets, shoes, belts, kerchiefs, and fans. At that same time the tiny rose de Mai was put under cultivation, and in 1670 the voluptuous tuberose was brought from Italy. In their modest *ateliers* the *gantiers-parfumeurs* clustered on the rue Sans-Peurs in Grasse and became a rich and powerful element in the economy of Provence during the reign of Louis XIV.

Perfume-making was a secret art. In the laboratory the master and his assistants were surrounded by vapors coming from a row of converters on the great brick furnace. Close by were wooden tubs full of thick, strong-smelling matter in which gloves were soaking. Hides and skins of all descriptions lay piled in the corners. Sewing, cutting, rolling, and molding tools could be found everywhere. Shelves along the walls held whiting, turmeric, umber, lacquer, red and yellow ocher, myrtle, and other colorings of the finest quality.

Every fine lady had to have a special personal fragrance by which she was recognized; her clothes, her cushions, her wigs, even her beads and rings were scented.

To become a master required three years of apprenticeship, three years of service as a journeyman; a candidate for guild membership had to present an original, highly complex "masterpiece" to the jury to prove his skill in preparing and cutting skins, in perfuming and coloring them, and in dressing them to the point of highest pliancy. By the year 1700 there were twenty-one such masters, and to limit competition they formed a guild in December 1724 which was accepted and registered at the Court of Aix in 1729, separating them from the tanners' guild. The twenty-one manufacturers of Grasse were directed by four trustees, assisted by four deputies. Their meeting place was in the convent of the Augustinian monks. Every three months the trustees visited all the masters, examining their finished products, their tools, looking into any claims of fraud and, above all, protecting the financial interests of the masters in the trade, exacting huge fines for the infraction of any regulation. By 1745 the guild had seventy *gantiers-parfumeurs*. No one could practice the art unless he was twenty years old and had the six years of required training. There were five classes of *gantiers-parfumeurs,* depending upon their gross sales. Their names appear in the records of the eighteenth century, names which still produce the world's finest essential oils for perfume.

Extremely prosperous, very astute as the fashions and economy of the times changed, the masters of Grasse turned away from the perfuming of gloves. The exorbitant tax on tanned hides and the disenchantment of their clientele with perfumed leathers led them to turn their interest to perfume-making in and of itself. This movement crystallized by the year 1789 when delicate fragrances came into style. Strong perfumes were the object of criticism, and women of refinement shunned their use

Perfumers began to offer to their customers beautiful flacons, trinkets, and decorated boxes for pastes and perfumed powders. Gloves were worn for night beauty treatment only, while cosmetics took the cosmopolitan centers of the sophisticated world by storm.

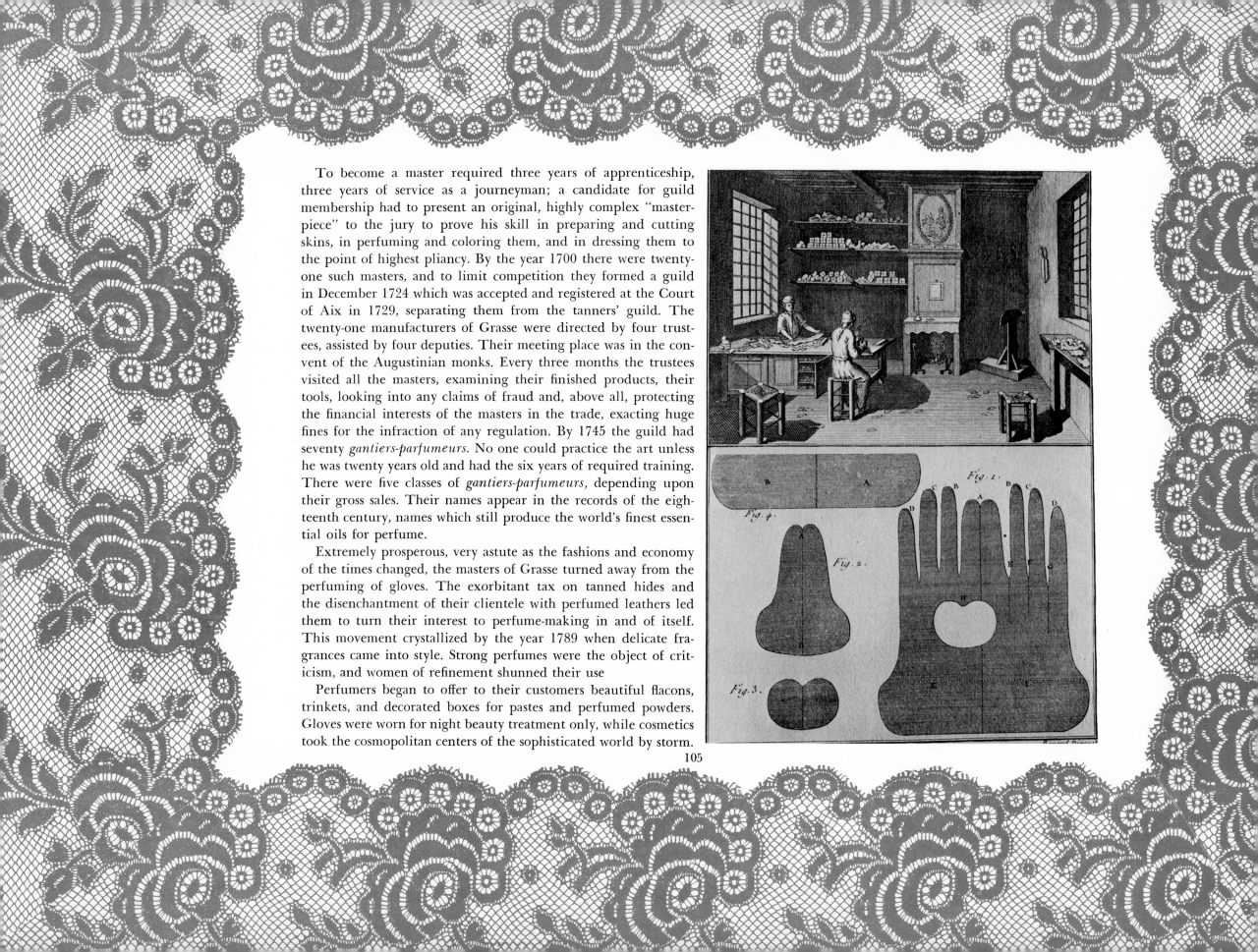

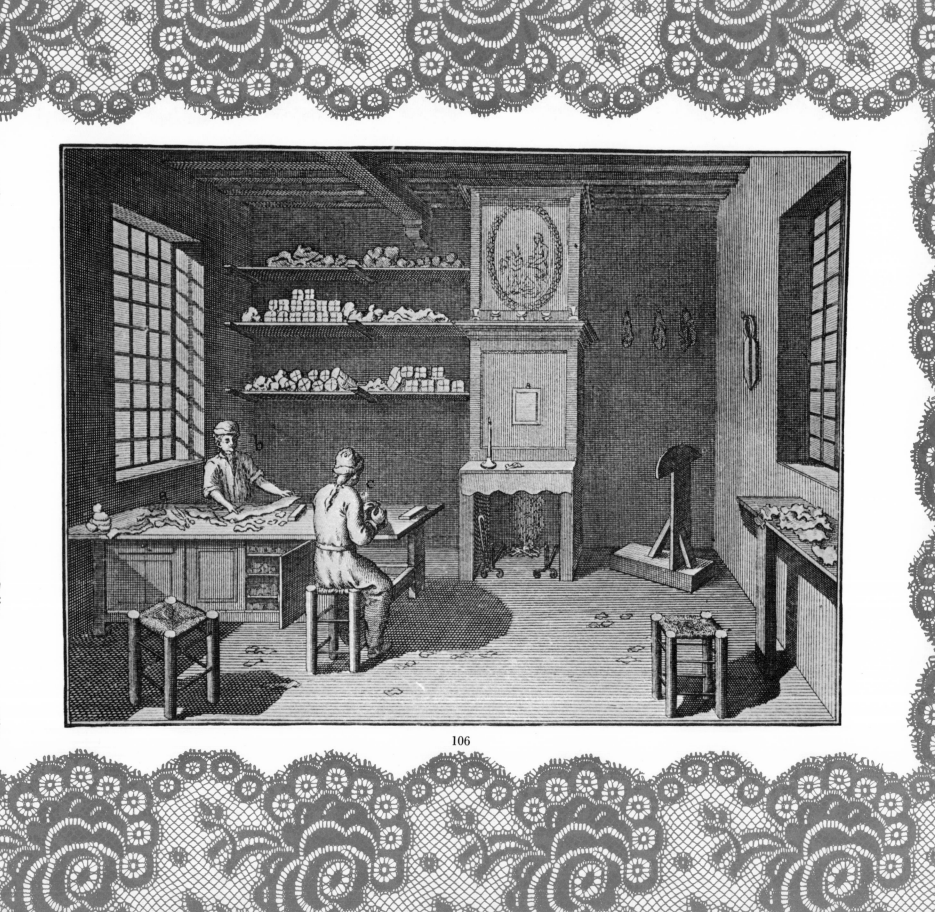

106

The influence of the perfumers of Grasse became more considerable in the eighteenth century, and the perfume masters opened flourishing boutiques in Paris. One of their number, Monsieur Fargeon, was perfumer to Queen Marie-Antoinette, and just prior to the Revolution half of all Europe purchased essences from Grasse. The revolution saw the last of the *gantiers-parfumeurs,* and only the deluxe perfume trade survived.

If the eighteenth century marks the transition from glove manufacture to perfume-making, the nineteenth century witnessed an even greater change—from individual craftsmanship to the industrial expansion that has given us the broad gamut of today's great and glorious perfumes. In this present era of interest in fragrance we may see the return of the beautiful, colored, well-cut glove impregnated with the sweet, fresh smells of the herbs of the plains, the fragrance of aromatic plants of the mountains, and the voluptuous scents of the flowers of the world.

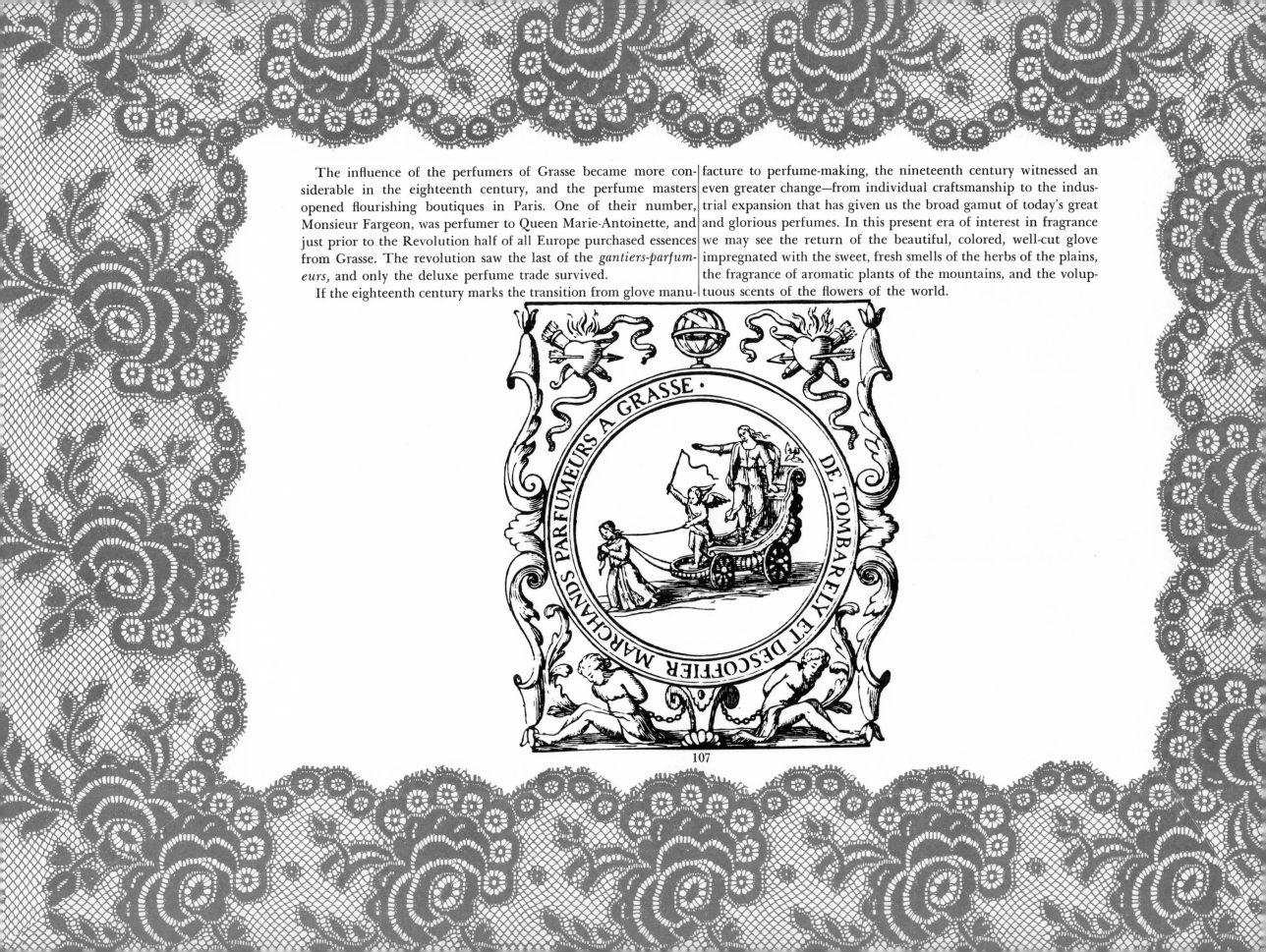

107

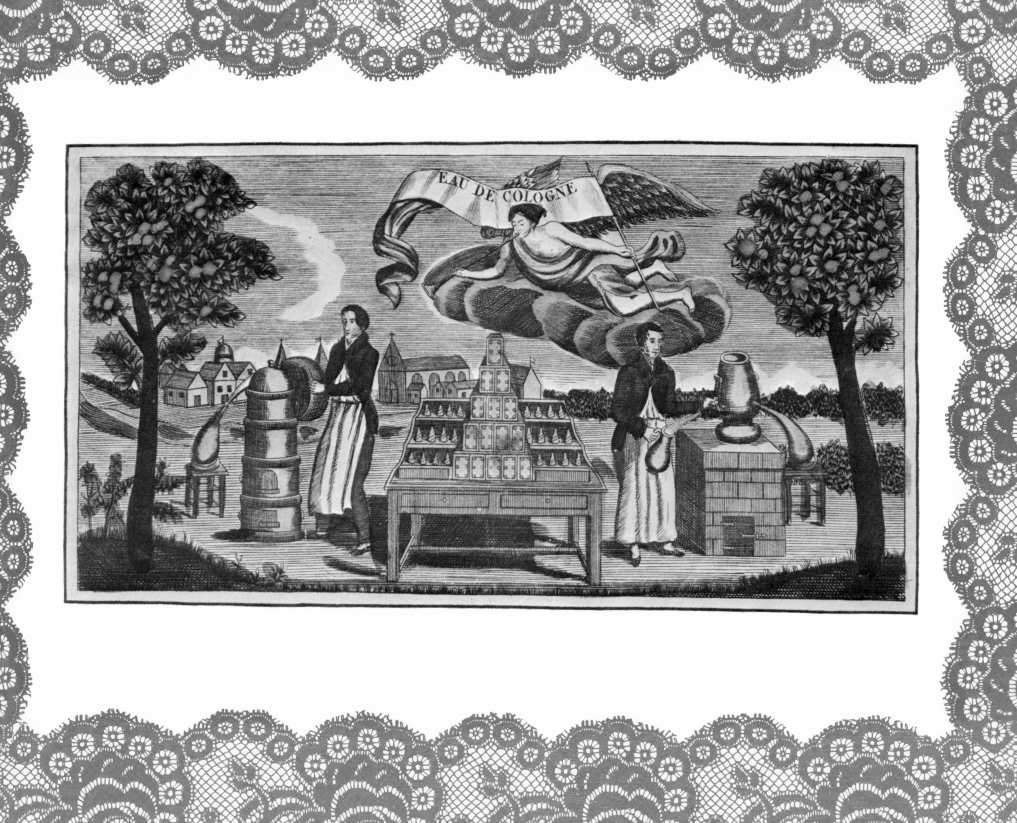

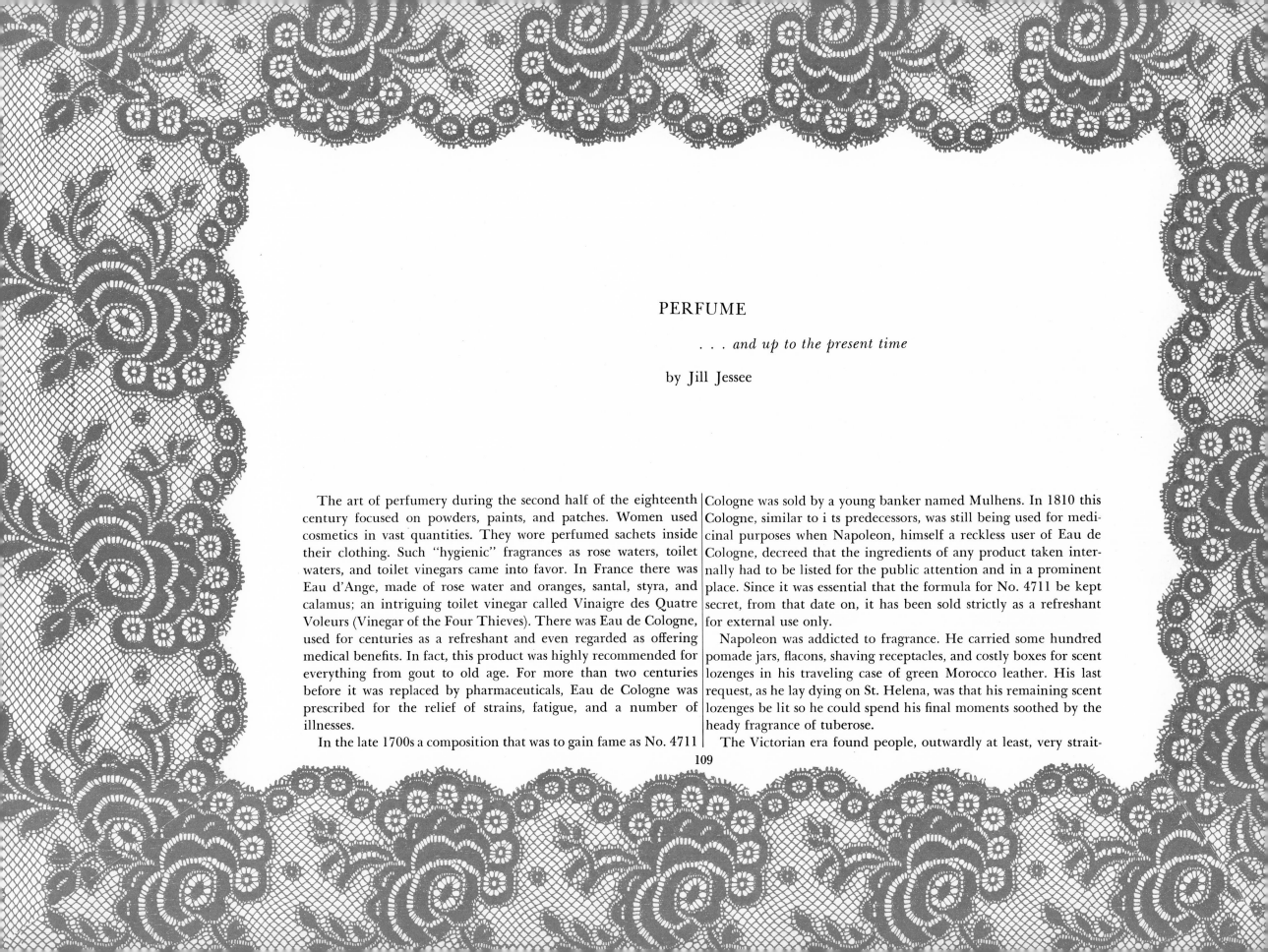

# PERFUME

*. . . and up to the present time*

by Jill Jessee

The art of perfumery during the second half of the eighteenth century focused on powders, paints, and patches. Women used cosmetics in vast quantities. They wore perfumed sachets inside their clothing. Such "hygienic" fragrances as rose waters, toilet waters, and toilet vinegars came into favor. In France there was Eau d'Ange, made of rose water and oranges, santal, styra, and calamus; an intriguing toilet vinegar called Vinaigre des Quatre Voleurs (Vinegar of the Four Thieves). There was Eau de Cologne, used for centuries as a refreshant and even regarded as offering medical benefits. In fact, this product was highly recommended for everything from gout to old age. For more than two centuries before it was replaced by pharmaceuticals, Eau de Cologne was prescribed for the relief of strains, fatigue, and a number of illnesses.

In the late 1700s a composition that was to gain fame as No. 4711 Cologne was sold by a young banker named Mulhens. In 1810 this Cologne, similar to i ts predecessors, was still being used for medicinal purposes when Napoleon, himself a reckless user of Eau de Cologne, decreed that the ingredients of any product taken internally had to be listed for the public attention and in a prominent place. Since it was essential that the formula for No. 4711 be kept secret, from that date on, it has been sold strictly as a refreshant for external use only.

Napoleon was addicted to fragrance. He carried some hundred pomade jars, flacons, shaving receptacles, and costly boxes for scent lozenges in his traveling case of green Morocco leather. His last request, as he lay dying on St. Helena, was that his remaining scent lozenges be lit so he could spend his final moments soothed by the heady fragrance of tuberose.

The Victorian era found people, outwardly at least, very straitlaced. The prim Queen of England, who herself liked "Ess. Bouquet," set rigid standards for society. Only persons of the demimonde were to be seen attired flamboyantly. Lipstick and powder were considered "fast," the clothes, makeup, and scent of "nice" women being therefore, of necessity, simple and unobtrusive.

Nevertheless, fastidious women clung to their favorite fragrances. Dainty lace-edged handkerchiefs were scented, and icy Eau de Cologne was used to bathe the brows of delicate females who fainted on the slightest provocation. It is significant that even though obvious cosmetics were frowned upon during Queen Victoria's reign, perfume advertisements were much in evidence and not at all subtle.

When Victoria's son, Edward VII, took the throne with his beautiful consort Alexandra, elegance became the watchword. From the moment of her marriage Queen Alexandra is known to have had a preference for Essence of White Rose, a perfume she used to the end of her days. Her sister, the Czarina of Russia, preferred Essence of Chypre, a fragrance also known to have been favored by Queen Olga of Greece.

In colonial America the typical Puritan response to anything as frivolous as the use of fragrance was probably either a good, cleansing ducking or an airing out in the stocks. However, as the rigors of life abated, the use of scent increased. Perfumes were imported with cargoes of Calcutta seersucker, Kashmir shawls, China silks, and other luxuries. Ladies took hours to prepare their elaborate toilettes, to be tortured into their corsets, to add petticoat upon petticoat, to arrange their coiffures, and to apply precious scents to throat, wrists, and elegant lace handkerchiefs.

Smelling salts were not the only refuge from "disturbances" in the Colonies or in England. Sachets and "waters" were popular. "Toilet Vinegar" was considered by connoisseurs of the time to be superior to the venerable traditional floral fragrances, as the formula contained balsams and vinegar in addition to traditional ingredients used in Eau de Cologne. Lavender Water was favored,

and though its origin goes back to the twelfth century in Europe, Florida Water was perfected in America. It resembled a mixture of Lavender Water and Eau de Cologne to which a dash of oil of cloves, cassia, and lemongrass was added. Not only can Florida Water be remembered as being very fashionable in days gone by; it is still being sold.

By the time of the Civil War American perfume sales had reached the million-dollar mark and American fragrances were beginning to give foreign perfumers some competition. In those days it was considered quite ethical for an American manufacturer to imitate a French perfume outright, and in fact the French often sent their own concentrates to the States for that purpose. Despite these practices, original creations were also being composed by native perfumers. Few survive.

The early 1900s ushered in a quaint, stuffy, but colorful and charming epoch when women were clinging vines and kept dizzy spells under control with Eau de Cologne. Many floral perfumes were in vogue, but there were some popular items that had names that sounded in that ladylike era quite naughty.

The aftermath of World War I actually marked America's entrance into beauty as a big business. With hundreds of thousands of doughboys returning from overseas with Parisian perfumes, American enthusiasm for fragrance zoomed.

Typical of the time is that the fine Fifth Avenue department store of B. Altman offered a Book of Styles for the 1919–1920 season which included none of such present-day items as lipstick, nail polish, or eye makeup, but which *did* feature prominently toilet water, creams, sachets, powder, rouge, and astringents.

In *A History of Cosmetics in America* by Gilbert Vail we find the following excerpt from an address made in 1905 by the president of the Manufacturing Perfumers' Association:

*The taste of the perfumery-consuming public appears to be for coarser and ranker odors. The day when delicacy of*

110

*odor and richness (not strength) were demanded appears to
have gone, and the cry is for something strong, rank, and
lasting. . . . Once an odor lasting for twenty-four hours
on a handkerchief was deemed satisfactory. Now, unless the
odor will last a week, it is thought weak and ephemeral.*

Mr. Vail's comment on the president's remark is as follows:

*President Dalley may have deplored the taste of the day,
but his distaste had no effect whatsoever in lessening the
demand for heady, exotic perfumes. More and more women
were casting off the yoke which had bound them to moderation in makeup for so long, and by 1915 it was no longer a
stigma attached only to "fast" women. The entire feminine
world had become cosmetic conscious and was directly responsible for the greatest boom the industry has ever known.*

Harriet Hubbard Ayer, a pioneer in the beauty field, published
a book in 1902 which has a great many interesting things to say
about perfume. The following abstract from an extremely serious
section titled "The Abuse of Perfumes" might be considered amusing today in view of the profusion of "heady scents" preferred by
the modern fragrance buyer:

*Some of us, in these days of artificial musk and suffocating
rose, who have stifled in the theater and have been overcome in cable cars and restaurants by the heaviness, have
fervently wished the promiscuous use of these powerful,
enervating, and sometimes nauseating odors might be re-
stricted to the boudoirs and drawing rooms whose queens
elect to vulgarize all their surroundings by this and kindred
extravagance.*

*Fastidious women (with here and there an exception) are
as delicately refined in their selection of sweet odors as in
every other personal appointment. A high-bred woman does
not associate herself with musk or patchouli. She may select
the most delicate of violet extracts, and so assimilate her
personality with the flower as always to recall it, or her*

*linen may be fragrant with the faintest odor of Florentine
orris. The shadow of the clear pungent lavender may pre-
cede her, but the most sensitive and refined women shrink
intuitively from the odors that attract the parvenu.*

*Few people outside the scientific world know the hygienic
value as well as the danger lurking in flower scents. The
effect of musk, rose, saffron, and almond flowers is almost
hypnotic to some sensitive organizations. To others the
heavy odors are like strains of sensuous music and in their
results the reverse of elevating. Hysteria is inevitably aggra-
vated and frequently caused by the odor of musk, and the
use of this perfume should be forbidden delicate girls and
women.*

What more marvelous commentary could we have, what greater
insight could be given us into the perfume thinking of the time!

Recent study of perfume patterns shows that there are twin
trends. On one hand, the classics in perfumery are still very strong.
A classic is a perfume that has kept a devoted audience for twenty-
five years or more. Such a fragrance has certainly proved its appeal
and its quality when it has sustained its popularity for that length
of time.

Not only is this true of a number of fine perfumes, but many
newer scents have been patterned on the classic style (most often
French in origin), for when a certain odor is a success, one that is
similar to it will surely be well received. As a consequence, one
can expect many new scents to appear that follow one or another of
the accepted classics.

On the other hand, some perfume buyers have reverted to using
the simplest, most elementary types of fragrance, a trend that no
doubt relates to the current interest in ecology and the desire to be
in close touch with one's natural, earthy environment. Such pur-
chasers—men and women—would rather smell like a strawberry or
a lemon than like a gardenia, a rose, or a spice.

Concurrently with these twin trends there are persons drawn
only to the sexiest animal scents—musk, ambergris, and civet.

Long-ago favorites, these pungent odors have once more captured public approval. Only time will tell how long these enthusiasms will endure, but they have stimulated new thinking in the marketing of perfumes.

Our rapidly changing life styles, the influence of the Women's Liberation Movement, the desire to return to nature and the natural, the influx of mystical Eastern philosophies, all have led to new approaches in the naming, advertising, and promotion of fragrance. In general, we shall probably see less stress on sex (except in the case of a sensual animal scent) in perfume advertising, less accent on women as sex symbols, and more of an approach to "women as people," active and constructive members of society. Again, time will be the arbiter of fashion as perfume for men is presently making a strong and important re-entry into the arena.

This is the creative age in perfumery. Never before in the long history of the art have perfume composers had such fine opportunities to blaze new trails. Much of this we owe to the marvels of science, the development of synthetics. After having suffered undeserved opprobrium and wide misunderstanding, synthetics in perfumery are now being valued for what they truly have to offer.

First of all, let us not equate the word "synthetic" with the word "cheap." Some synthetics cost more than some naturals. In fact, most perfumes contain some synthetics no matter what their proportion is to natural oils. They are invaluable in the creation of modern fragrances and contribute to their originality. Nor do all synthetics merely imitate naturals. Sometimes the laboratory can duplicate a natural by analyzing the composition of an oil and reproducing that composition; sometimes a synthetic is made wholly of naturals by utilizing various derivatives, and sometimes it is a compound that has never existed before.

We must acknowledge and accept certain deficiencies in nature and certain changes in the course of agricultural practice. There are flowers and other botanicals that simply refuse to cooperate with the large-scale needs of today's perfumer. Their yield is so infinitesimal and therefore so costly that it is totally impractical to use them in large quantity. So were it not for science, there might be many familiar much-appreciated fragrances that we could no longer enjoy. Synthetics are not subject to floods and droughts, wars and pestilences for a supply and thus they are stable, uniform, and dependable.

The most important attribute of the synthetic is that it goes beyond nature in making possible completely new and different scents, scents that do *not* exist in nature, first-time-ever scents. Synthetics add nuances, give original twists and interpretations. Scientists are launching and perfecting new synthetics with every passing day so we have much to anticipate and look forward to in the realm of perfumery.

Since the latter part of the nineteenth century, sweeping innovations in the art and science of perfume have brought undreamed-of delights to users of fragrance. Creative imagination in scent and perfumes has rocketed. We can now breathe perfumes with life and elation, perfumes that sing and soar, that defy any of the trite descriptions. What would a Madame Du Barry give to sample some of our perfume wealth!

Where once nature was our sole source of fragrant raw materials, she now has science as her ally. Nature has, by no means, been replaced. But science lends new depth, new scope, new potential. They make a beautiful pair.

And what a pleasure it is to know that, as a result of this marriage, fine perfumes, so often the privilege of comparatively few in the past, can be enjoyed today by many.

*Vive le parfum!*

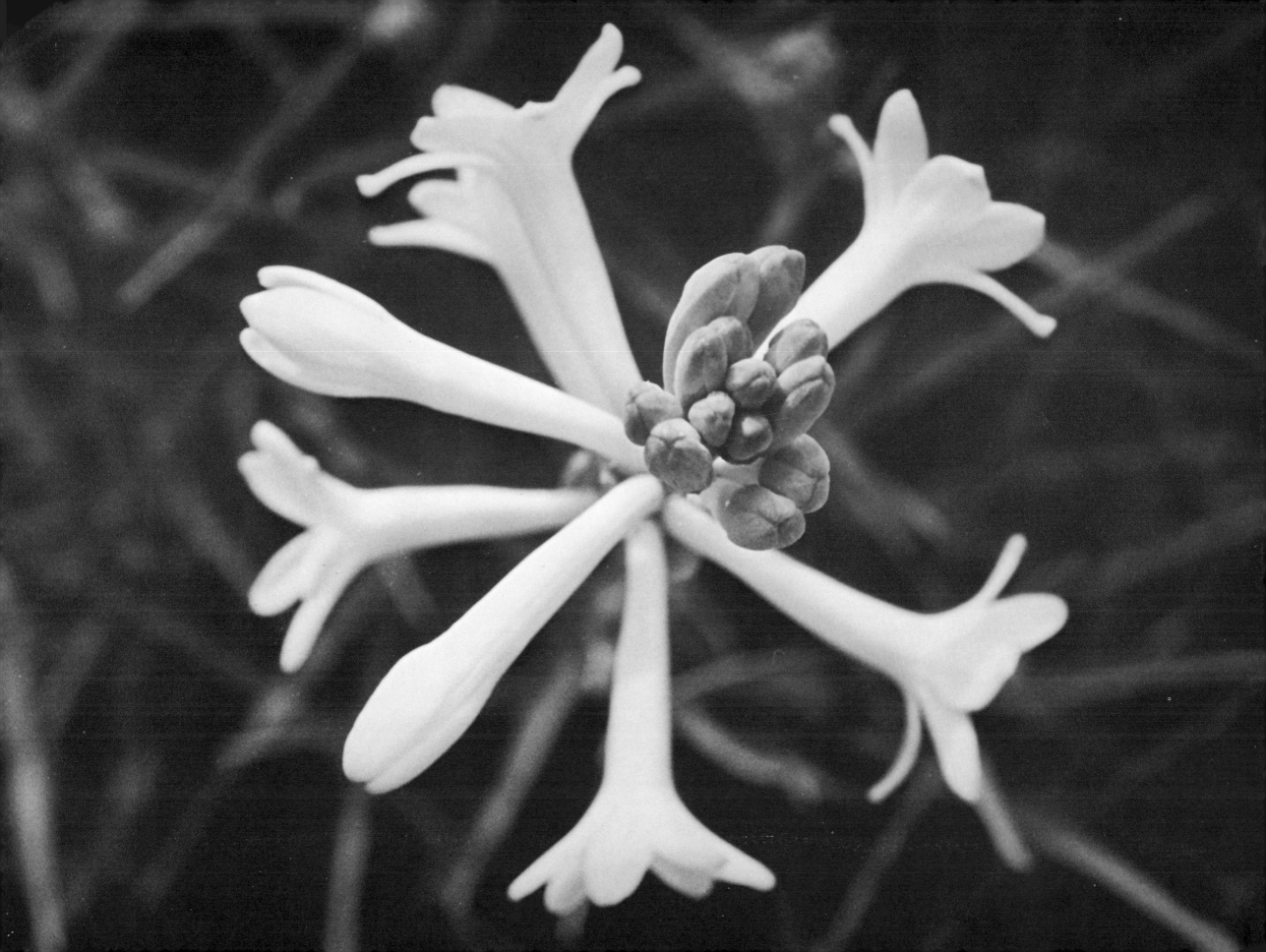

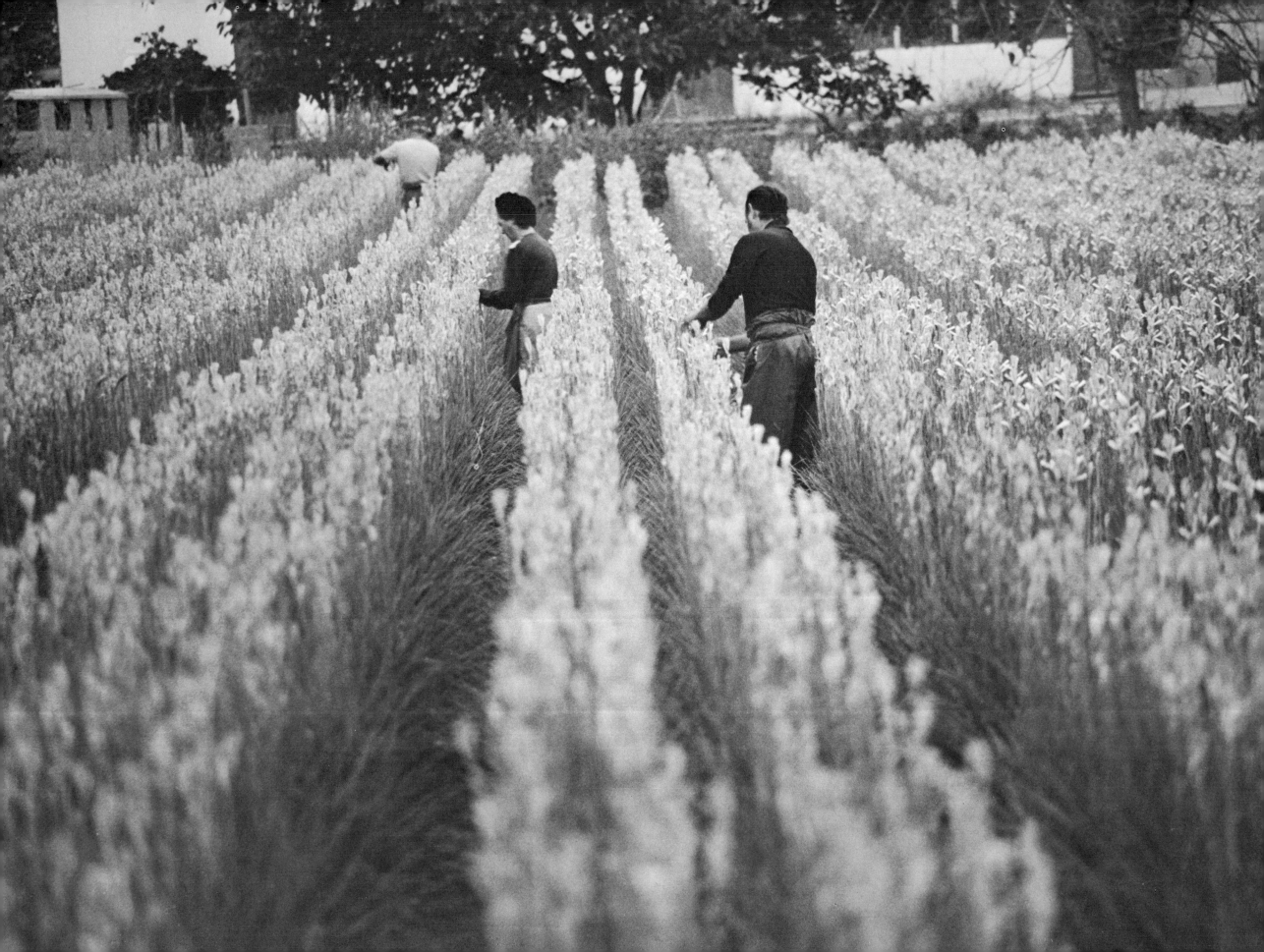

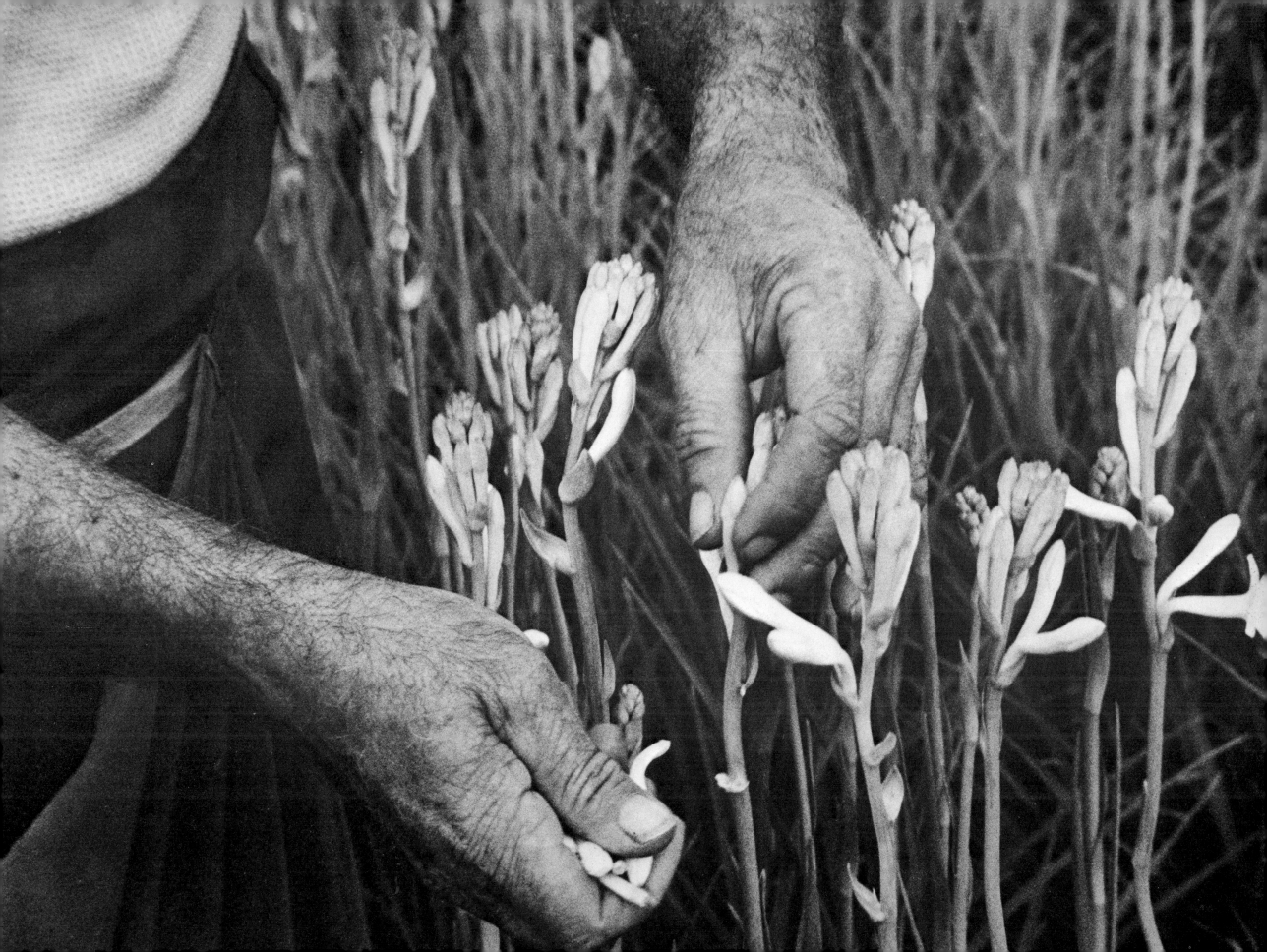

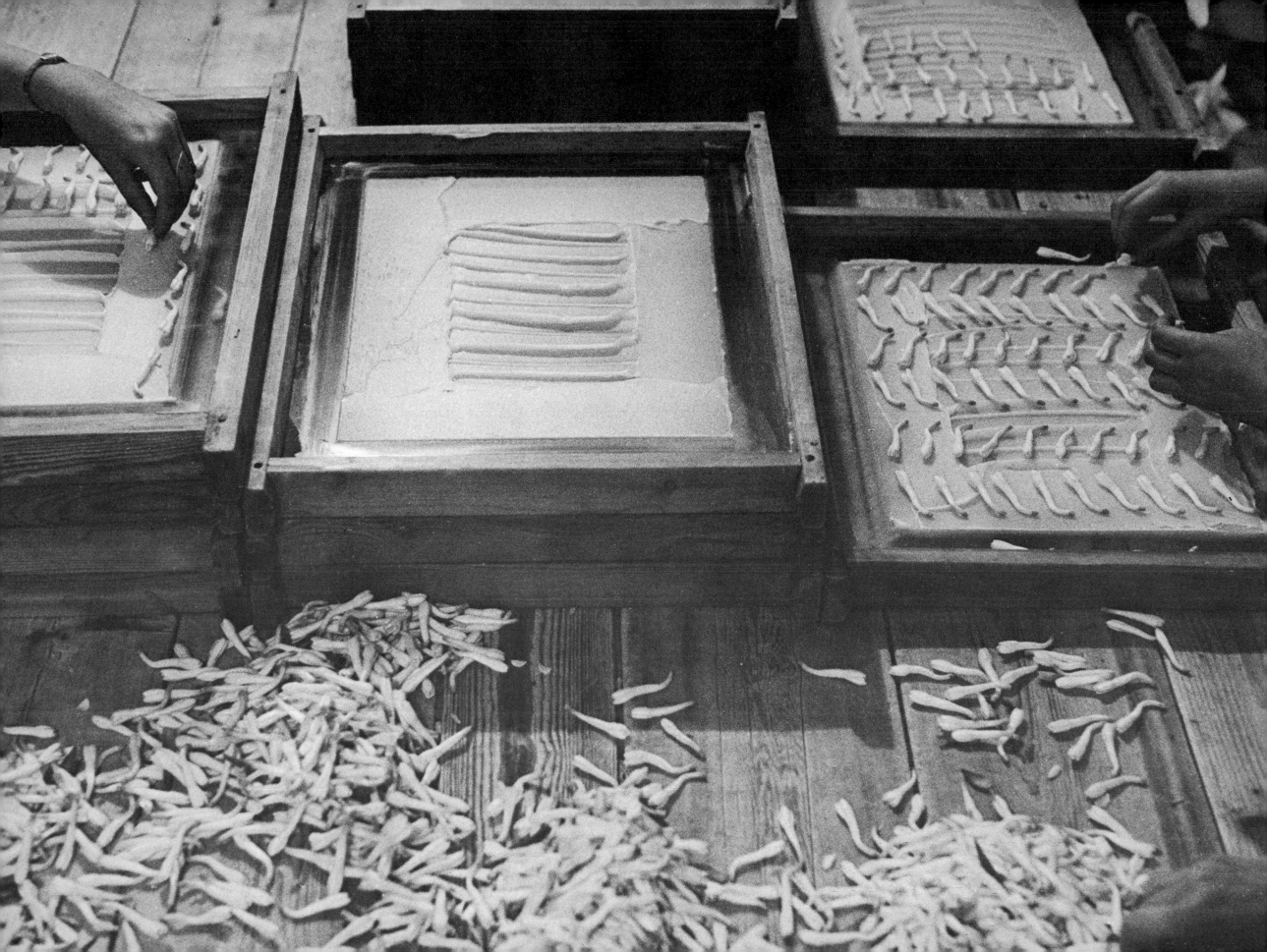

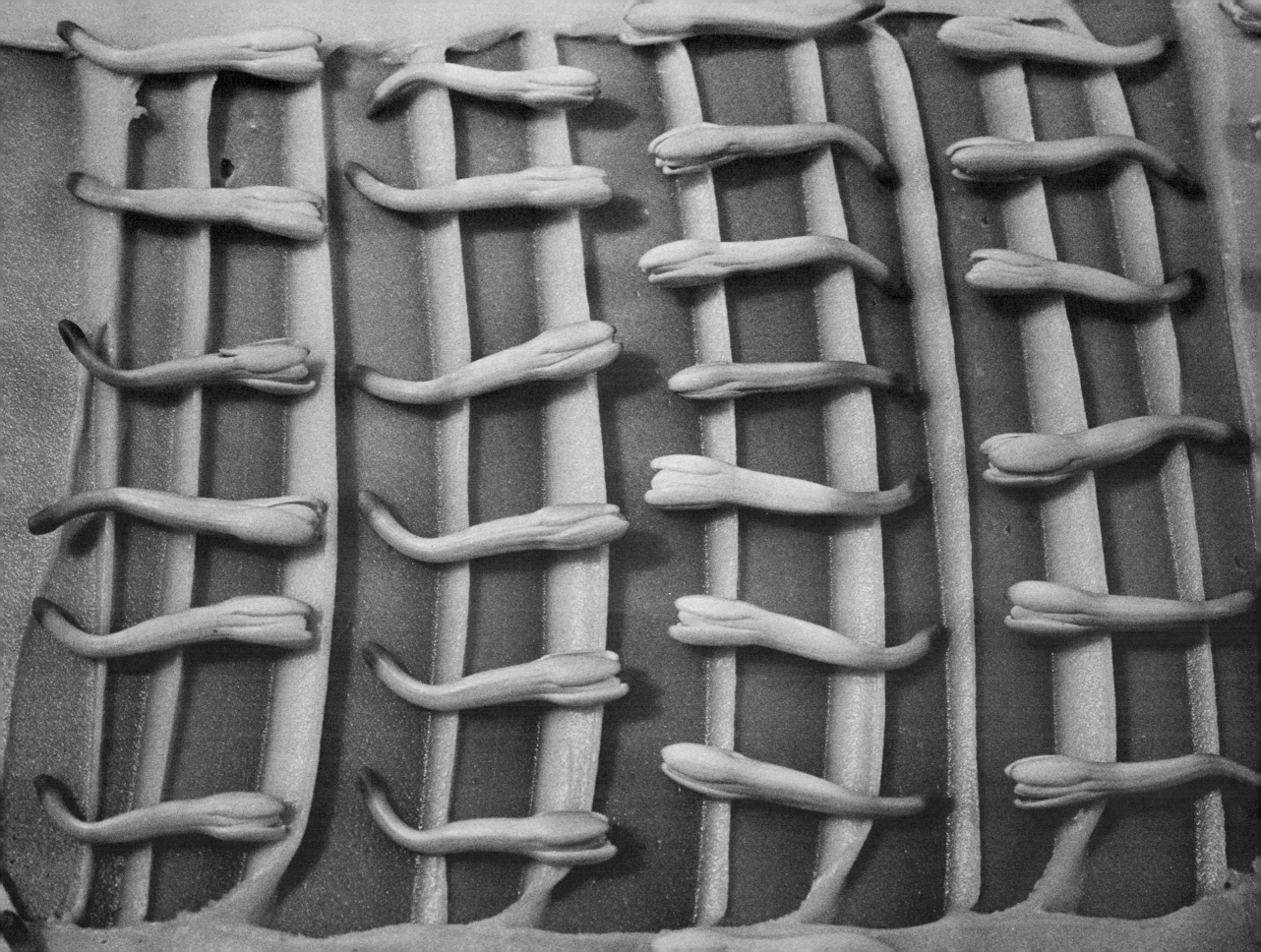

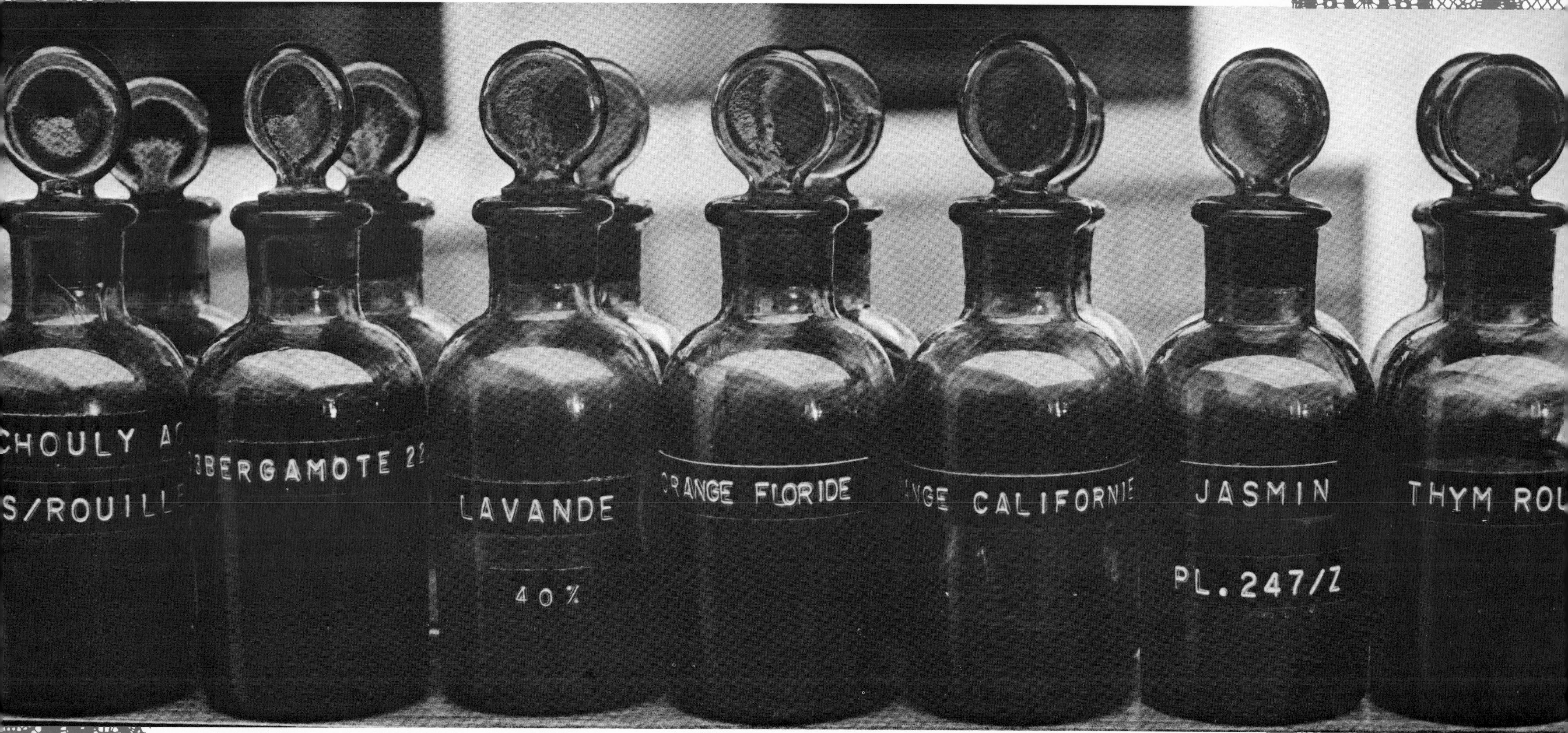

CHOULY A
S/ROUILLE

BERGAMOTE 22

LAVANDE

40%

ORANGE FLORIDE

ANGE CALIFORNIE

JASMIN

PL.247/Z

THYM ROU

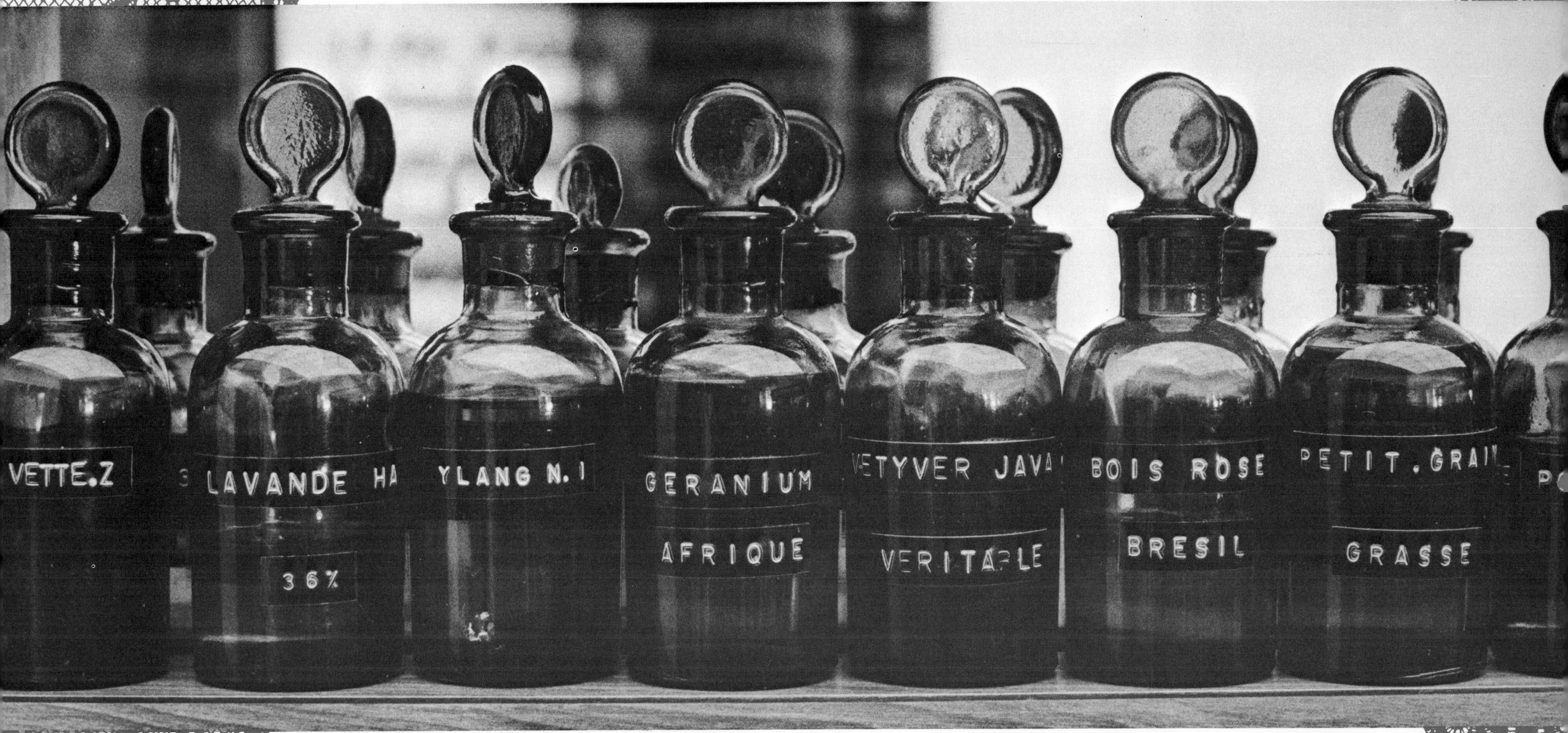
VETTE.Z
LAVANDE HA
36%
YLANG N.1
GERANIUM
AFRIQUE
VETYVER JAVA
VERITABLE
BOIS ROSE
BRESIL
PETIT.GRAIN
GRASSE

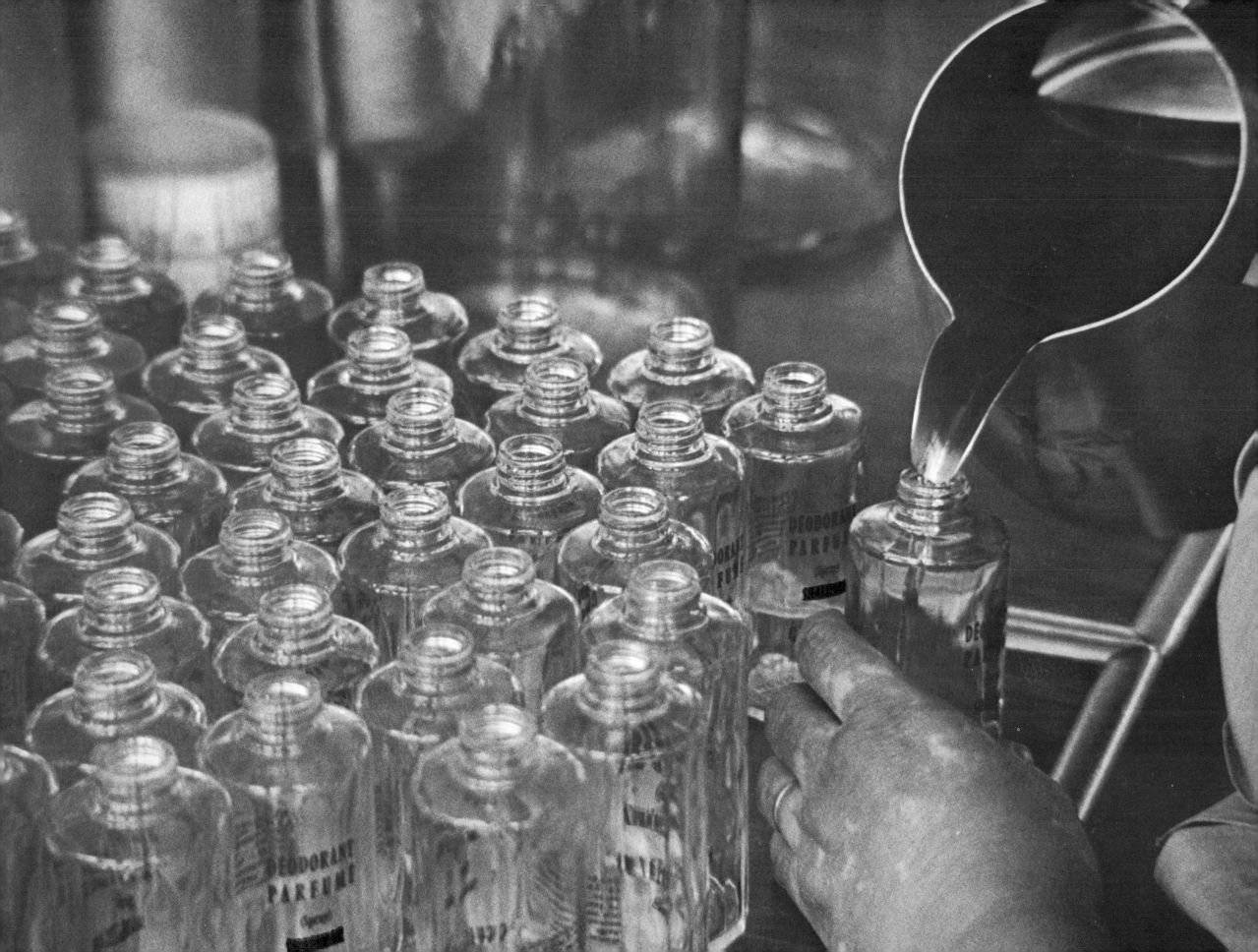

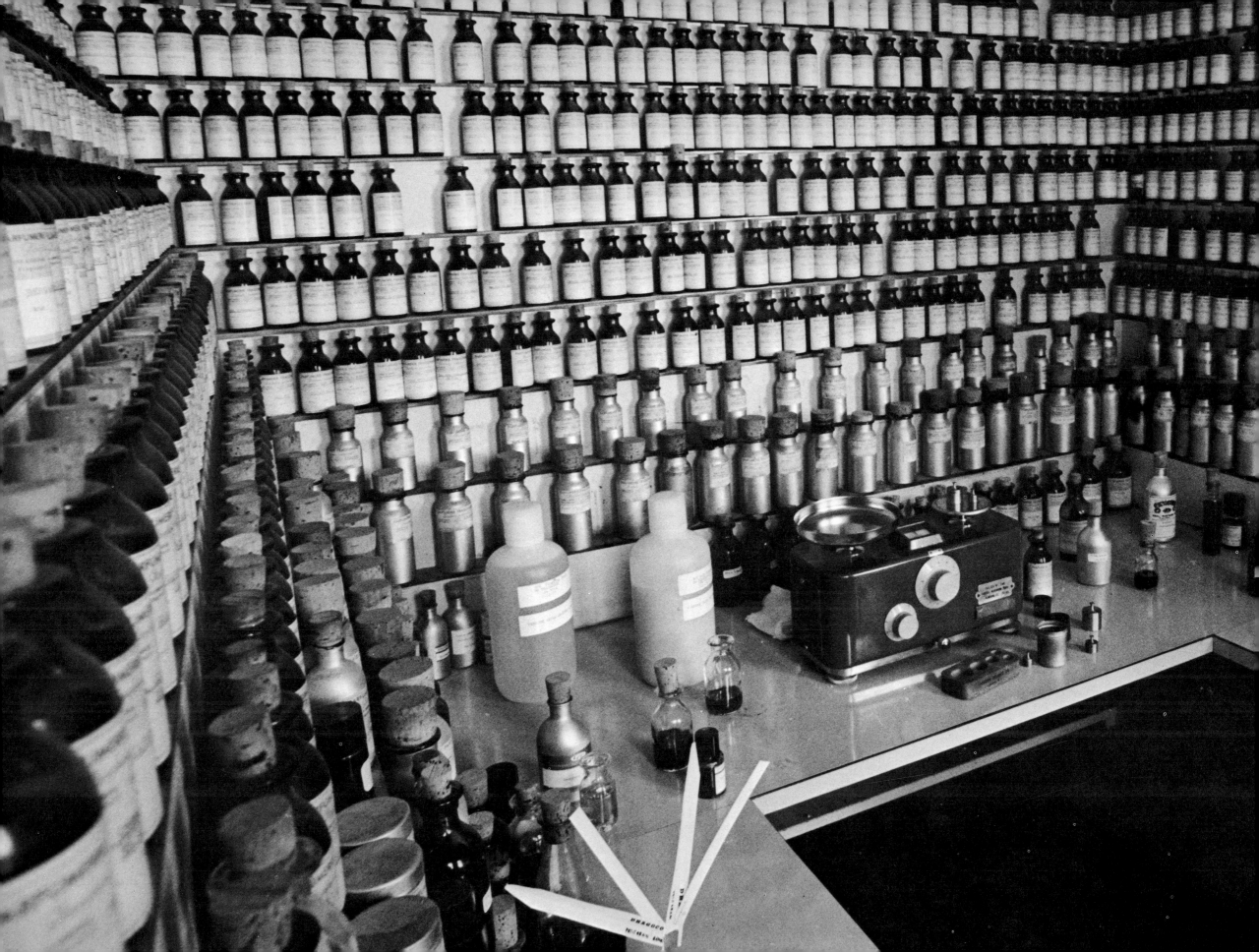

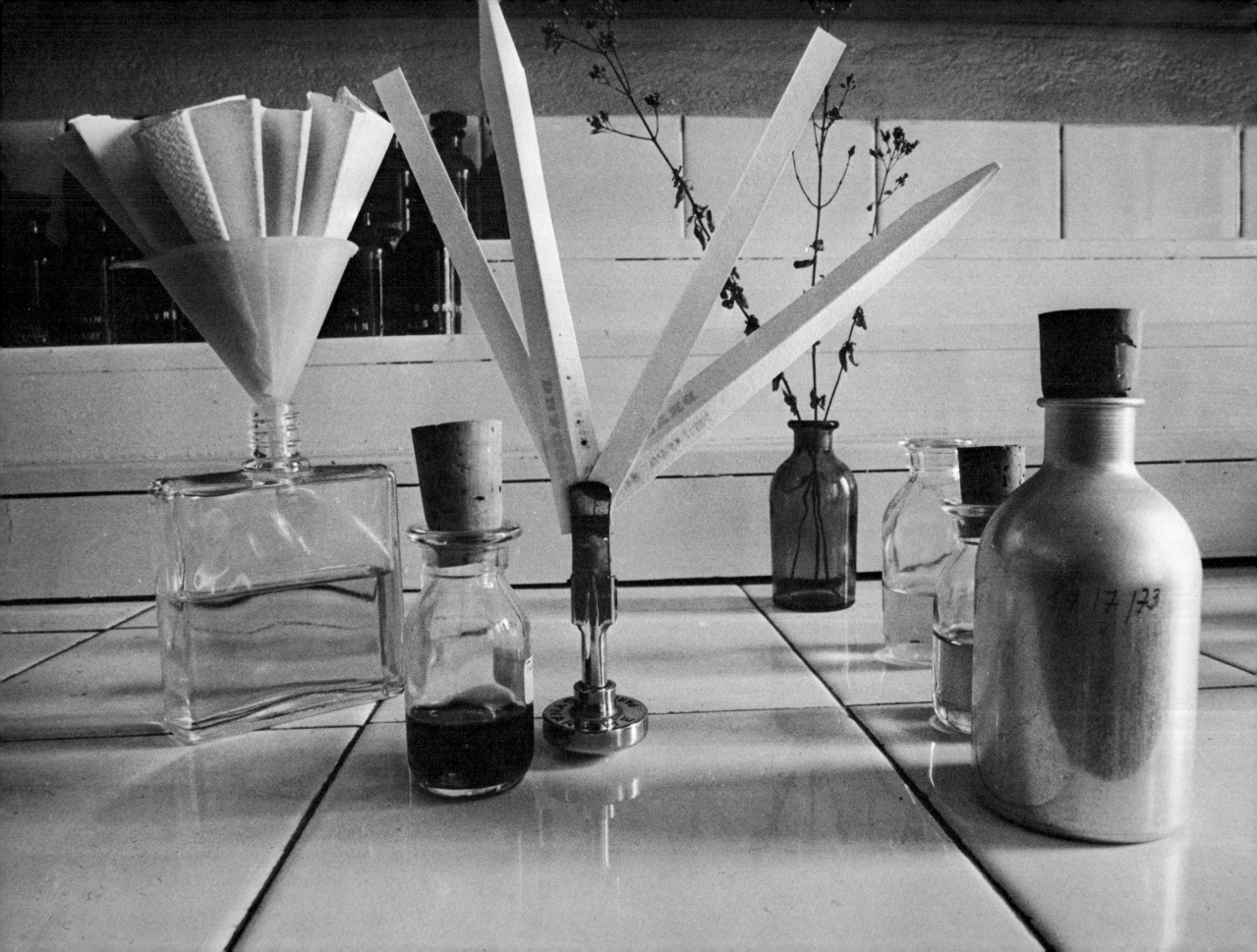

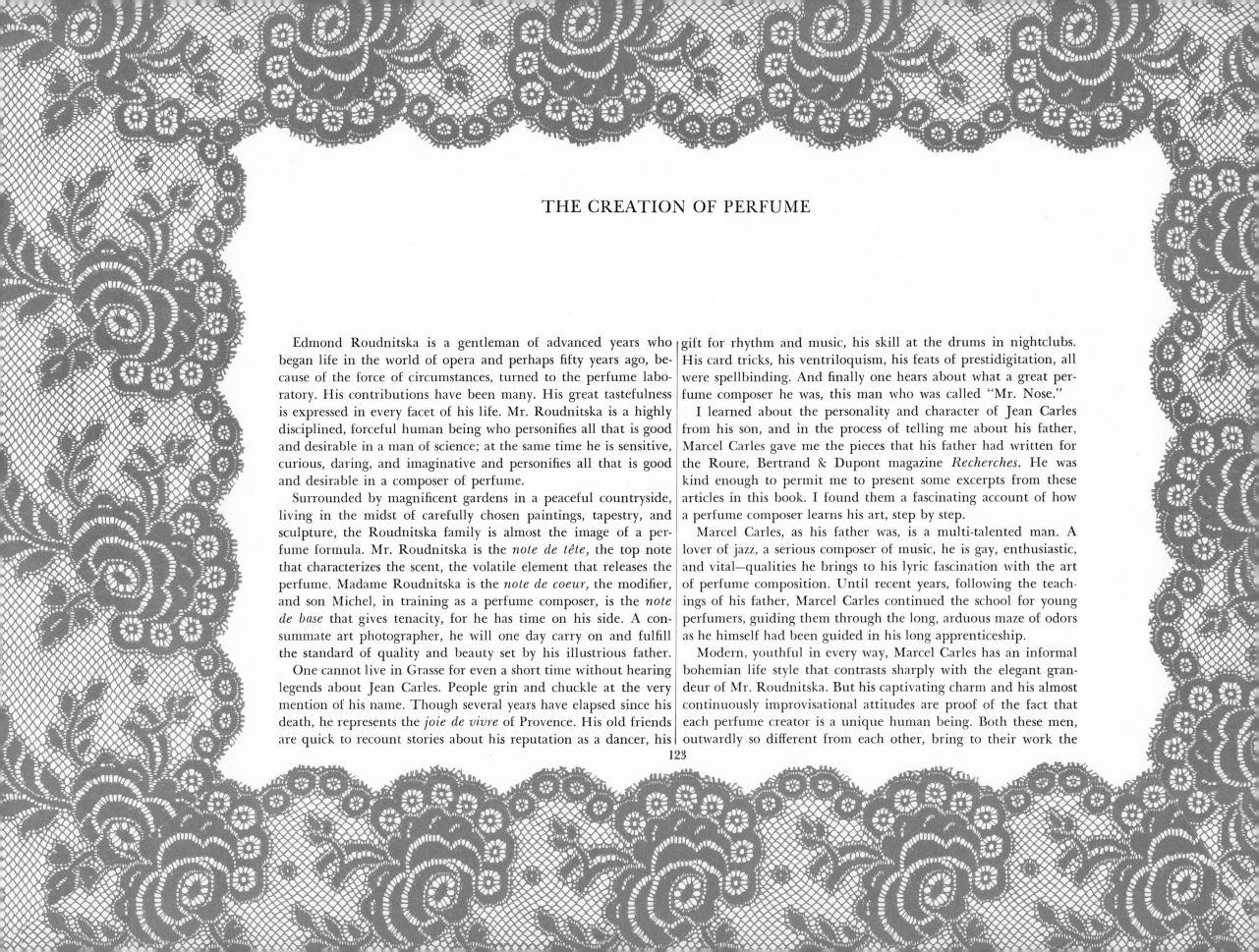

# THE CREATION OF PERFUME

Edmond Roudnitska is a gentleman of advanced years who began life in the world of opera and perhaps fifty years ago, because of the force of circumstances, turned to the perfume laboratory. His contributions have been many. His great tastefulness is expressed in every facet of his life. Mr. Roudnitska is a highly disciplined, forceful human being who personifies all that is good and desirable in a man of science; at the same time he is sensitive, curious, daring, and imaginative and personifies all that is good and desirable in a composer of perfume.

Surrounded by magnificent gardens in a peaceful countryside, living in the midst of carefully chosen paintings, tapestry, and sculpture, the Roudnitska family is almost the image of a perfume formula. Mr. Roudnitska is the *note de tête,* the top note that characterizes the scent, the volatile element that releases the perfume. Madame Roudnitska is the *note de coeur,* the modifier, and son Michel, in training as a perfume composer, is the *note de base* that gives tenacity, for he has time on his side. A consummate art photographer, he will one day carry on and fulfill the standard of quality and beauty set by his illustrious father.

One cannot live in Grasse for even a short time without hearing legends about Jean Carles. People grin and chuckle at the very mention of his name. Though several years have elapsed since his death, he represents the *joie de vivre* of Provence. His old friends are quick to recount stories about his reputation as a dancer, his gift for rhythm and music, his skill at the drums in nightclubs. His card tricks, his ventriloquism, his feats of prestidigitation, all were spellbinding. And finally one hears about what a great perfume composer he was, this man who was called "Mr. Nose."

I learned about the personality and character of Jean Carles from his son, and in the process of telling me about his father, Marcel Carles gave me the pieces that his father had written for the Roure, Bertrand & Dupont magazine *Recherches.* He was kind enough to permit me to present some excerpts from these articles in this book. I found them a fascinating account of how a perfume composer learns his art, step by step.

Marcel Carles, as his father was, is a multi-talented man. A lover of jazz, a serious composer of music, he is gay, enthusiastic, and vital—qualities he brings to his lyric fascination with the art of perfume composition. Until recent years, following the teachings of his father, Marcel Carles continued the school for young perfumers, guiding them through the long, arduous maze of odors as he himself had been guided in his long apprenticeship.

Modern, youthful in every way, Marcel Carles has an informal bohemian life style that contrasts sharply with the elegant grandeur of Mr. Roudnitska. But his captivating charm and his almost continuously improvisational attitudes are proof of the fact that each perfume creator is a unique human being. Both these men, outwardly so different from each other, bring to their work the same kind of devotion, discipline, attention to detail, knowledge of materials, and interest in the marketing of perfumes.

In Edmond Roudnitska we have the consummate master; in Jean Carles we have the tradition of the past; in Marcel Carles we have the new, the vibrant, the feel of the future. But in all we have the beauty that is perfume.

---

*Interview with Edmond Roudnitska*
*Cabris, August 1973*

*Mr. Roudnitska, what is a nose?*

I think people have very much exaggerated the importance of a nose in our profession. One often calls the perfumer a "nose," putting the word in quotation marks, but it is nevertheless quite exaggerated. A painter, for instance, doesn't do much painting with his eyes. He composes [creates] with his brain, and he composes [creates] with his hand, his brush, you understand. For us, the nose is, above all, a means of control, but one cannot say that one composes with the nose. One composes with memory, the memory of [olfactory] sensations, and with these sensations one imagines the perfume, and then, in a way, one tries to carry it out. But the nose is only a means of control, as the ears are a means of control for the musician. For example, the musician doesn't need to have a piano to compose. It is sufficient that he grabs some paper, makes some lines with his pencil, and then he writes the notes, but it is with his memory, his memory of the sounds, that he creates, and for the perfumer it is the same thing.

*It's a bit like a chef . . . .*

Oh, you mean a *chef de cuisine*. That's an appropriate analogy, but to advance our idea, it's a little like Beethoven; at the time he created the Ninth Symphony he was already very deaf, and he created the Ninth Symphony uniquely from memory, the memory of sound. He created perhaps his greatest masterpiece.

*A composer starts young with the study of an instrument, an artist starts with his palette and brushes and colors, a chef de cuisine starts in the kitchen itself, but a perfumer—where does he start?*

He starts in the laboratory too. Just as the chef starts in the kitchen, the perfumer starts in the laboratory of a perfumery. He starts by studying the odors, smelling one after the other, and when he has practiced this a great deal, he begins to make small experiments and learns to combine the odors as a *chef de cuisine* tries to make different combinations of tastes and as a painter makes combinations of colors. It is very analogous, all of this.

*You yourself, did you start in the laboratory?*

Yes, I started in a laboratory making analyses at twenty-one years of age. I stayed there a year and a half.

*What background did you have?*

I started a program of Arts et Metiers [Arts and Professions] but I couldn't continue, for family reasons. Then I took courses in a school in Paris and finally entered a perfumery at twenty-one. When I started to work I had no idea what perfume composition might or might not be. But I was in the lab to earn my living like everyone else. And then—perhaps it was by luck, if you will—I was observed, noticed by the director of the company, and

124

at the end of a year and a half he placed me in perfume composition and I left and went to Paris at that time. . . . [Pause in tape.]

I want to add to something I said before apropos of the music of Beethoven when he was deaf. Not only did Beethoven write the Ninth Symphony while he was deaf, he conducted the orchestra, which is something considerable to note, because he couldn't hear the orchestra, and he conducted all the same without any guide lines other than his full score and his observations of the gestures of the musicians. And this is an important point when one thinks of dynamics. Secondly, one talks a lot about abstract art, nonfigurative art, and so on. But no one ever realizes that perfume creation is essentially an abstract art. The composition of perfumery, except when one imitates lily of the valley, when one imitates a rose and other such things, is all relative because one takes only a certain aspect of lily of the valley, a certain aspect of the rose. But in general, when one is making a perfume, by the very nature of the thing it is an abstract perfume that corresponds to an abstract form. . . . "Chypre," "Femme," "Chanel No. 5"—these are abstract perfumes. They correspond to nothing. They are not anything real. They represent nothing we have known about before.

When, as I told you, I lived in Grasse in 1926, I stayed in the laboratory for a year and a half, which gave me an opportunity to learn about all the raw materials very rapidly; then I went to Paris where immediately I began to work in perfume composition. I remained in the neighborhood of Paris for twenty-five years, making compositions, and in 1946 we created, my wife and I, Art et Parfum S.A. In 1949 we came to live in Cabris, and here we are. And it is a simple enough career.

*Is your wife also a perfumer?*

In a small way. Above all, she takes care of the manufacture, the administration of the company, and thus she participates a great deal in the work. We composed Moustache for Marcel Rochas together.

*Are you free to tell us the names of other perfumes you have created, or is it a secret?*

It is a *polichinelle* secret. Do you know what a *"secret polichinelle"* is? It is a secret that everyone knows. You see, it's not even a secret at all. The perfume for which I was first known was Femme of Marcel Rochas, and then I started to create the perfumes for Christian Dior. That is to say, Diorama first, then Eau de Cologne Fraîche [also Dior], Diorissimo, and then after that Eau Sauvage and then Diorella. And for Hermes, I made L'Eau d'Hermes, and several others that are less significant because they do not enjoy great success.

*  *  *

Our son has been with us for two years. He has studied very hard. He has a good solid background, and of course he has been studying the various raw materials, and that takes a long time.

*Especially now with the enormous number of synthetics?*

Oh, yes, there are thousands more materials than there were forty years ago when I started. It's not comparable.

*How many natural products are actually in use now?*

About one hundred over-all, but there are fewer than that in *constant* use. However, in contrast to that, there are several thousand chemical products.

*Do they come from many countries?*

Well, natural products come from all the countries of the world . . . really from all the continents, not all the countries. From India come the palmarose, the lemongrass, things of that nature; from Java we have the patchouli, the vetiver. From America we have the juniperus . . . you call it cedar, but it is

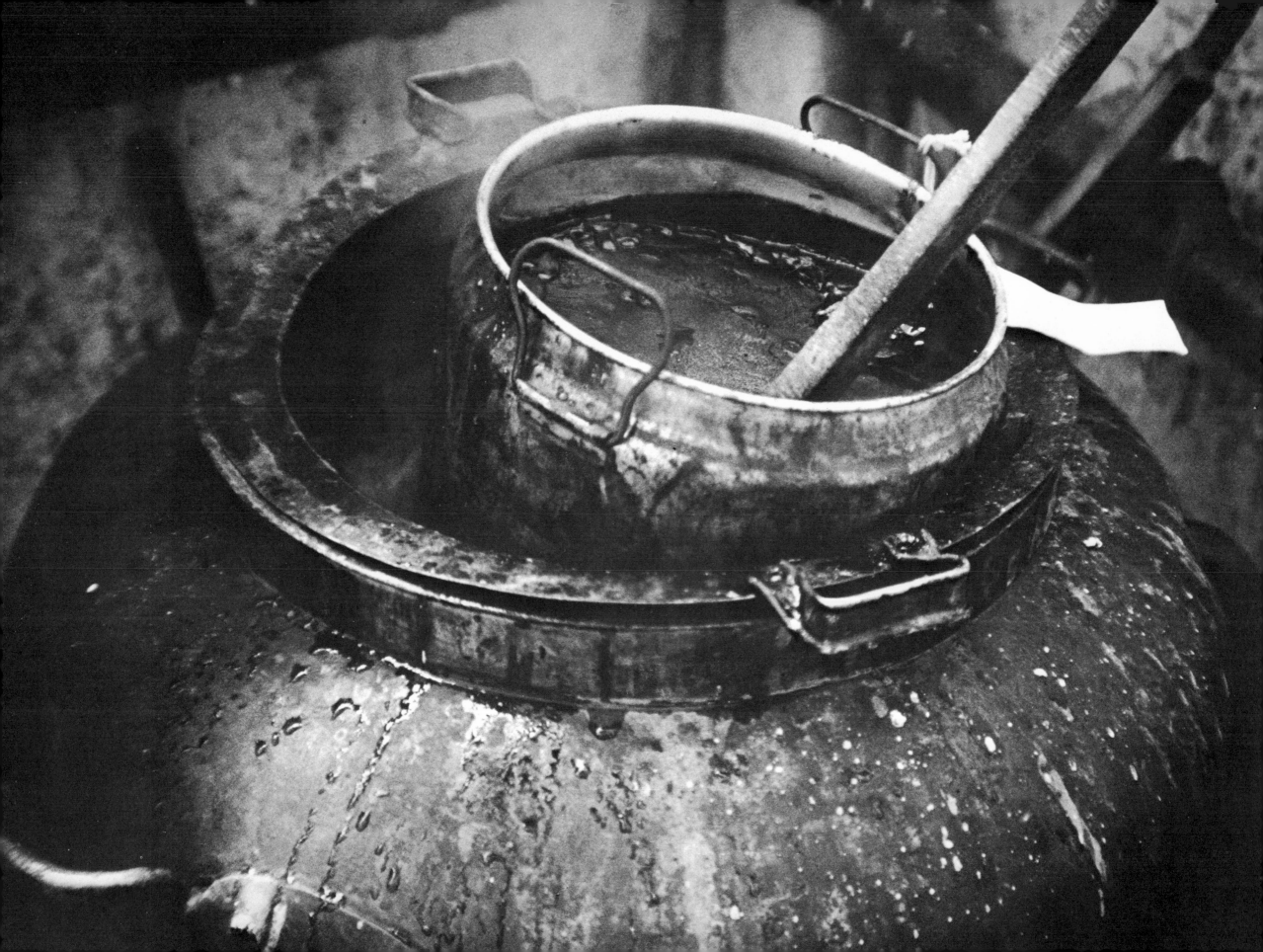

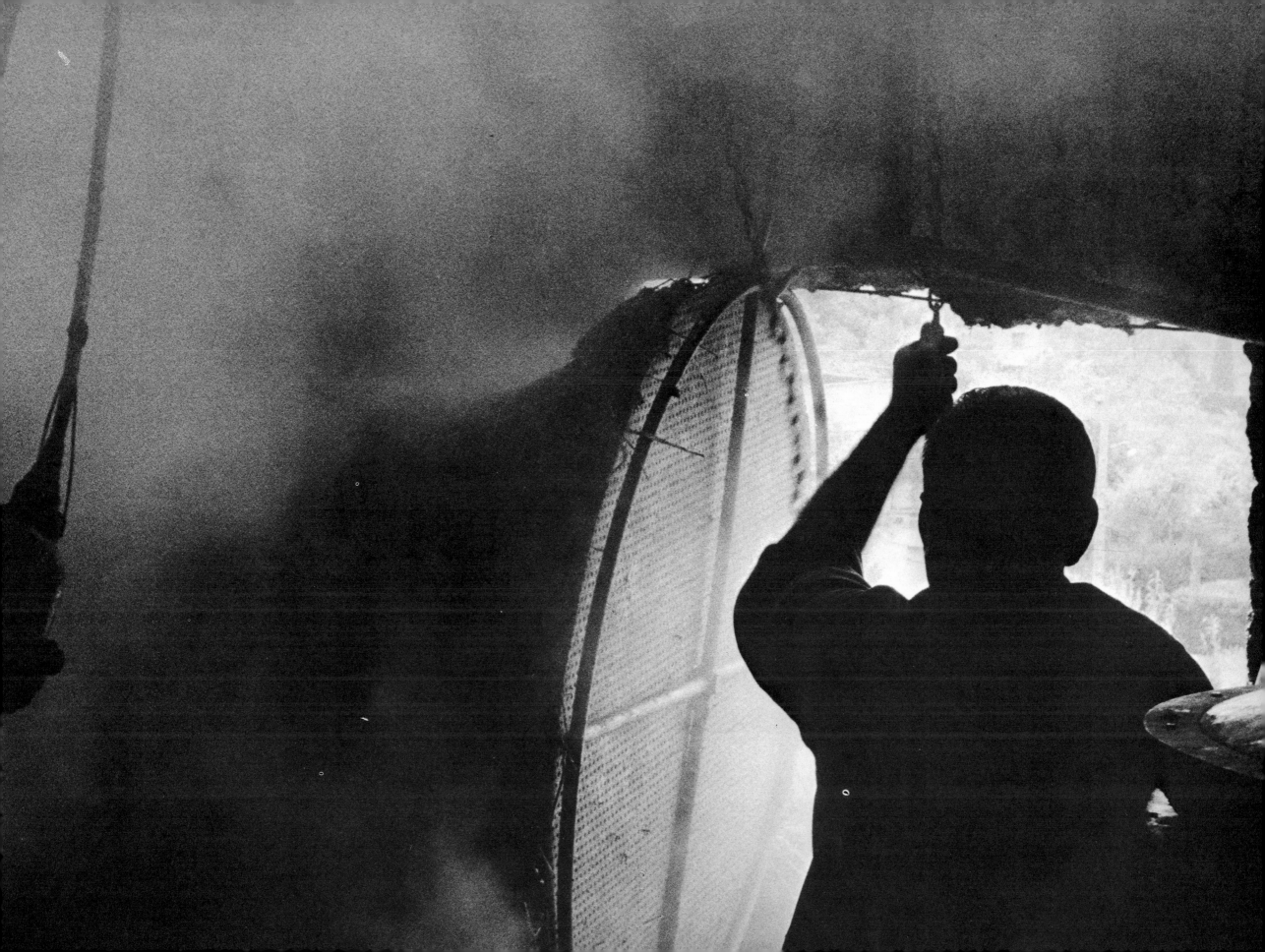

juniperus from Texas, from Virginia. From France, from the region of Grasse, with all the essences it produces, which you already know about. There is sandalwood from India; there is another sandalwood, not quite the same, that comes from Australia. From China, from Formosa, from Japan, there are certain essences. From Russia and from Poland carui. From Spain, the essence of sage, caldamum gum. Italy, it is understood, everything citrus. Everything such as bergamot, lemon, orange, tangerine, jasmine also, to be sure, grows in Italy. Jasmine also comes from Morocco and Egypt.

*Does the jasmine that grows on the heights in Africa have the same odor as that which grows in Grasse?*

The jasmine of Grasse is a jasmine that comes from plants that grow in the mountains of that region, which are wild jasmine plants onto which are grafted the jasmine grandiflorium. In Italy, in Calabria, they plant grandiflorium directly, without passing through the grafting stage. In Morocco I don't think they graft it either. I think they do the same as in Italy. They plant it directly.

*Is the essential oil the same?*

Yes, jasmine gives the same oil.

[Michel Roudnitska] The quality of the oil is different.

*Inasmuch as there are now about a hundred natural products and many thousands—let's say thousands—of synthetic products, does this pose additional problems, fewer problems, more problems than you had in making compositions formerly? What do you think? Is it more difficult or less difficult now?*

Above all, we have many more possibilities. Consequently—well, I don't exactly know how to put it—it is much more difficult for those who don't really know how to work, because they are in over their heads, they are overwhelmed by all these products, but for someone who really is skilled there are ever so many more opportunities. It's therefore more interesting. For people who are not connoisseurs it is difficult to understand, for example, what you mean when you say an essence is a "head," or another is a "body," or others are "modifiers."

*You are speaking of the notes of the head [notes de tête]; the heart [notes de coeur]; and the base [notes de fond] [depth]?*

Yes, and these correspond simply to the process of evaporation in these products. Products that are most volatile evaporate the fastest—they are the *notes de tête.* Less volatile products, which come afterward in the heirarchy, are thus the *notes de coeur,* and those which have relatively little volatility come afterward and are therefore the *notes de fond.*

*What inspires you to create a perfume?*

It's very variable. It's never actually done twice in the same manner. It depends on the idea one has. I work with ideas, an idea for a perfume. A thought comes to my mind. I foresee, I visualize a certain form for a perfume. I try to construct it. I try it with the raw materials I lay out for myself. I try first to outline or sketch out the form with products that are most familiar to me, and then I try to modify it, and, step by step, this study goes along, because a study of this nature can last several years, and as it does, I might have my hand on some new raw material, and I say to myself, "Well, now, this might be just the thing I need to complete the form." And that's how the experiment progresses.

*And when are you satisfied?*

Never.

*When you create a perfume in certain of your concepts do you think of a certain personality, a certain character, a typical thing, something in nature?*

No, no . . . to really create a perfume you have to think perfume, you have to live entirely in the universe of odor, think in that universe and, being in it, visualize forms . . . do you see what I mean? . . . and it is these forms one has to try to construct. It is very abstract . . . that's why I said it is truly abstract.

*If natural products continue to diminish—by that I mean if the source of supply continues to diminish with its present rapidity—do you think there will be a day when we won't have natural products?*

We have already entered into that era. We have been in it for several years. Consequently we are well prepared. Little by little we are going toward a perfumery that is more and more without natural product, or I should say with much *less* natural product than before. Here I must insert a small parenthesis—I must tell you because I don't want to forget to do so—that we must really fight against the belief that is in the mind of most perfume users, newspaper people, writers, even certain persons in the perfume trade—a belief that synthetic products and chemical products are inferior to natural products. This is absolutely false. This is almost the opposite of the truth. It has become actually the reverse of the truth, because on one hand there are natural products that are very inexpensive and cost only a few francs per kilo, and on the other hand there are some raw materials that are definite synthetics that cost several tens of thousands of francs per kilo. Thus they are very costly, but they are beautiful. There are others that are less expensive that are also very beautiful. Consequently we work with the scents as a painter works with colors without asking ourselves if we are working with chemical or natural raw materials. Do you understand? It's exactly the same thing. When you see a beautiful painting you don't question whether the artist who painted it painted the sky with natural or chemical colors. You don't ask the question. One should not ask that question about perfume either. This is very important.

*Do you use synthetics by choice, or are you forced to because of the limited supply of natural products?*

I'm not forced to do anything. I am not obligated to anyone, nor has anyone ever thought to place me in a position of obligation to purchase this or that product. I pick my own raw materials, and as far as I am concerned, whether they are natural or not natural, they are simply raw materials to me. They are odors, scents. If they come from here or from there, it makes no difference to me whatever. I work with raw materials that please me, with raw materials that I think will give me a certain result. That is all, irrespective of its origin.

*Like an artist.*

Yes, but with a synthetic it is easier to judge its behavior during its period of evaporation because, in a natural product, in an essence, there are five hundred constituents—thus there are some that are more volatile, some less—you understand. So it isn't easy to say why an essence is doing this or that, why it is volatile or not, inasmuch as evidently the volatile constituents dominate, but when you have a defined product, there you can know immediately the part it plays in your study.

*Do you have to be a chemist to be a "nose"?*

Certainly not—frequently it's injurious. If you're a chemist, there are certain rules with which you must comply. But if you're an artist, your horizons are so broad that nothing stops you.

*Can the purely scientific mind understand all these abstractions of which we have been speaking?*

Listen, it is not a rarity to find that men of science are very much attracted to the arts and have a taste for them. Sometimes they even practice them, and consequently I don't see at all any contravention to the kind of open thinking associated with the artist. I don't think that a scientific education blocks understand-

129

ing of art. It's not that. But in the course of an education in chemistry there are a certain number of prohibitions that a scientist must accept, whereas the artist cannot abide by or accept prohibitions.

*As you have lived in perfume, there are perfumers such as Guerlain who have also lived in it. They are not chemists. If there is a person who doesn't work like you, who doesn't have the possibilities that you have technically, but who has an idea and who comes to you and wants you to create something based on his idea for a perfume, is it possible for you to do that?*

Everything is possible, but it is not the most stimulating way of working—to work on the ideas of someone else, first of all. Furthermore, as far as I myself am concerned, I have never worked in that way—mostly because I never do business with people who impose their ideas on me. However, most certainly you can have this kind of communication.

*In asking the original question I'm thinking of couturiers, for example.*

I have some studies which I instigated myself, and then I have a certain number of things that are ready, or more or less ready. And when someone requests a perfume from me, I offer one of these, but they are composed from ideas of my own. Ideas that such and such a perfume should go to such and such a company, because that company projects a certain image—a certain approach.

*Ah, now we're getting at it.*

It is the reverse of what you asked me in your question. Actually it is *I* who choose the perfume, and the people [clients] are free to accept or reject it, of course.

*Translated: Grasse, 1973*
*Rosamond V. P. Kaufman*

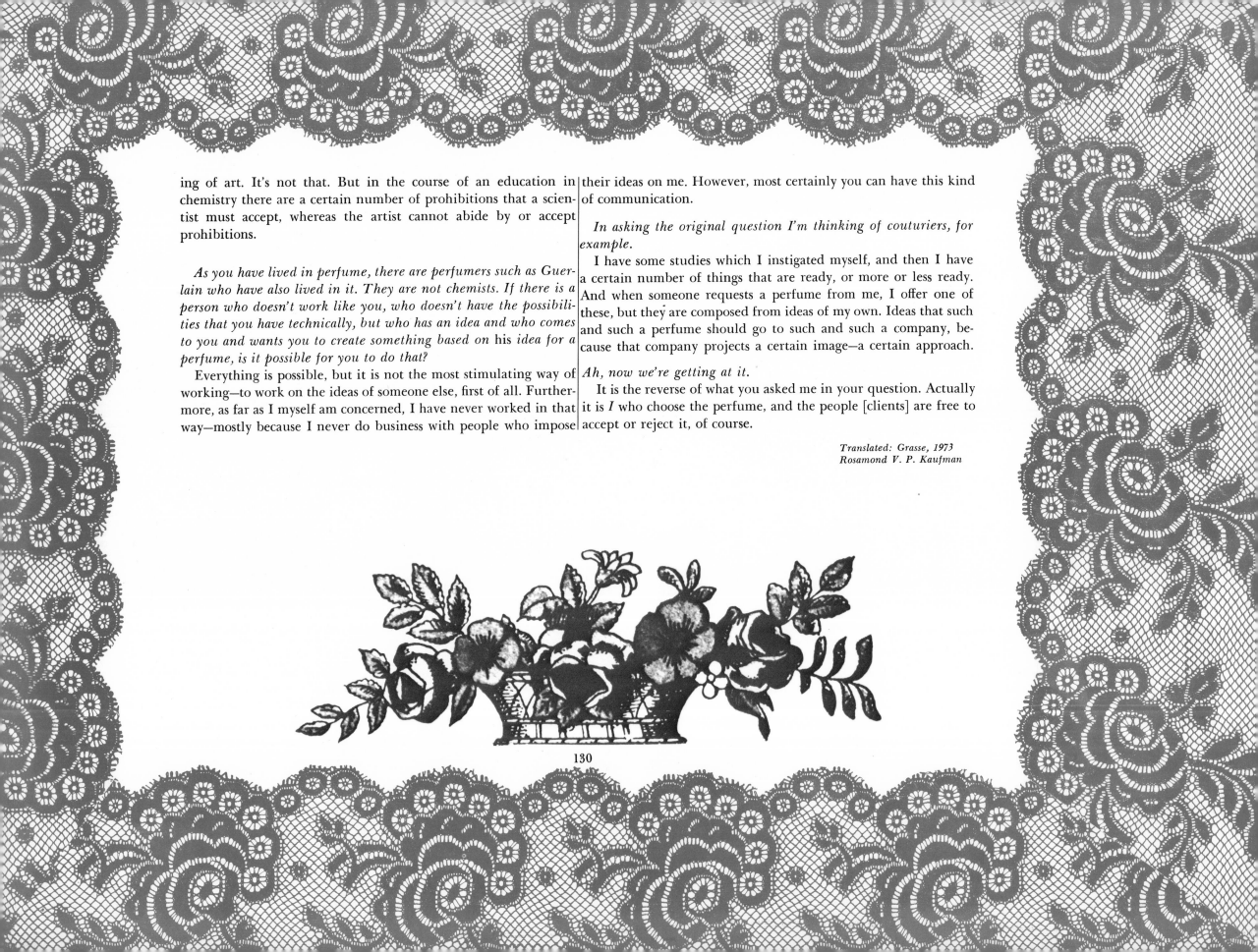

130

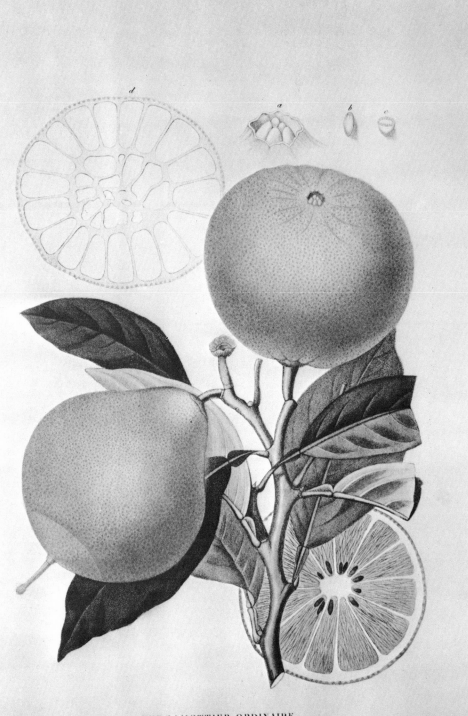

BERGAMOTTIER ORDINAIRE.

*Bergamotta Ordinaria.*

Tab. 55.

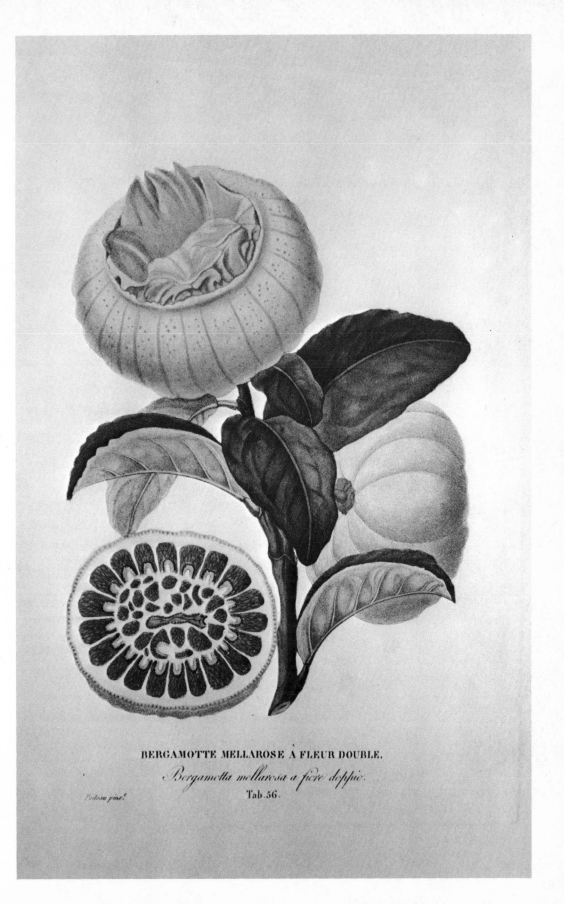

BERGAMOTTE MELLAROSE À FLEUR DOUBLE.

*Bergamotta mellarosa a fiore doppio.*

Tab. 56.

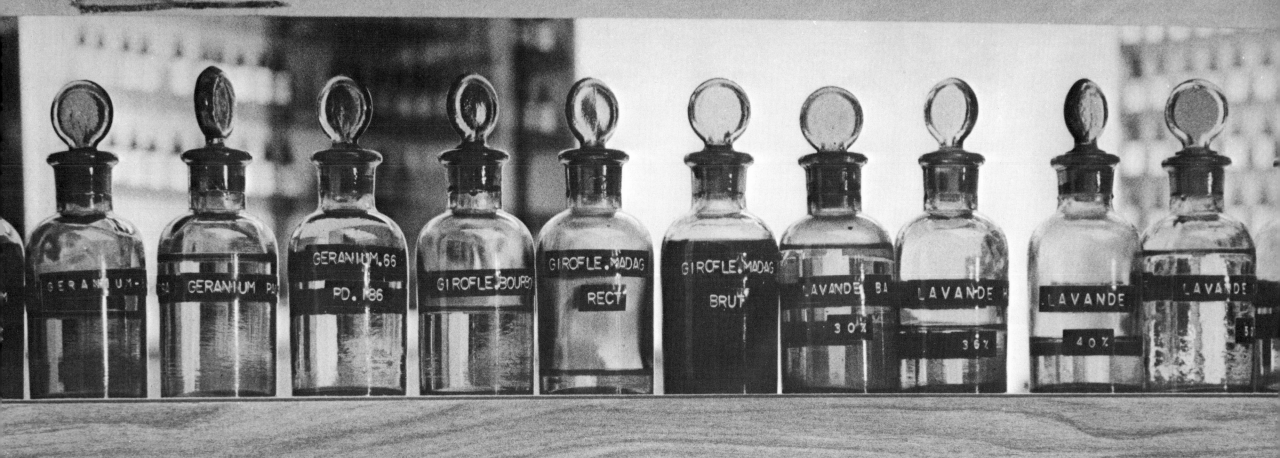
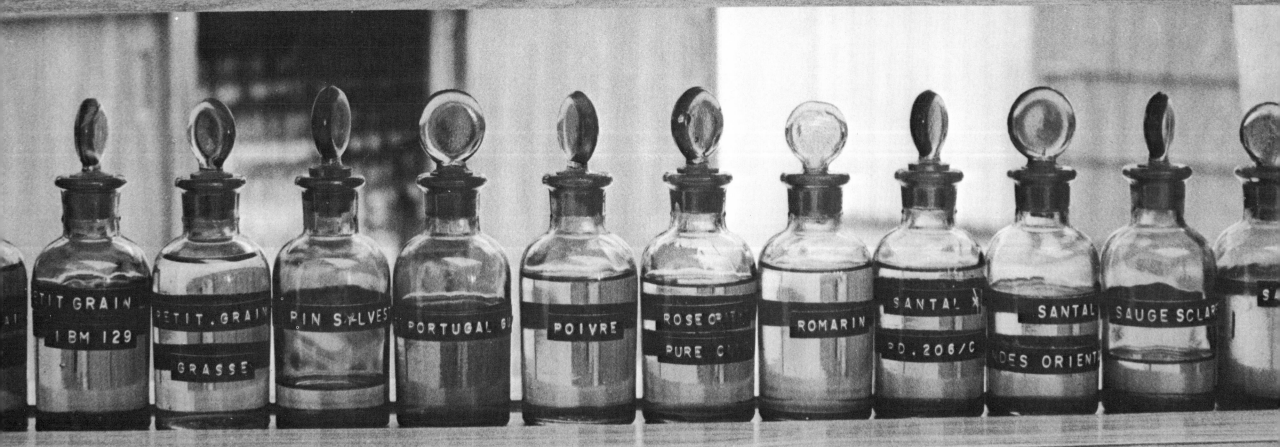

# CREATIVITY IN PERFUMERY

*Lecture given at the First International Perfumery Conference,
Paris, June 15–19, 1969*

by

Edmond Roudnitska

At the Sixth Mediterranean Symposium on Olfaction held in Monaco, Professor Marcel Guillot posed two interesting questions.

1. *Is there a way of teaching creativity? Or is creativity an innate gift that cannot be modified or influenced in any way?*
2. *What is the normal process of creativity? Is it stimulated by a dream, or is it a concept inspired purely by imagination? Can one compare creativity in perfumery with that necessary to other forms of artistic endeavor?*

1. Personally I think that the gift referred to in Professor Guillot's question is imagination itself. The capacity to create is essentially the ability to imagine. For someone gifted in imagination everything is a reason for exercising that special faculty—that is to say, everything stimulates him to carry out the projects that his mind conceives in the area or areas to which he is particularly drawn.

This quickly becomes a sort of game, for the more the creator practices this kind of mental gymnastic, the more successful he is at it, and thus the greater his sense of satisfaction.

The most seemingly insignificant detail can set off his first association of ideas; this carries him forward to another thought, which in turn stimulates a third and so on. Furthermore, other accidental circumstances may present themselves during the same period of time, giving birth to new associative ideas of such a kind that the link between the first idea and the final result is no longer visible. Nevertheless, there is always, from the beginning to the end, a certain logical thread of thought that is woven to a large degree out of the fabric of knowledge and experiences—that is to say, out of his acquired personal resources.

All the preceding comments are not confined only to creativity in perfumery, but that is exactly the reason why, if a minimum of imagination seems necessary at the start of a career in order to activate free association of ideas, and in order that the future educator can count upon the presence of this skill when choosing proper exercises for the progressive developments of this technique, it is obvious that since the enormous mass of our raw materials and combinations of these materials induce an inordinate risk of reckless usage, the education and work of the perfume composer can be neither fruitful nor enriching if it is not methodical.

The method, in broad terms, should consist of educating the olfactory sense by systematic study and review of raw materials; by classification of these materials, which classification must be merely suggested by the teacher and left to the final personal but orderly choice of the student-perfumer; by thorough study of the traditional harmonies of odor which, as we have just implied, can singularly be achieved by exercises ranging progressively from the very simple to the extremely complex.

When the training of the sense of smell, of the olfactory memory, and of the creative imagination have been carried on simultaneously in numerous practice sessions with these raw materials, these disciplines must be followed by the study of recognized classic perfumes, proceeding from the most elementary to the most difficult.

If, in the course of this formation, the teacher has consistently taken great pains to stimulate the student's imagination, encouraging him to explain his sensations and describe them in pictorial terms, if he furnishes his pupil with numerous instances of the use of the association of ideas and inspires his pupil to train himself in this way, the novice perfumer will then have, upon completion of his apprenticeship, the tools he needs to carry on alone. It will only be necessary for him to become more alert to his own senses in order to conceive ideas for perfumes of his own creation later on.

Today everyone is convinced, and certainly Professor Guillot is the first among us, that, irrespective of the area of interest, if a student is to achieve success, innate talent alone is not sufficient. The talent must be cultivated and developed if it is to be effective in the pursuit of a knowledge and a technical skill, without both of which he can only harvest a bad crop, so to speak.

Inasmuch as perfume composition demands a firm foundation based upon an in-depth knowledge of an extensive number of raw materials, as well as a perfect understanding of the proportions in which they must be brought together, it seems clear that fine results in this field can be obtained only when one is willing to work with complete dedication over a protracted period of time. Furthermore, it is the responsibility of educators to tell the truth to prospective perfume composers and, recognizing those who have aptitude, to develop in them the necessary moral fiber that will permit them to pursue a career in a thankless job, but which, on the other hand, is the only highway to their success.

2. In responding to the first question, I have already set about answering the second. Assuming that the method of education for a future creator is based purely upon the same mechanisms as creativity itself, the two questions are inseparable.

I have had an opportunity to say that artistic creation in general proceeds from inventiveness and originates with an idea or an emotion. I believe that all forms of artistic invention have numerous traits in common. The interrelationships between artists working in different mediums give ample proof that this is so. That which distinguishes one art form from another is mainly the raw material from which it has been fabricated. Ordinarily one doesn't handle the different impulses—auditory, visual, olfactory—with the same techniques, but the artistic problems of bringing the idea into reality are comparable, and it is this factor that gives all artists a common language and causes them to use varied but similar terms.

To say that creation grows out of an idea or an emotion is to indicate that a sensitive human being, which the artist is by very definition, is constantly stimulated by all that surrounds him, by all that attacks or assails him, and by the unceasing play of his imagination, which gives him no surcease. The difficulty lies not only in having ideas but in carrying them out, in knowing how to sort them, to arrange them in an orderly manner, and to choose which of them is worthy of effort in a long search for accomplishment that might extend over many years.

Almost since the beginning of my career, it has been my custom to mark down in a little notebook all the ideas for perfumes that come to my mind. I am now at number eighty-eight. Less than ten of these thoughts have been utilized or put into production; the rest are still undeveloped.

Fortunately, most of these ideas are timeless and remain worthwhile. I often congratulate myself on the fact that I take time, because year after year I profit from the appearance of new materials and from increased knowledge in my field. For example, currently I am at work on two compositions, one of which was started in 1946, the other in 1947. They have been set aside on occasion and periodically re-examined, always benefiting, thanks to my withdrawal, from my renewed enthusiasm when I return to them. I am well aware that these compositions would have suffered greatly if they had been perfected and launched twenty-five years ago. Even though it is a question of dealing with the same two ideas and in the same forms suggested to me by two raw materials of that early period, I am working today with two totally different elements, not entirely new, you understand, but about which I hadn't thought previously. Due to the fact that my skill has also improved in twenty years and that I can expect much more than I dared hope for when I began, it turns out that perhaps I am preparing with twenty-year-old ideas perfumes that will be worn twenty years from now.

The point of departure can thus be the raw materials themselves or an adaptation of these raw materials in a way that brings out some special accent that allows the perfume composer to construct a product that he certainly imagined to begin with.

The idea could be even more conjectural. In 1945, while walking on a road in Normandy, I smelled a woody odor that attracted me very strongly. I have never really known to what exactly I should attribute this odor, which has haunted me ever since. But I had visualized, or foreseen, if you will, a combination that would translate my sensation into perfume. In this same fashion, the odor of tanned leather was developed and translated into the language of perfume.

The principal quality of imagination is that it must be without limits; it must be boundless.

An idea can also be a challenge—the solution of a technical problem, such as the difficulty inherent in adding highly concen-

trated aldehydes to a lovely Chypre without disturbing it and thus getting Crêpe de Chine; or getting a good reproduction (never perfectly successful) of a certain pretty smell in nature; or, even better, a scent of something in nature serving as a pretext for all sorts of stylized fragrances; and here we see this skill orienting itself toward that of the painter who takes from nature only those specific models that strike his fancy or capture his interest. This sometimes, as in the case of the artist Jacus, transforms a landscape into a fairyland.

The muscian, too, is able to compose a piece of music based on association of ideas, the inspiration for which might be drawn from nature or from Heaven knows what.

This establishes a fundamental factor common to all forms of artistic activity. The inspiration is the pretext, the pretense, if you like . . . the excuse to paint a picture, the excuse to combine musical notes, the excuse to create a perfume for beautiful women, which is doubly pleasant. It is indeed true that one day a perfumer used the pretext to create Pretexte.

To compose perfume is to combine certain scents deliberately and create a perfect unity from them. The creator has an infinite number of ways to bring this about. And even though I may think it conceivable that a perfume composer can dream of a perfume (on condition that he can remember it the next day), personally no such thing has ever happened to me. I dream frequently but never about perfumes. Undoubtedly it is because I think about them quite enough all day long.

Apropos of the index cards on which I have noted the ideas relative to perfumes that come to my mind, I can only answer briefly one of the questions that were put to me at the Sixth Mediterranean Symposium on Olfaction: How do you write down these ideas for perfume?

This question assumes that this notation of thoughts is pertinent only to me personally.

The manner of this writing-down of a perfume idea depends

on the kind of idea it is. If it is a matter of a sort of over-all visualization of a perfume (and this doesn't happen often), surely the transcription of this mental image poses a difficult problem due to the vagueness of our present means of identification. The olfactory form (the anticipated perfume, as it were) being perceived in a more or less elusive way, it can only be described by a very personal and imprecise vocabulary. Above all, the description must be such that it permits me later on to recapture the exact same mental set or a similar state of mind appropriate to my setting up a research program which eventually can bring into being on a practical level the perfume I imagined.

I do not allege that another person, reading my notation, would necessarily plunge into the same set of thoughts. But if the other person is imaginative—and that *is* an essential prerequisite—the reading of the notation in question may very well evoke in him another image capable of setting off his own creative mechanism. The result will be different from that which I visualized but just as valuable and perhaps better.

If the idea is of a kind that poses a technical problem—for instance, adding the aldehydes to the Chypre—then I can foresee one or several solutions. Consequently my description might include a detailed statement of the problem—that is to say, traps that should be sidestepped, obstacles that must be surmounted, errors that must be avoided, precautions that must be taken. But I might also give attention to the solution with a list of appropriate or possible products that favor the new combination, and I might also indicate for future reference some proportions certain of which might be rather unorthodox—in brief, a copying down of all the ideas that pertain to the principal thought.

In this case, it would be much easier for another person to participate in this concept and interpret my notation because the entire idea will have been transcribed in readily accessible words, all of which are in common usage. However, the perfume developed by the other person would then either be the same as the one I myself would make or notably different if, starting from the same point of departure, the same pretext, the same stimulus, the pattern of association of ideas that takes place in his mind during the entire period of experimentation flows along lines different from my own.

The original idea can be one or several orientations of the raw material, with observations being made of the corresponding forms; this is frequently the case. It can be the fortunate but calculated coupling of two apparently contradictory scents, or the substitution of one material for another in a medium where the change plays the decisive role in the creation.

One can also start from an idea suggested by the work of an artist or a musician. The title of the Pastoral Symphony alone can stimulate the idea for a perfume. It is idea number twenty-six in my index. I leave it to your own imagination.

The fragrance of a natural product can set off thoughts about its composition; perhaps an infinitesimal amount may serve as the base upon which one can see an entire scaffold to be built—a project of long duration, but the structure of which can be described (and written down).

In addition, one can set about creating a classic scent—lilac, for example—disciplining oneself so as not to use traditional raw materials and combinations.

But in every instance the notation of an idea has to be extremely explicit and sufficiently detailed for an intelligent, alert, tasteful reader to find therein something important to think about and a motivation for personally putting the perfume idea into effect.

It is in this spirit and with this goal that, as a father, I mark down my ideas, regretting all the while that I cannot place them in the care of a perfected machine like the "living memory" of Dr. Sauvan.

*Translated: Grasse, 1973*
*Rosamond V. P. Kaufman*

# EDUCATION IN PERFUMERY
*An Interview With*
*Marcel Carles*
*Argeville, August 1973*

*We would like to have your ideas on the method of your father, which you yourself follow.*

Well, it is a very vast subject and requires a lengthy explanation. In the beginning of systematized perfumery a great number of perfumers created perfumes by accident. They smelled the raw materials, they mixed them, and once in a while as a result they got a good perfume . . . often a bad one. My father tried to create a method that would allow a perfumer to conceive the perfume first and then to compose it, with certainty and exactly as he meant to, without any idea of a hit-or-miss approach. That is to say that the idea for a perfume form was conceived prior to its actually being composed.

Starting with my father, perfumers proceeded to conceive of a perfume consciously, although they had been doing so *unconsciously* for centuries—in effect, to smell their perfume creations in their mind, write down the formulas, and then work them out in the laboratory, using their original concepts as a guide.

*If your father realized that perfumers couldn't continue to work by accident, what did he do to carry out his own idea of how they should go about correcting the situation?*

The first thing he did was to classify the odors into several families in such a way as to determine the natural and the synthetic odors. Then he observed the accord between these odors and classified *them*.

Next, he exercised his olfactory memory by smelling these odors, committing them to memory, and after that he worked on research experiments in the accords of these odors. There are hundreds, if not thousands, of simple raw materials, natural and synthetic, and there are also a certain number of accords or harmonies between these raw materials which are very important. Often these accords are perfect harmonies—that is to say, they are balanced accords. For example, if you take three raw materials of the same volatility and of similar strength and mix them in such a fashion as to fuse them so that the power of one compensates for the power of the other, you have a balanced accord. Because they have the same volatility, three products, the odors of which are going to come forward at the same time, are not just three products that are opposed to each other but rather a new kind of unified raw material. For example, patchouli, *mousse de chêne*, vetiver. In certain proportions we shall no longer say they are patchouli, *mousse de chêne*, vetiver. We shall be able to say that we have an accord. We have a woody note. And that is very important because it is, in fact, creating a new raw material. One cannot say a priori exactly what the components of this raw material are—it is just as though a child looked at a blotter seeing green but not recognizing it to be also yellow and blue. Do you understand? Just as though you played the chord do-mi-sol on the piano, hearing the chord. You could not identify it as do-mi-sol unless you were trained to do so. It is a perfect harmony, and if you have never heard such an accord before, you cannot recognize it. It is important to know all these various accords in perfumery, and we are compelled to do continual research in accords in order to create new raw materials for the perfumer.

*When your father started his research how did he begin his classification?*

To begin with, he separated the natural from the synthetic products to simplify matters, but that is not essential because he could have put both types of products on the same chart without mishap. It was easier, in his view, for the young student to start with the natural products, which are more definite in character, and then go to products made by chemical synthesis. He classified the different odors into notes, such as woody notes, fruity notes, jasmine notes, floral notes, animal notes, spicy notes, anise notes, mint notes, rose notes, orange notes, and other very definite series.

*When did your father realize that you had a talent for perfumery and when did he begin teaching you? Did he start to train you in a broad way or uniquely in perfumery? Did he think that your whole culture should touch on perfumery, and what method did he choose for training you in the techniques of perfume creation?*

Perfumery, in every sense, demands great general culture and knowledge. The question of good taste is applicable to art, music, and to perfume, and I think, at the beginning of my life, it was a broad cultural background that my father tried to give me. When I was sixteen he gave me the choice of continuing my studies, orienting myself toward law, medicine, or perfumery, all of which he considered within my grasp, but his main reasoning was, "If you go into perfumery you will inherit all my knowledge and all my clientele, and it is a shame to leave unused all that I have learned in so many years."

In the beginning I don't think I had a natural talent, nor did I evidence an inclination toward it, but I recognized that perfumery was fascinating the minute I touched upon it. I was full of enthusiasm and set to work seriously.

*So then we understand that your father started you out using the charts of his method. How did you perceive that you could make the definitions between odors?*

Well when you smell lemon it contrasts with sandalwood, sandalwood contrasts with cloves, cloves with orange—you are smelling very contrasting odors. It is much easier to memorize the smell of each of these products individually. If you note the charts of my father you can see the progression of this kind of study. So you study these contrasts the first day, the second day, and so on. Then when you have finished the study of odor by contrast, you start over again with the study of odor by family. But here it is very difficult to distinguish lemon from bergamot, from tangerine, from bigarade, from portugal, for instance. The student whose olfactory memory has been trained in elementary things can go on to the more difficult exercises of studying the odors both by contrast and by family. One can start with both studies simultaneously but it is too difficult for a beginner to do so, and for that reason we separate the natural products from the synthetic products in our exercises, as well as separate the contrasts from the families. The method is very old now, but it was perfected all through the years of my father's career and became final in the years 1955–1960.

My father became the Director of the Roure Laboratory at the age of thirty-three. And from that time on he worked at his own method, but he had been thinking of it and doing the necessary research long beforehand.

*Did you add all of the synthetic raw materials to his plans and to his exercises? Is that what you have personally given to the method?*

Obviously the method is not complete on the basis of this research we have here in our hands. It is rather a sort of résumé because the method of study is extremely complex. In the final stages one has to work on charts and sketches of perfumes, one has to study the accords, make imitations of existing perfumes. To tell you the truth, it would take me about three months to go over all the steps in the method with you, to explain them adequately. One of the major things is the principle of volatility, because this brings us to another type of classification that is very important: the classification between the notes of the greatest volatility (*notes de tête*), modifiers, which are of medium volatility (*modificateurs—notes de coeur*), and notes of great tenacity (*notes de base*). When one makes a perfume, one must make a perfect balance among these three classifications of notes.

The *notes de tête* are always agreeable—for example lavender, lemon, bergamot, mint, which are very pleasant but do not hold. The idea is to get a pleasant odor that holds. The modifiers make the link between them and the *notes de base,* which are the most tenacious, which give the real character to the perfume. Often they are unpleasant smelling—vetiver, patchouli, *mousse de chêne,* and various others. They are quite disagreeable at first encounter, but in the course of several hours they become pleasant smelling. Thus the entire art of the perfumer is to balance these three types of raw matrial. Let me explain it to you further.

First we have a harmony of *notes de tête,* which is very pleasant. To the *notes de tête* we add the odors of the modifiers, which may be a bit nauseating and unpleasant in and of themselves, but which are most acceptable when covered by the pleasant odor of the *notes de tête* to which they had been added. When the modifiers enter into a pleasant stage of their own, they in turn cover the initial unpleasant odors of the *notes de base.* Finally the *notes de base* themselves will enter into their own pleasant-smelling stage, which is extremely tenacious and fixes the entire perfume. In the creation of a perfume it is really the *base* that keeps it from evaporating, but the originality of the perfume comes from the total composition, not from any one of its components.

There are several ways of giving a perfume originality. Originality can come about through the use of a new raw material. For me, this is the most interesting challenge. Originality can also come about through a harmony of *notes de base* known but used in a way that no one else has yet thought of. Originality can also come from the influence an accessory product exerts upon a classic perfume. An accessory product is one which by its strength and by its character cannot fit into an accord but which can add something definitive to an accord. As an example of an accessory product, suppose you are wearing a yellow dress today, but tomorrow you can change the belt, use a large bag, put on a big, startling leather hat, and by using leather accessories you have transformed your yellow dress. You will have created a new outfit. Another time you may remove the present belt, place flowers at the waist, neckline and wrists, and you will give the impression of having created a new outfit. But in no case can you go out in the street wearing nothing but your belt! That is the usefulness of accessory products in giving originality to perfume. That is the case of such materials as galbanum, mint, certain products like cumin, which are too powerful used in an accord but which are good when used merely to modify an odor.

*If I understand you, Mr. Carles, the real study comes from being able to conceive of a perfume mentally and then transform it to this type of triangular balance on paper and then into its liquid form. How long does it take to become a perfumer?*

That is a very difficult question to answer. It depends on the capacity, the talent, the intelligence, the general culture of the individual. I have had several students who were just mediocre in the beginning but who became extraordinarily good perfumers after a number of years. One must think of the method as a tool that gives the student the kind of technical knowledge that permits him to express himself—his personality, that is to say—in the artistic sense. But the method, in and of itself, is not a substitute for the student's imagination.

On the other hand, one can be a good student and a bad perfumer. One needs a year in a special laboratory where one can confine oneself exclusively to exercises following the studies of the

139

method. The method requires time, and the student needs training in the use of his imagination without any thought of the price of the material, of the commercial aspects of the future, or of any extraneous matters. He must work in an atmosphere of "art for art's sake" so as to become erudite on the subject of perfumery, to know perfumery from inside out, and to be able to create something original. Then one must have another year to work with other perfumers as part of a team on practical problems. The problems I speak of are those of commercial perfumery: aerosols, soaps, flavorings. These are all commercial problems that must be dealt with by the student in his training. And probably he needs another year or two in order that he be able to work alone. He has to have time enough to develop ease and confidence in his own work and in his own ideas. One must allow about three or four years for a perfumer to "earn his keep."

*I want to give you a word so that you can demonstrate for me the way a smell stimulates your imagination in terms of odors and certain of your ideas that you would like to express.*

That will be an exercise for me because it is a very personal matter.

*But that is what I want. I want to have an example of your subjectivity as a perfumer. What comes to your imagination when I say the word "pine" to you?*

Pine is very complex. I think of a vacation, the sea, the mountains, summer—for me it is an odor that is always associated with summer.

*Did you ever think of using it in a perfume?*

That is paradoxical. We are conditioned—90 per cent of all the pine odor we use is in bubble bath preparations or bath salts, so we think of it primarily as perfume for those purposes. Only on occasion do we think of it as an element in an elegant perfume.

*Would you give me your impression of mimosa?*

I don't like mimosa very much. It is a little nauseating to me and makes me a bit queazy. I don't think of it as being very clean-cut. It makes me think a little of a woman of doubtful reputation.

*Hyssop?*

Hyssop is a plant that is used very little, but I see it in a perfume for men, such as a *note* in a tobacco scent.

*Neroli?*

Neroli is very distinct because it always gives a feeling, a sensation of fullness. It is the type of odor that permeates everything with which it comes in contact. It gives the notion of opulence. It is very, very rich and has several uses: the classic use in Eau de Colognes to which it gives a fresh odor, a little orange note, but I personally prefer to use it in an extract. I find that in certain harmonies, from the very beginning, it brings out a very pleasant and a rich smell. This can be a drawback, not when one is making an eau de toilette, but when one is making an extract or a perfume, one has to have the courage to control this early odor of freshness while trying to keep the rich character of the perfume—the breadth of the *note de tete,* so to speak. I know that my thinking is against the trend, but personally I like heavy scents, and I find that neroli has what I like. It has fullness and freshness at the same time.

*Iris?*

Iris is a very fine raw material. It is very expensive. But it isn't used too often in commercial products because to get a real character of the odor, one must use a great deal. Most perfumers reason that if one uses an equal quantity of other fine absolutes, which are equally expensive, one can get an even better, finer perfume at less cost. For example, for an iris *note*—if you used an absolute of jasmine, with certain synthetic products, you could arrive at something finer in some ways than using actual iris. You would have a

140

perfume with an iris note, but it would be a richer perfume. Or you could start with an absolute of violet for example and go on from there.

*Geranium?*

Geranium is an irreplaceable product, irreplaceable. Above all for everything that has a "fern" odor. The *note* of fern is certainly the most important *note* for men's perfumes. It has always been the most appreciated scent for the male market and continues to be so. It is indispensable, for example, in all perfumed products other than perfume itself, such as soap, bath salts, household sprays, and you know that in some cases this is also part of our work. The odors of hay and fern are very important in this phase of our work. Even if we use very beautiful synthetic geranium, we have not as yet been able to arrive at elegant perfumes with the same fullness, the same personality, or the same character as those we create with natural geranium.

*Basil?*

Basil is an accessory product. It gives personality. It is generally used in very small quantities. But in certain eaux de toilette, one can succeed in having a lovely fragrance, thanks to accords. And if one is able to find things with which it harmonizes very well, one can even use an enormous quantity of basil— depending on the accord of course—in a product for men. It offers great originality. Recently I worked on a perfume for men that uses at least 20 per cent of basil. This is, of course, outside of normal procedure.

*What is the name of it?*

Oh, it isn't launched commercially as yet. I made it for myself as a study.

*Would you give me your impression of* genêt *or what the English call broom?*

*Genêt* is an odor I don't like to use because it is an absolute that is very heavy. I don't find it very noble in character. There are things I would much rather use, such as jasmine, rose, perhaps hyacinth—things like that. But *genêt* and mimosa—I don't care for them at all.

*Verveine?*

Verveine is very nice, very interesting. It has somewhat the fullness of neroli. It is difficult nowadays to launch a perfume of quality using verveine because so much of the odor of verveine is made from products that are cheap, not only in price but in the kind of odor they emit. They are used for deodorants and for household products and that is creating a wrong impression of this nice odor in the public mind and giving it an image that is vulgar, much to my regret.

*Patchouli?*

That is by far my father's favorite product. It has an enormous amount of personality, and one has to be very courageous to use it. For example, in Tabu, my father's perfume, there is 10 per cent of patchouli. Never before had anyone dared to use such a high proportion of patchouli. One has to be audacious. Before my father's time, perfumers thought patchouli to be incompatible with certain odors—jasmine, for example. What is important is to be bold enough to find the accord, to make a liaison between patchouli and the other products one wishes to use. Patchouli, carnation, jasmine make a fantastically beautiful accord. One must work carefully with patchouli because very often in a solution with alcohol the scent is spoiled. One has to be very skillful and find another product that harmonizes well with patchouli to mitigate against such a circumstance, but it is a marvelous product.

*Since we have talked a bit about the specific elements in perfume creation, do you think we shall see the day when the perfume creator will be recognized for the perfumes he creates, that he will be identified with them?*

I don't believe so. I will tell you why. If a number of perfumers work together and one of them leaves the team, the others can recreate his work when he goes. That is why there is doubt in my mind. A great number of perfumes are created by such collaborations, though it is true that some of our most elegant perfumes of today have been created by single perfume composers. I myself created Capricci when I was on a beach in Algeria. I conceived of the perfume form in my mind, wrote it down on a slip of paper, and sent it to my father. Taking the formula in hand, my father was able to put my idea into practical form, and that is the way Capricci was born.

*Why is it that you and your father are considered experts in "Spanish" perfume?*

Oh, that is because, even though my father did his work in Grasse, he was often a technical consultant to other perfume houses in other countries, and his particular area, the country where he was in most demand, was Spain. If he was an expert in any way, it was that he was an expert in merchandising. He really understood the consumer habits of Spain. Perfumes preferred in Spain have more pronounced character than those preferred in Paris. My father worked toward perfumes to be sold in both places, but with an entirely different approach for each market. He naturally reserved what he considered to be his finest perfume creations for the Spanish market because he found that financially that was more profitable for him, particularly such perfumes as Aqua Brava, Emir, Tabu. Please remember that there was a time when the perfumers of Grasse were not as highly paid as they are today and it was necessary for some of them to be "traveling salesmen" for the firms for which they worked to augment their incomes.

One of the reasons my father trained young people as he did was that he knew that they were unable to acquire a lot of experience in what people in different countries were purchasing, and the best way to acquaint them with the most popular products was to have the students understand exactly what these products were—from the creation to the consumer—so he insisted that they make chemical analysis of all existing perfumes. To enable them to do this, my father made charts of the components of every single perfume on the market. He classified all the commercial perfumes that were floral, woody, green, and so on. Then his pupils had to analyze all the existing perfumes for themselves so that they would come to know the market, to understand what sold, and to be able to anticipate important trends. The result was that at all times, resorting to my father's outlines, his pupils had an automatic, built-in recognition of every perfume line.

What is even more interesting for us is to compare the perfumes that really have sold a great deal. We can consider Arpege first. Charting Arpege, we find that the accord is rose, jasmine, acetate de vetyveryle. Then charting Chanel No. 5, we have rose, jasmine, vetyveryle, certain aldehydes being major in this perfume. When we go to Madame Rochas, we have methylionone, vetyveryle, rose, jasmine. Following that we can take Caleche—rose, jasmine, acetate de vetyveryle, santal. We take all or any perfumes that have had success and we find that they all contain rose, jasmine, and acetate de vetyveryle. This shows us that through the years the most commercial, the most popular, and the most desirable accord has been rose, jasmine, and so on.

So that when a student wants to compose a modern perfume he starts with this sketch, this accord. Then he dresses it up with other accessories, but he keeps this scheme because he knows it is very marketable. For example if you take Jickey, which was found in 1892 or thereabouts, the accord is patchouli and carnation. Tabu is patchouli and carnation, and All Spice is a woody note with patchouli and carnation. We can take Lavande, which is most popular in Spain and for which they use twenty tons of concentrate per year. It is a lavender base, but what gives it character is patchouli and carnation. So we can accept the fact that patchouli and carnation, although they may be very vulgar in the opinion of some, are two scents which when used in combination are very commercial. Every time the student uses the accord patchouli–carnation he can push it to any extent he wishes, he can embroider it as he likes, but he knows from the start of his creative idea that it is going to be commercial and marketable.

And so you see that my father's goal was to train his students so that when they became independent of him, they had a firm foundation of trained olfactory memory on which to build their hopefully marketable perfumes. He wanted them to carry out these ideas by writing them down first before composing in the laboratory the beautiful perfume forms that they conceived in their own very personal imaginations. And as you see, he reached his goal.

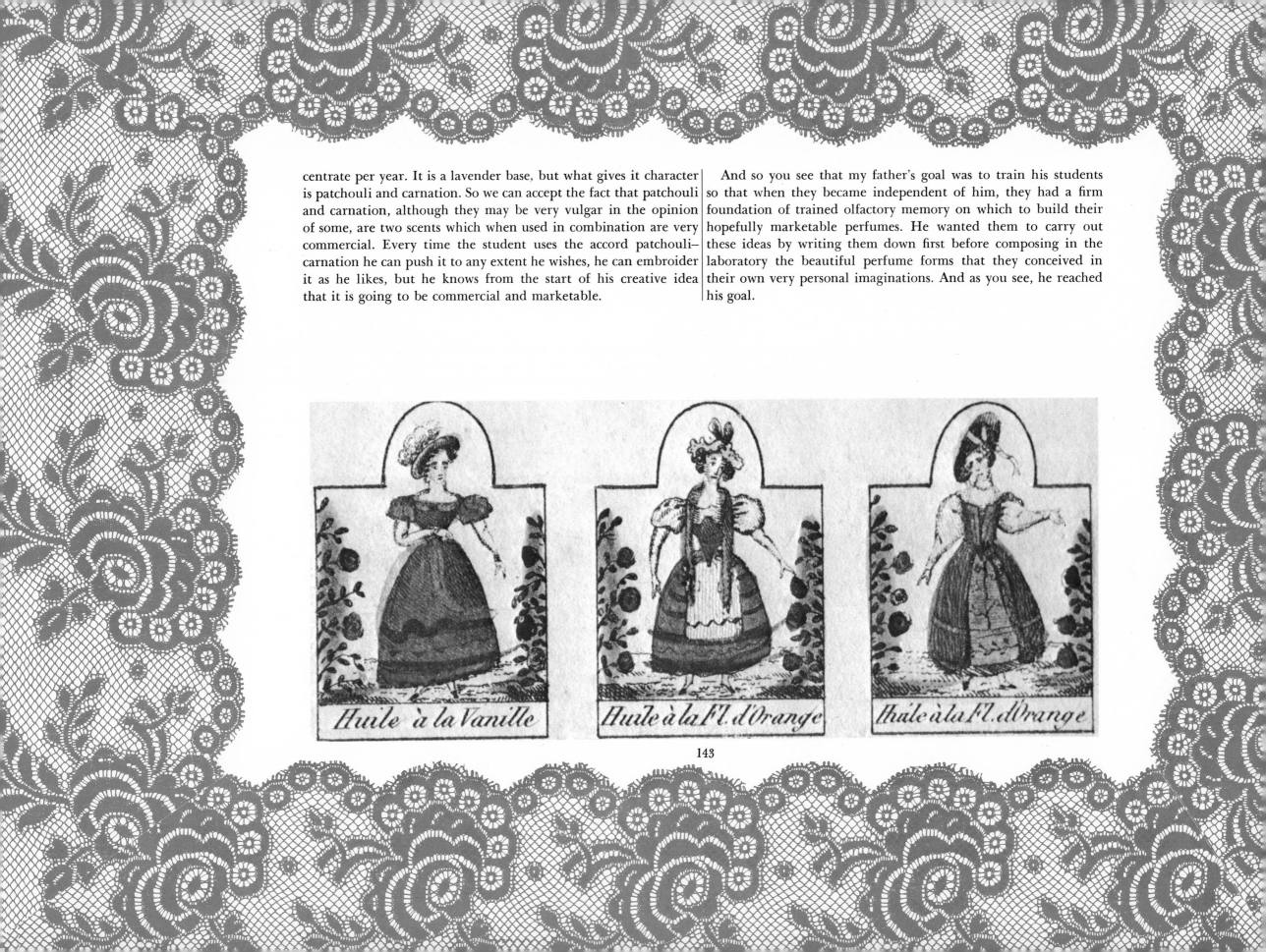

Huile à la Vanille    Huile à la Fl. d'Orange    Huile à la Fl. d'Orange

143

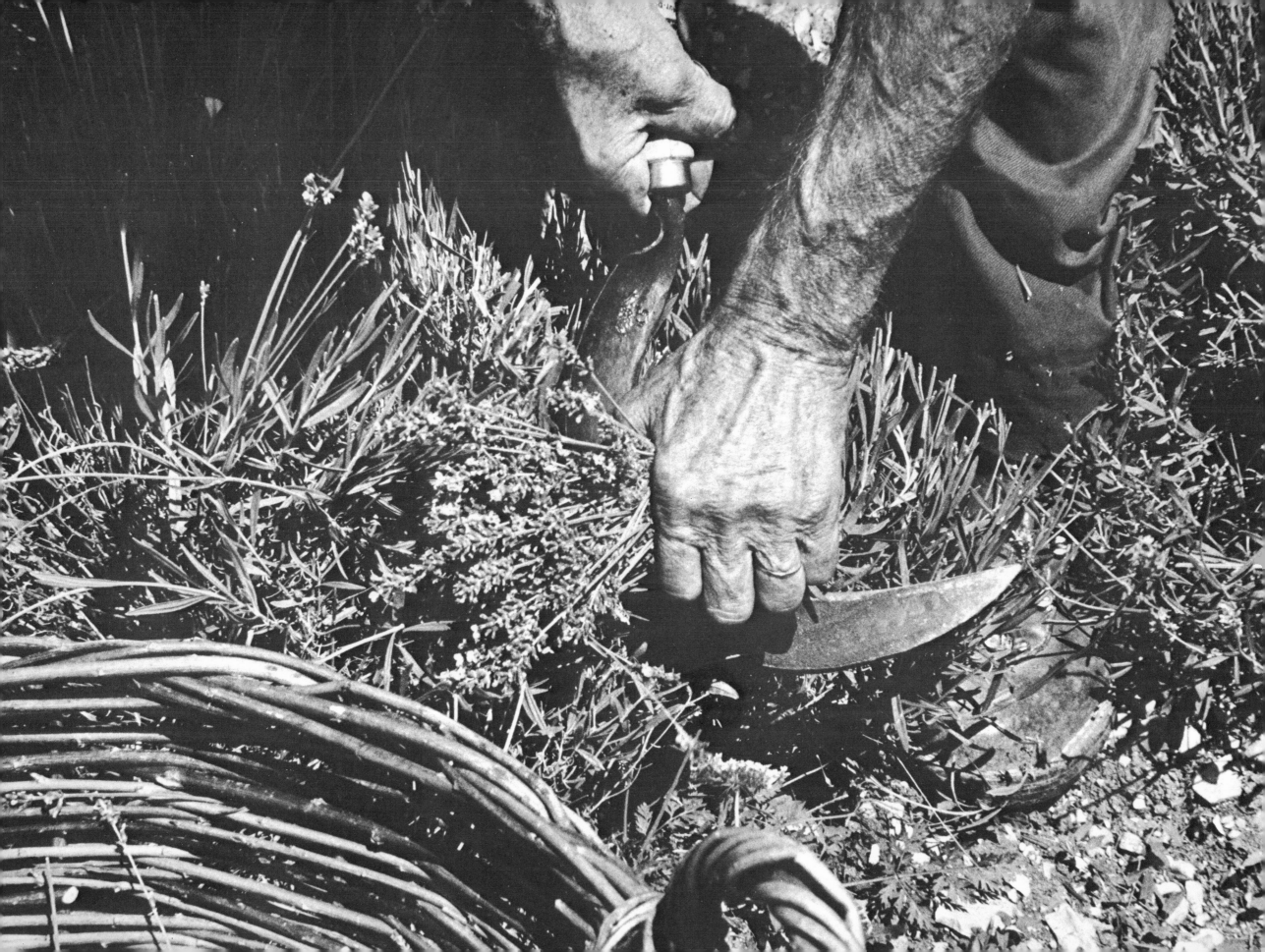

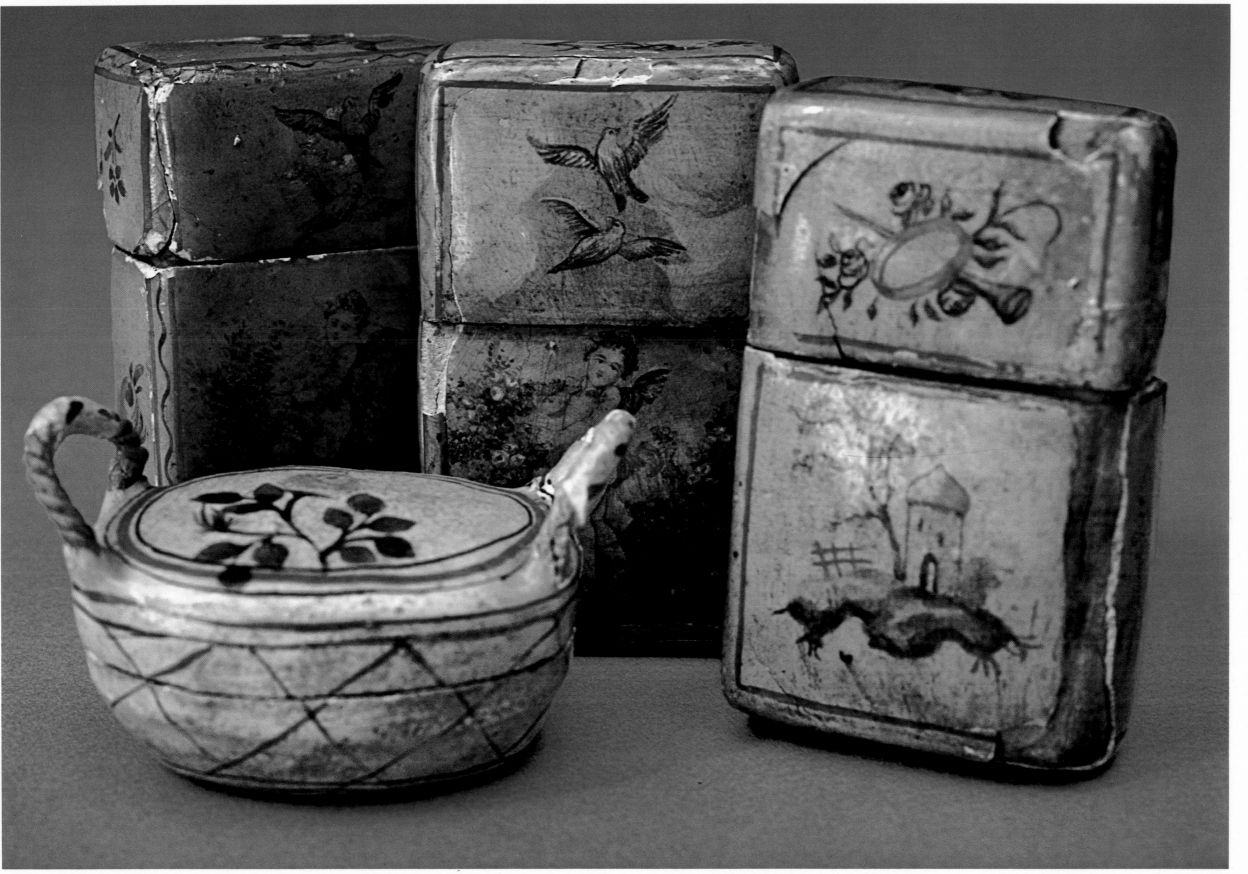

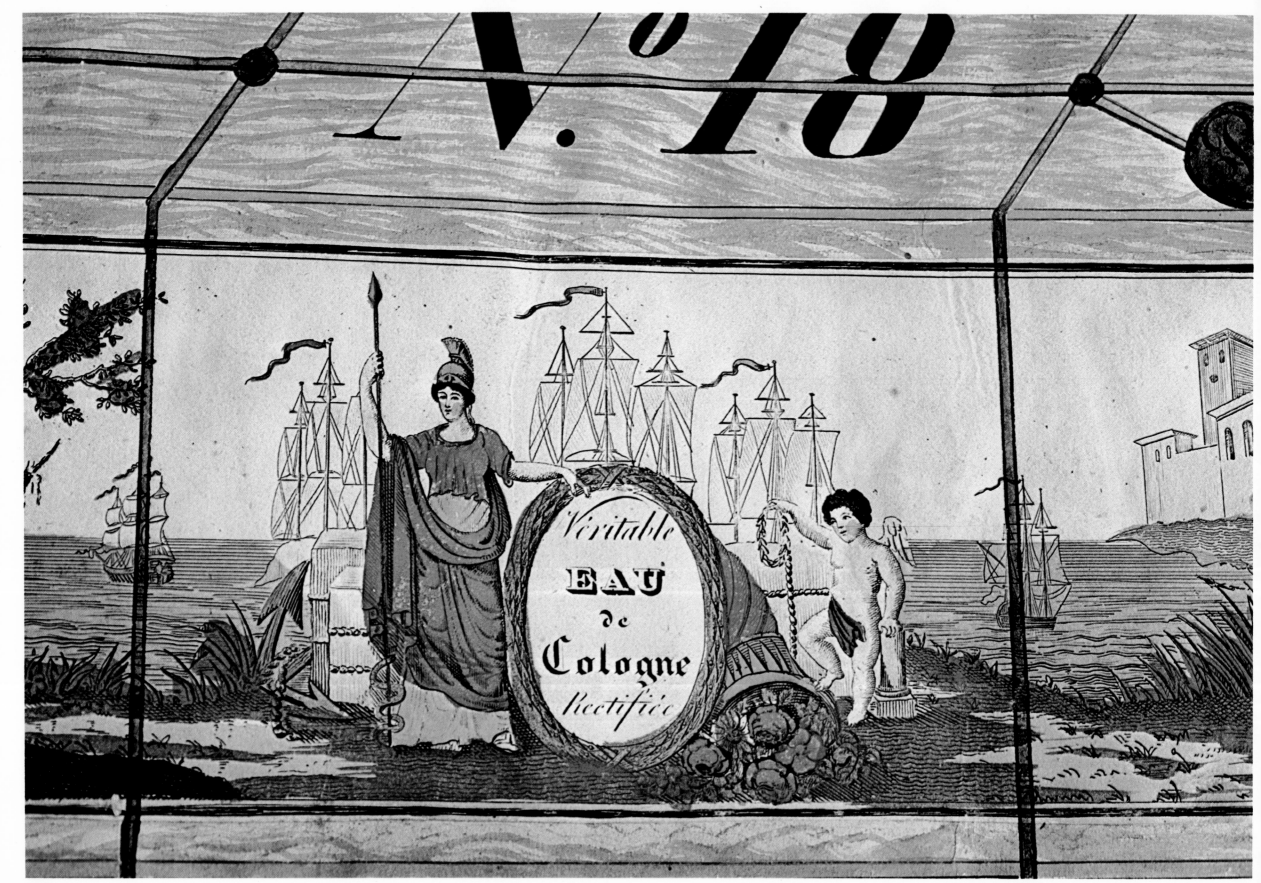

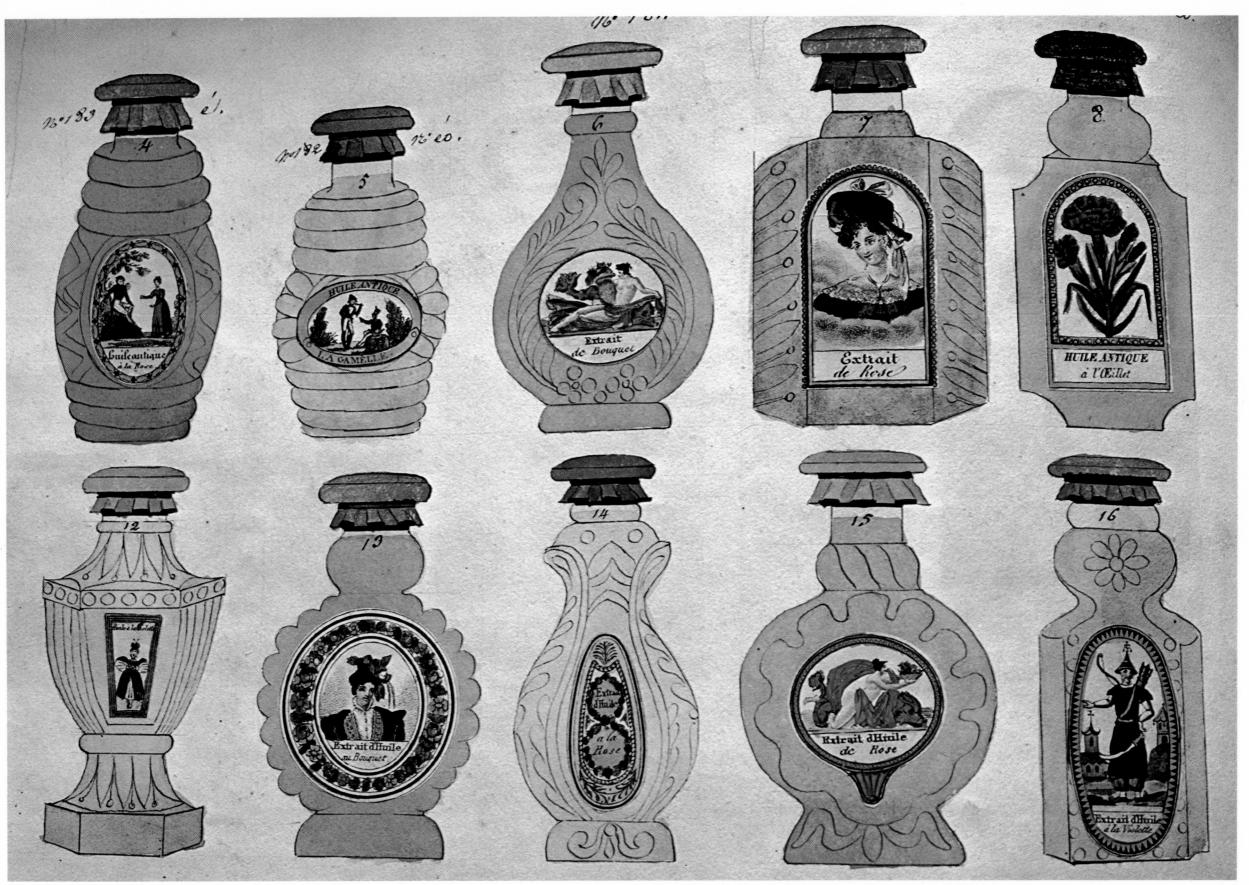

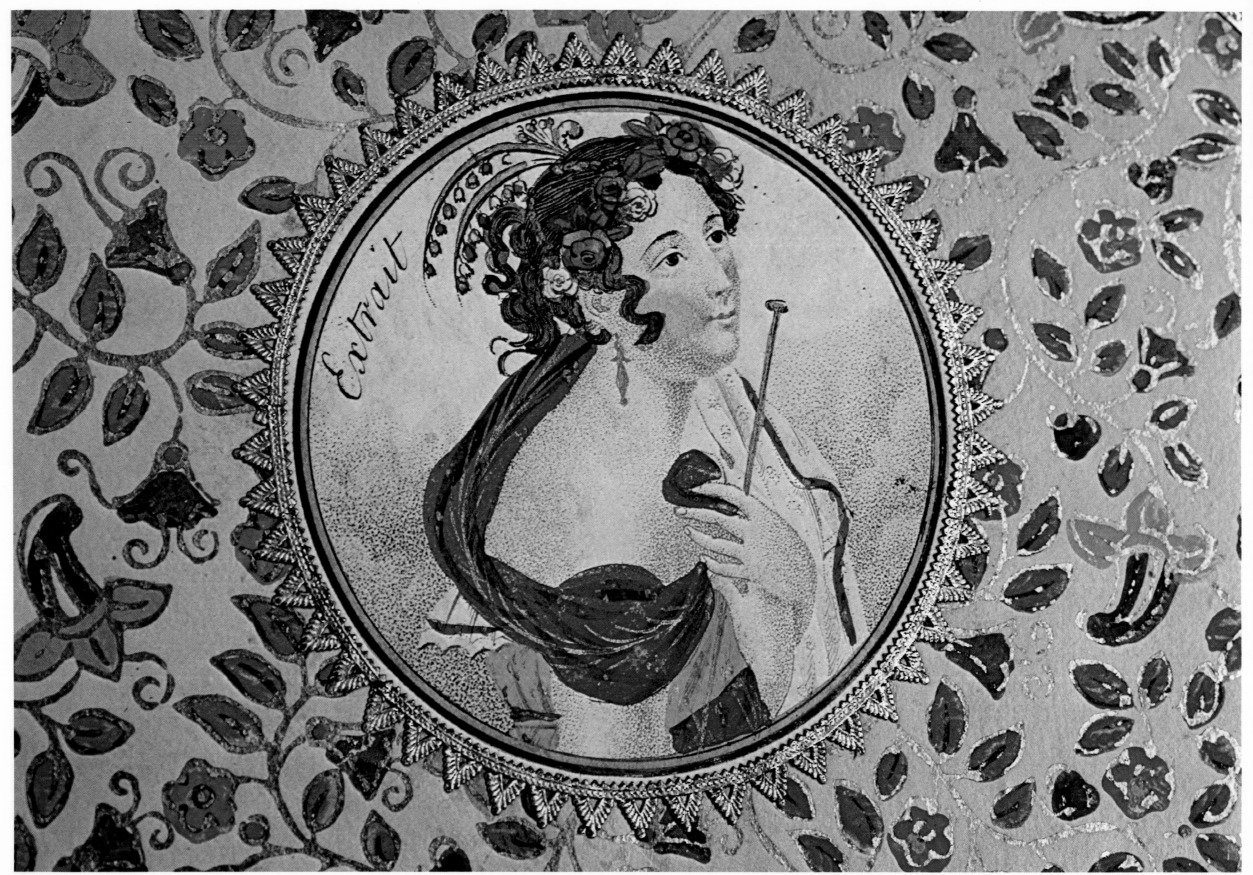

148

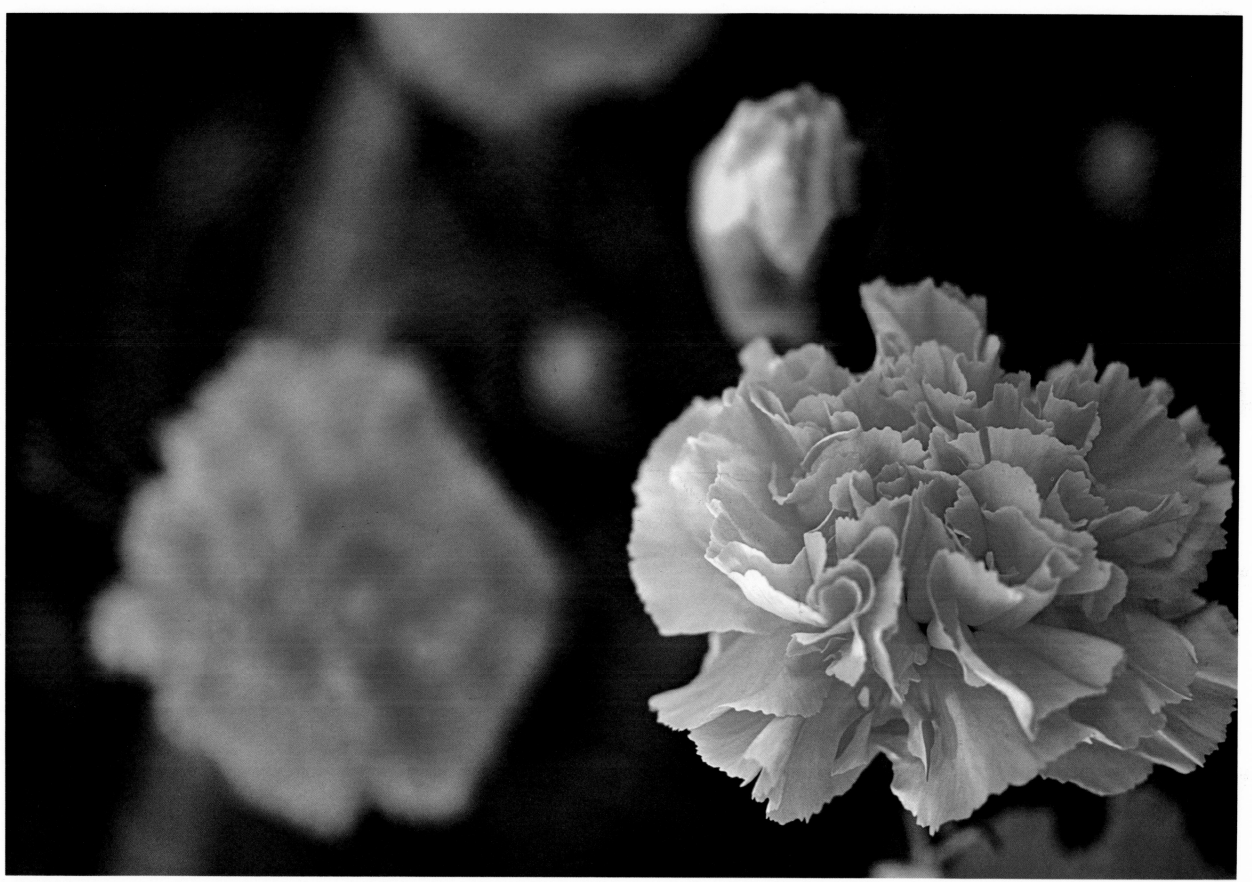

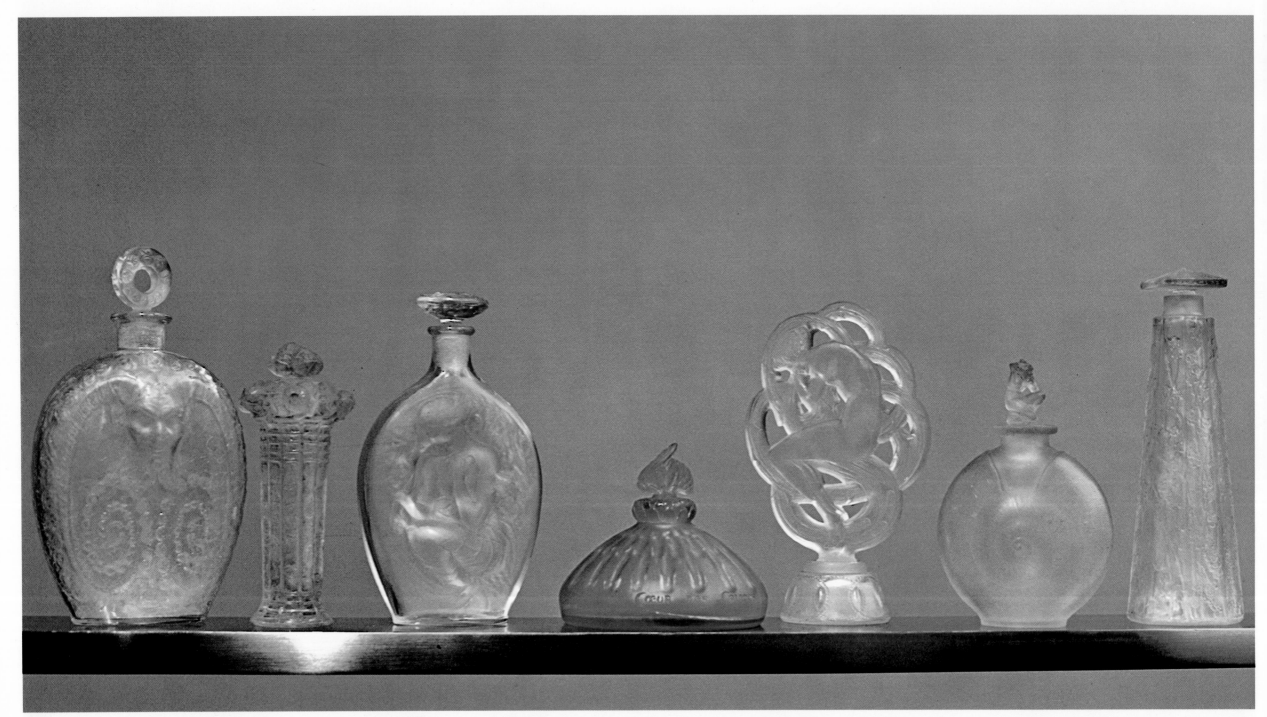

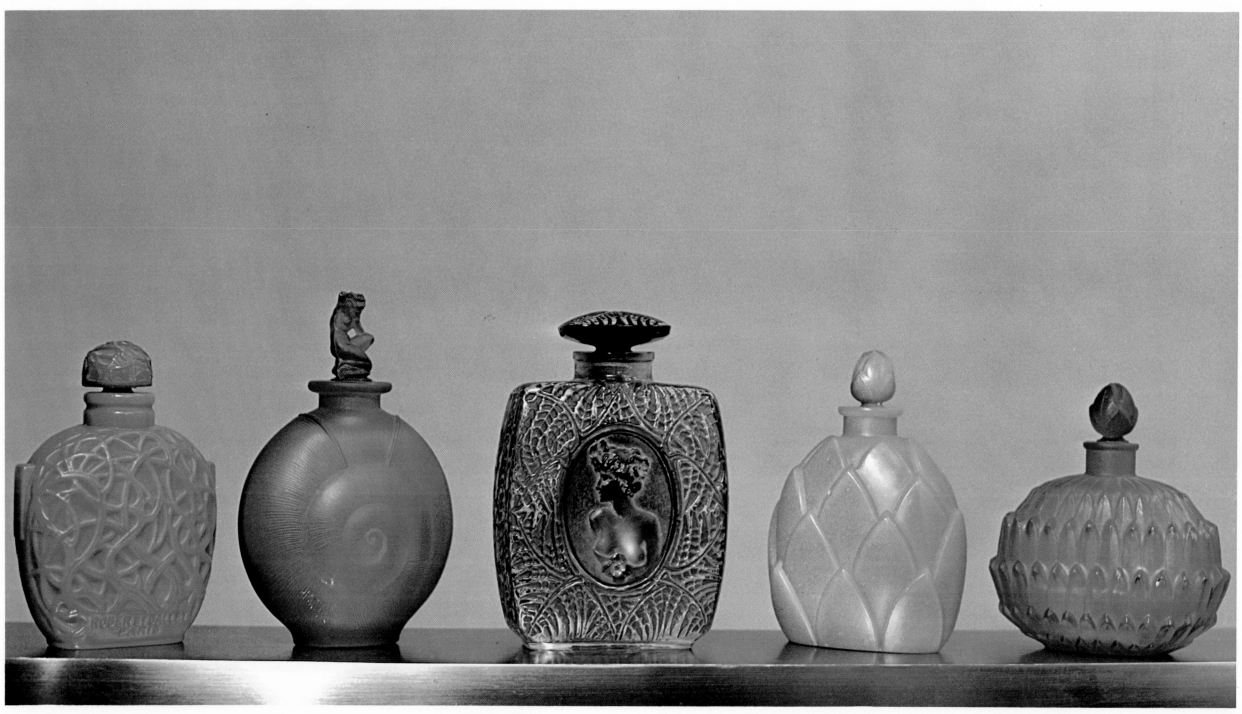

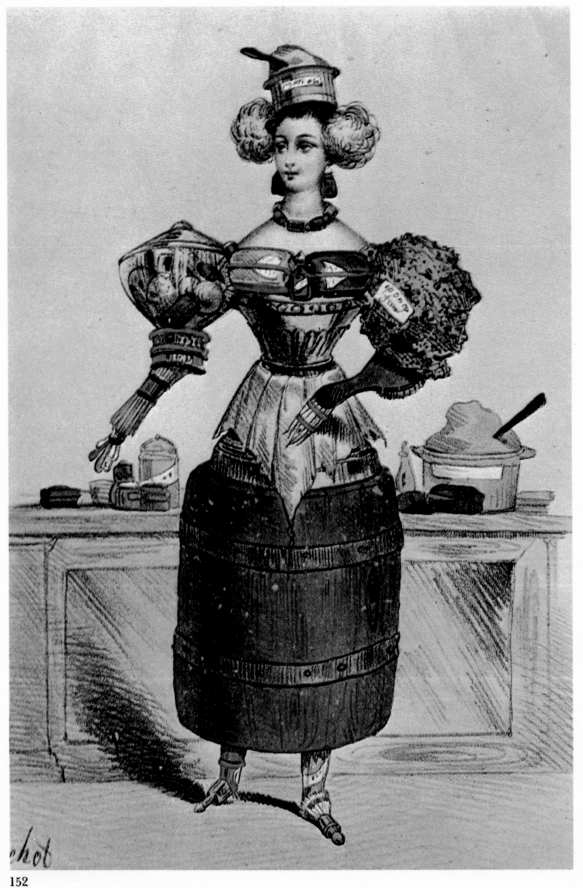

152

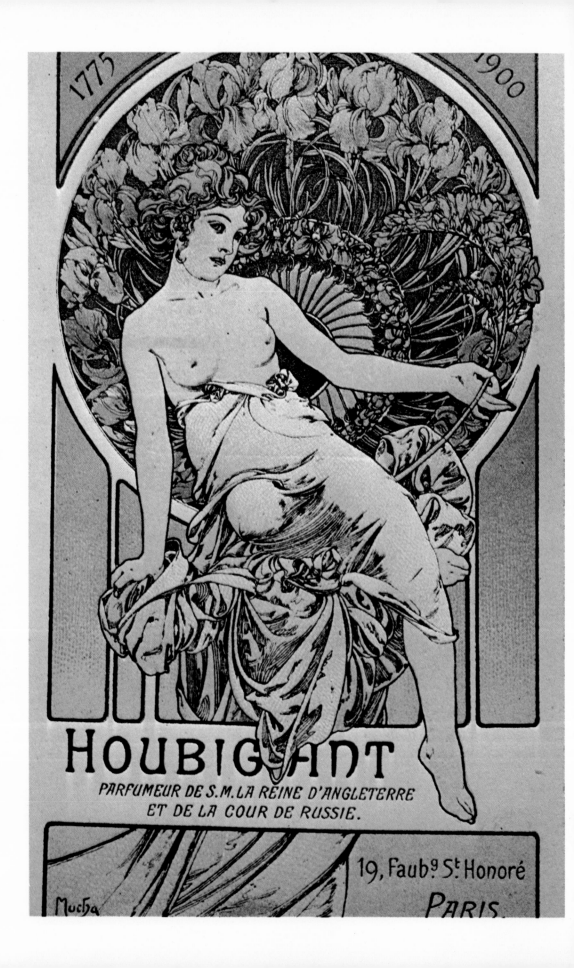

HOUBIGANT

PARFUMEUR DE S.M. LA REINE D'ANGLETERRE
ET DE LA COUR DE RUSSIE.

19, Faub.g St Honoré
PARIS.

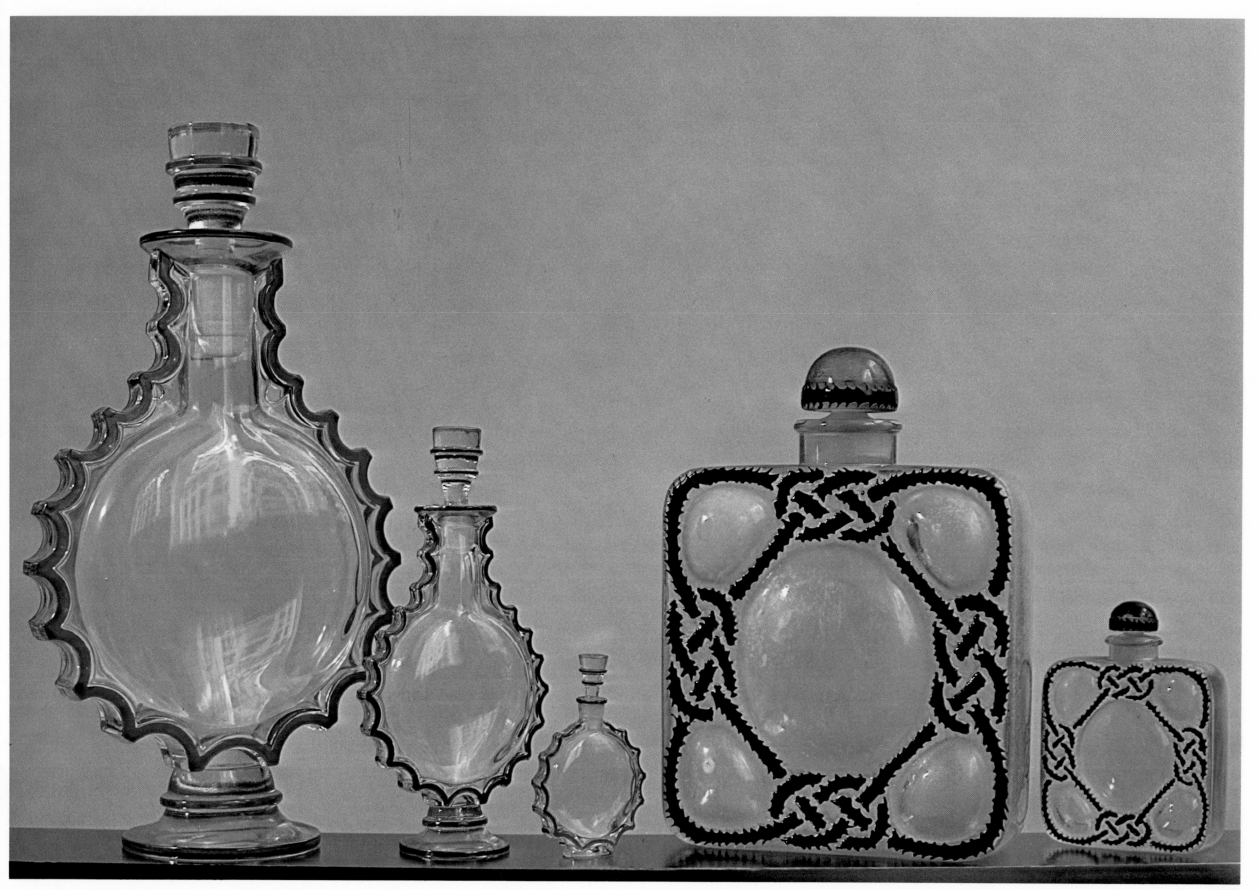

153

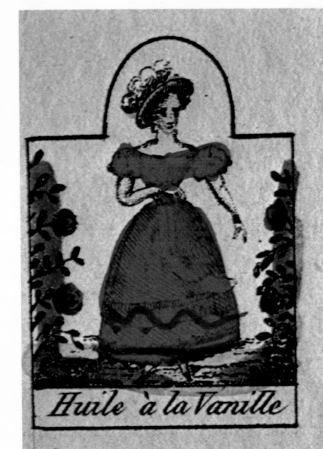

Huile à la Vanille

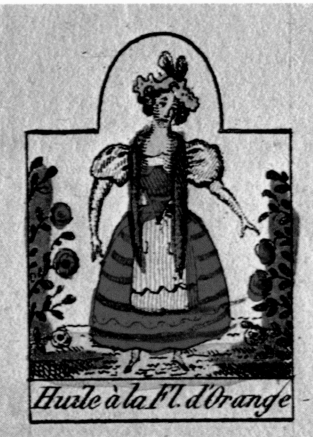

Huile à la Fl. d'Orange

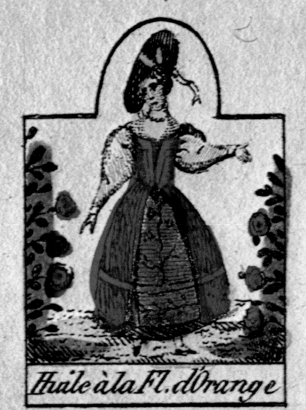

Huile à la Fl. d'Orange

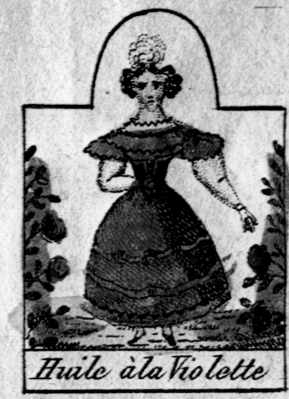

Huile à la Violette

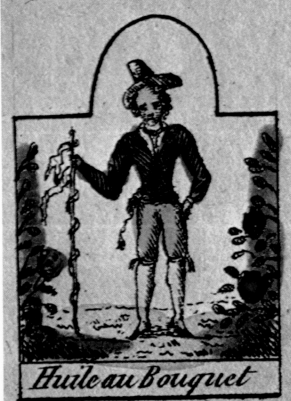

Huile au Bouquet

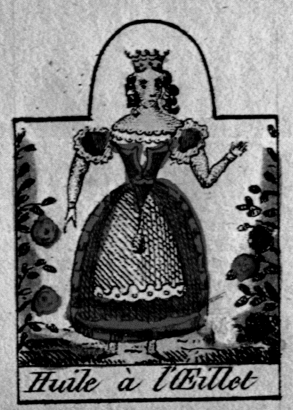

Huile à l'Œillet

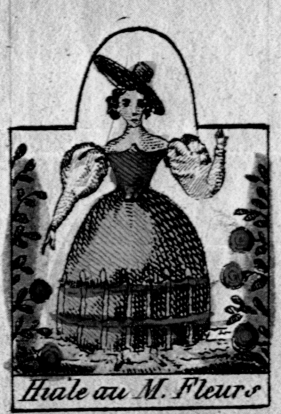

Huile au M. Fleurs

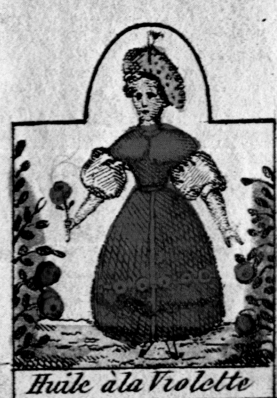

Huile à la Violette

154

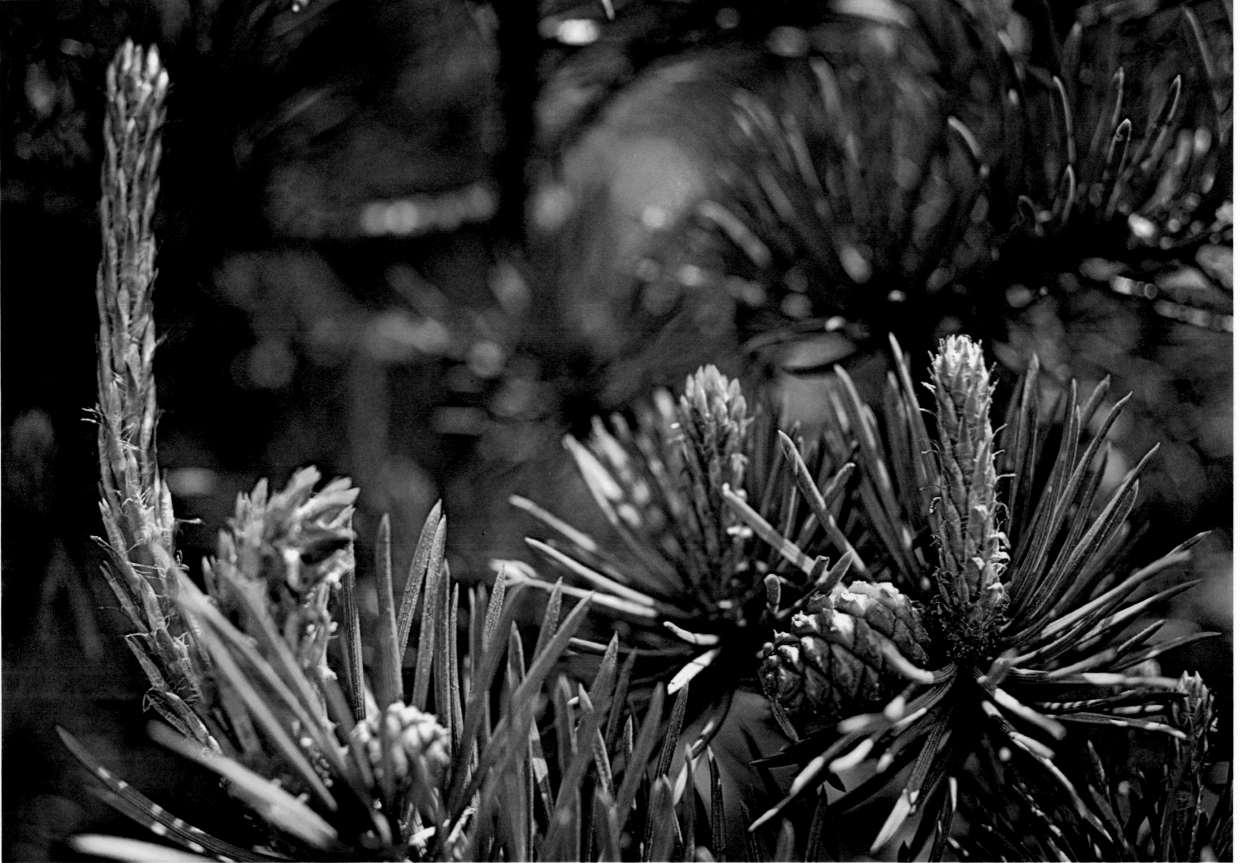

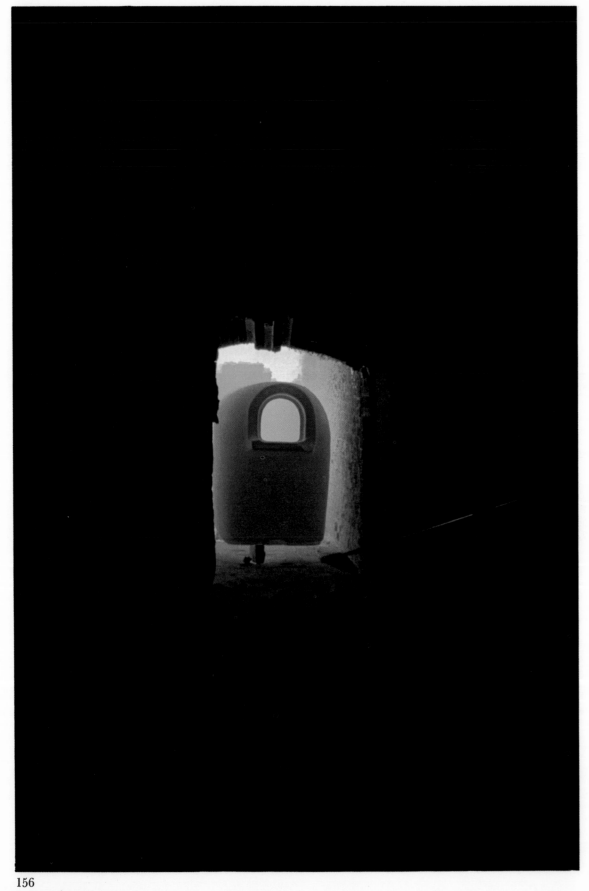

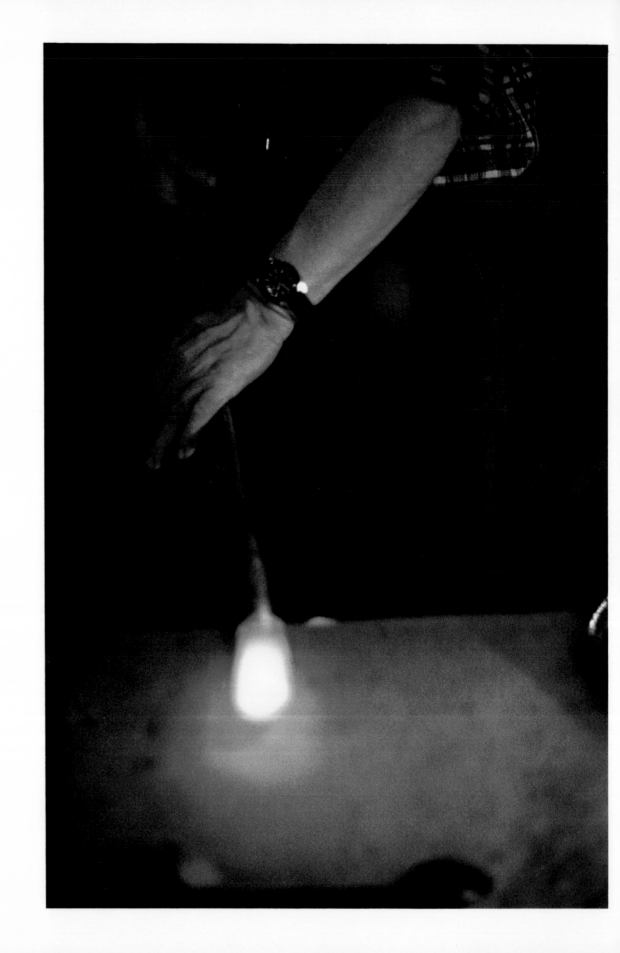

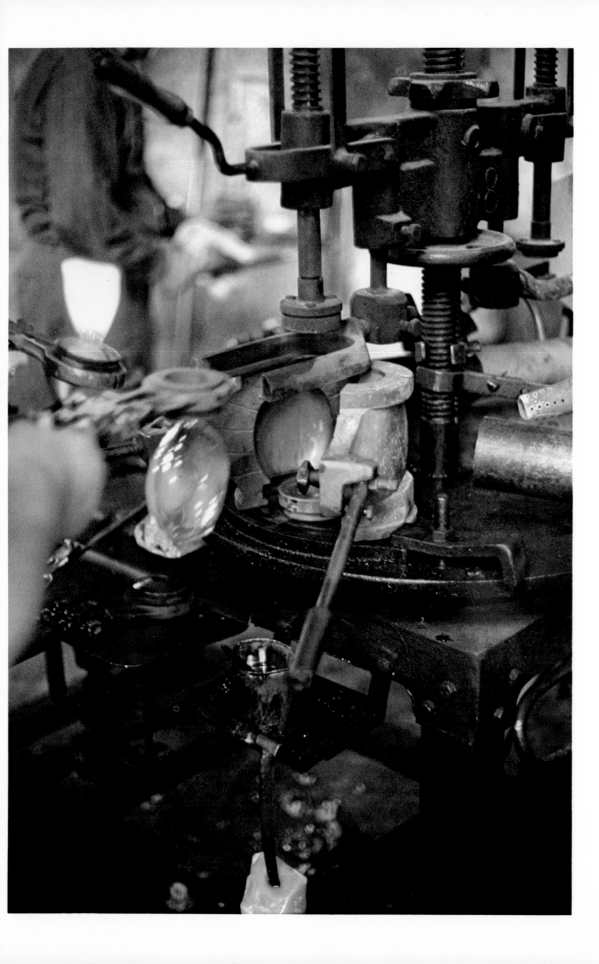

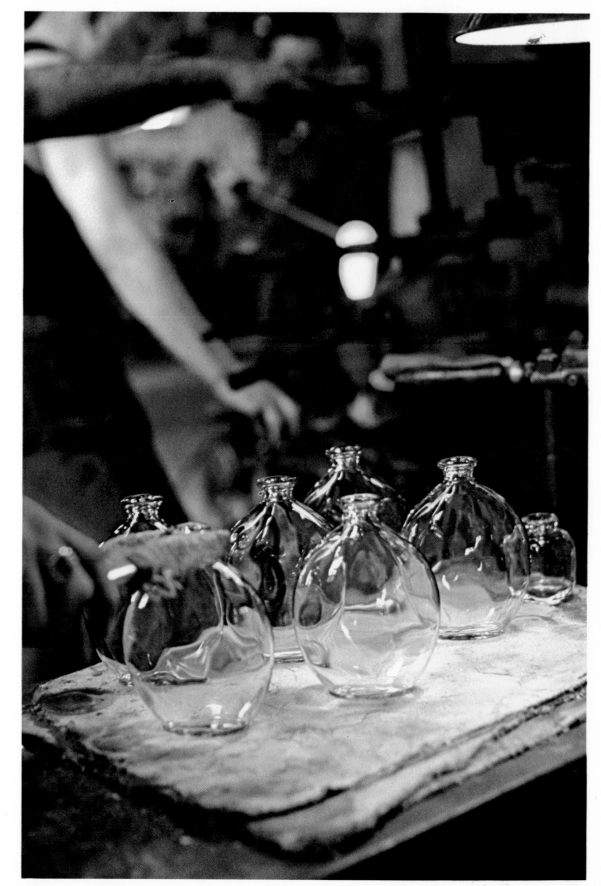

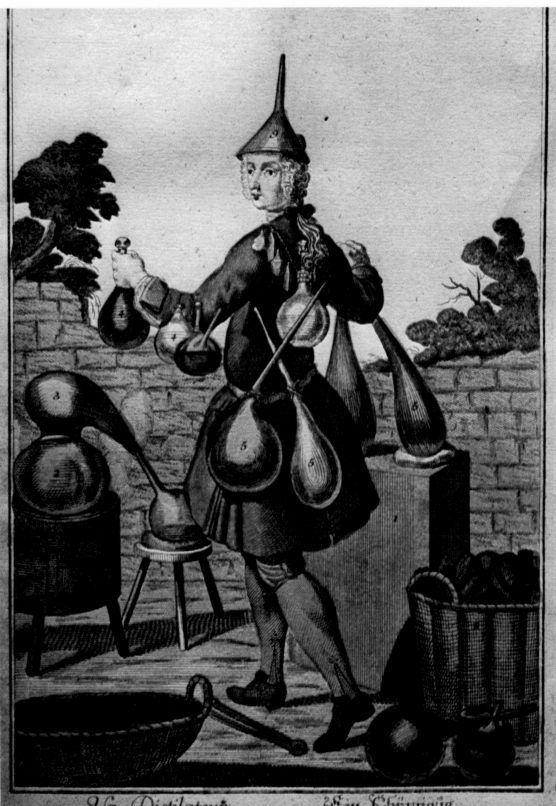

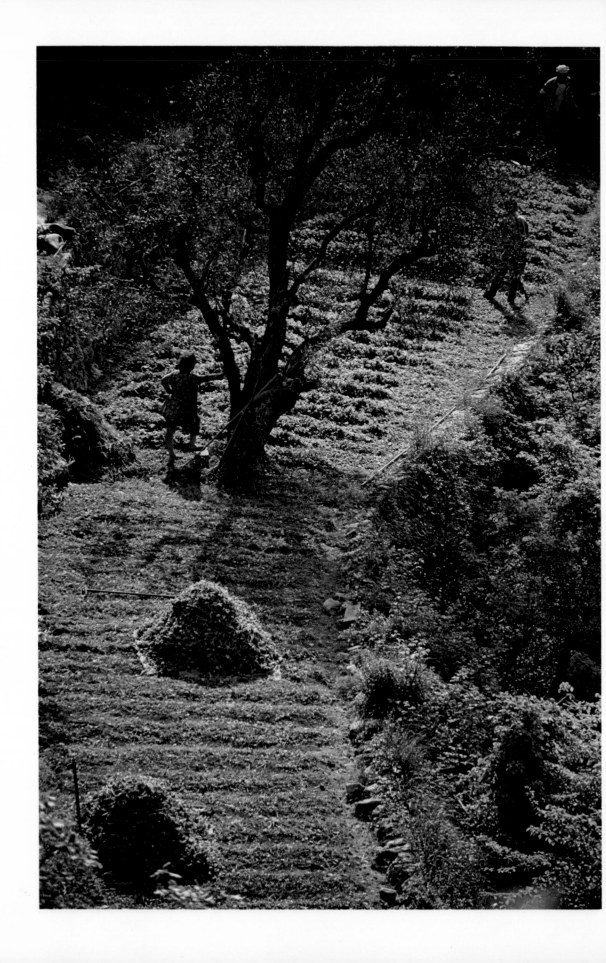

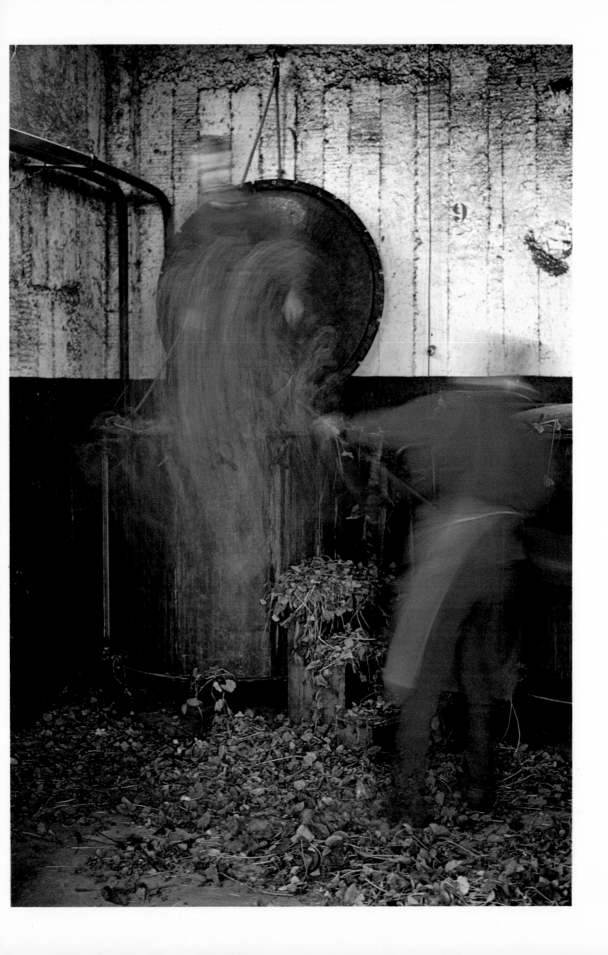

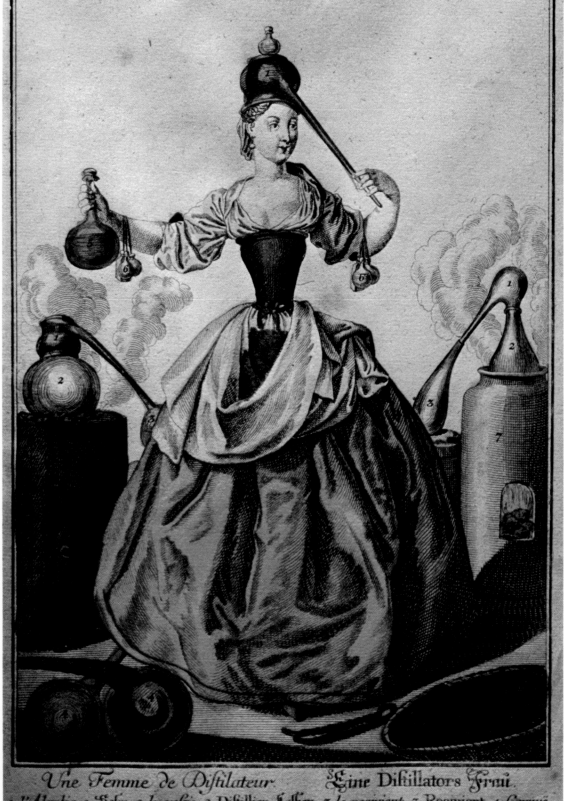

Une Femme de Distilateur. Eine Distillators Frau.
1. l'Alembic 1 Helm 2 la vesie 2 Distillier Kolben 3 le recipient 3 Recipient 4 Cornüe
4 Retortin. 5 flacon. 5 Glaß. 6 petite phiole 6 kleine gläser 7 fourneau à distiler 7 Distillier
Ofen 8 Simples pour distiler 8 Kräuter zum brennen
Cum Priv: Maj. Mart. Engelbrecht excud. A.V

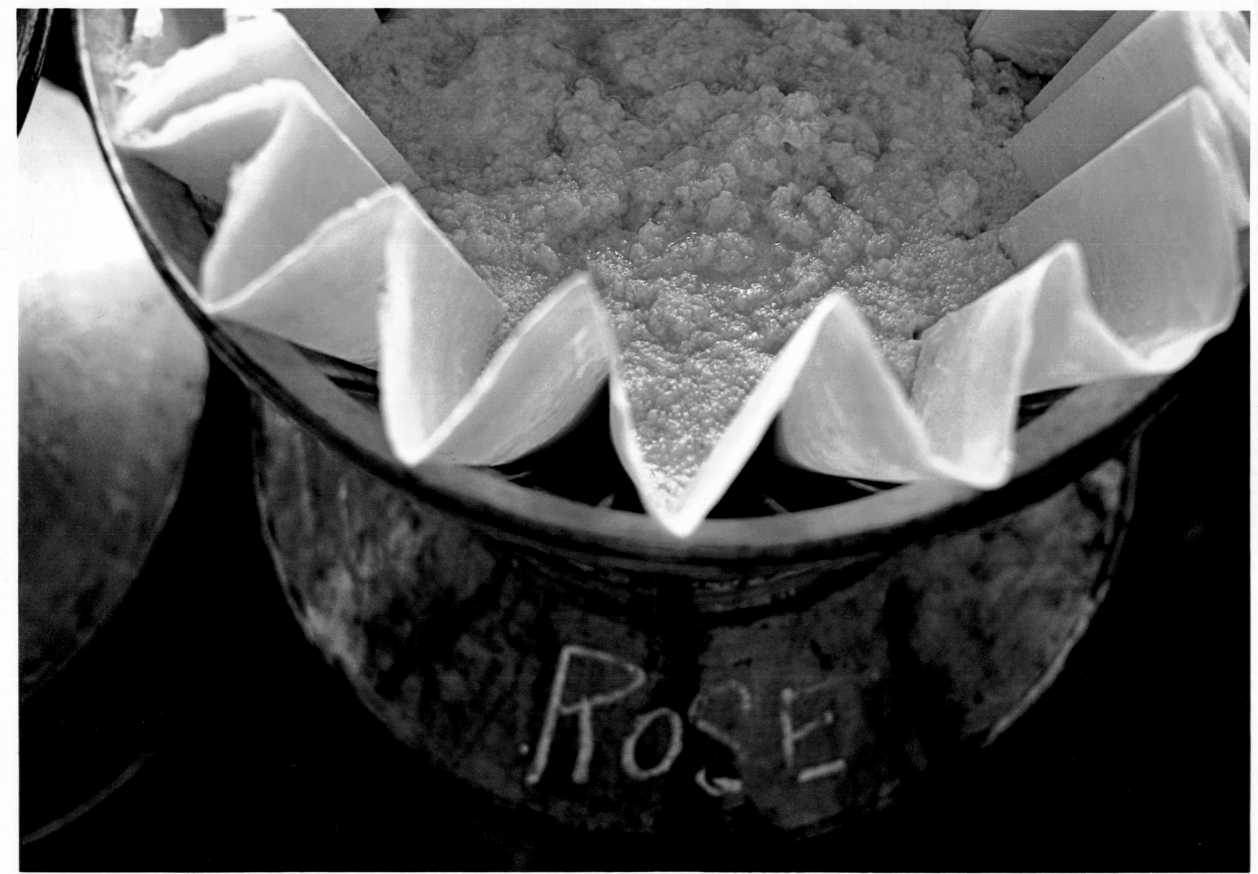

# A METHOD OF CREATION IN PERFUMERY
## By
## Jean Carles

*As reprinted from* **Recherches**, *1961, 1962, 1963*

The apprentice perfumer at the beginning of his career is like a ship without a rudder. If he is left to his own devices or badly led, his discoveries will lack organization and will lead him inevitably to wasteful and ineffectual use of his creative energy.

In my early days on this rugged pathway, I found myself in the presence of tutors who seemed to have disregarded the necessity for basic rules and whose interest in our futures was of the mildest. Watching how they proceeded with their own work did not make it seem particularly absorbing; they appeared to believe in a happy-go-lucky way of life, desultorily dipped smelling strips into the available samples of odorous materials, and thus their formulations progressed, small addition by small addition, and not according to some pre-established plan. Thus, in the past, most of the great perfume creations, or rather, of the commercially successful perfumes, were produced almost by chance, sometimes to the unfeigned surprise of their originators! Although such happy occurrences are always possible, a firm belief in them should not be the guiding rule.

Since the trial-and-error method held no appeal for me, I attempted from the very outset of my career—fifty years ago—actually to understand the whys and wherefores of the fascinating world I had entered for better or worse. This is why I feel I may now offer to share whatever experience I have acquired with my younger colleagues, many of whom still work undirected and create in a haphazard fashion, in the expectation of a potential miracle.

In perfumery, however, miracles are few and far between. From the outset, a perfumer should be able to tell whether a creation stands a chance of becoming a sales success. The technique I eventually worked out has made perfume creation surprisingly easy. Thanks to it I am never at a loss in creating new perfumes.

Although some sort of apology should be in order for the seemingly inordinate conceit of what I have just set forth, all my laboratory colleagues and all those who came to us for tuition can vouch that I have stated nothing but the truth. Also, I firmly believe that the simplicity and the ready applicability of my method will become fully apparent once I have disclosed my views on organized creative perfumery.

Perfumery at present is at a crossroads. The number of trained perfumers tends to decrease, since the long apprenticeship required appears an insuperable obstacle to most young people who cannot afford to wait long enough before earning their living. Such a situation should be remedied at all costs. While it is not to be expected that originality can be taught, nor that the potential sales appeal of a novel composition will be apparent to the young perfumer before he has gained the experience that only time will bring, it is nevertheless of prime importance that the apprentice perfumer be given help and guidance for coordinating his first attempts in the field of perfume formulation. There is no mystery in the way I work. Over the past thirty-five years more than one hundred students, both French and foreign, have taken courses in perfumery in the Company's laboratory at Grasse and have been taught according to the simple method I had devised for myself.

Thus is given [later] the result of fifty years of sometimes disappointing, but often most rewarding experiences, in the hope that my young colleagues will find therein new possibilities for future creations and will see their enthusiasm increase tenfold when their efforts are crowned with success, since without enthusiasm there can be no perfumer.

Actually, what is perfumery and how should it be understood?

Perfumery is an art, not a science, as many seem to believe. A scientific background and knowledge are not necessary and may even sometimes prove an obstacle to the freedom required in perfume creation. The creative perfumer should use odorous materials in the same way that a painter uses colors, and give them opportunity for maximum development and effect, although it is understood that potential reactions such as discolorations within the ultimate formulation and also the stability of the perfume should be given due consideration. This is about the only use he will be able to make of this scientific training, if any.

The perfumer's only tool is his nose. I was called "Mr. Nose" in the United States about twenty years ago. But any one of us is a potential "Mr. Nose," since in perfumery there just is no privileged "nose." Anyone may acquire a highly developed sense of smell, as this is merely a matter of practice. A good nose—that is, an excellent olfactory memory—is not enough to produce a good perfumer. By the term "a nose" is meant a perfumer who is able to distinguish a pure product from an adulterated product, who can tell lavender 50 per cent from lavender 40 per cent. I myself, in spite of my long experience, am only a beginner in comparison to the old "noses" whom I met at Grasse at the beginning of my career and who were able to detect olfactorily the geographical area where a given oil of neroli or of lavender came from.

Olfactory training is of prime importance and should never be neglected or interrupted. Our own perfumers make it a strict rule to test daily their knowledge of perfume materials, and this is why a half hour is set apart for this exercise which we all perform in true competitive spirit.

Let it be emphasized again that no "nose" can be said to be better than another, and that it is merely a question of olfactory memory, for which daily training is not only necessary but indispensable.

Thus the training of a beginner who knows nothing about perfumery should start with the olfactory study of all odorous materials, both natural and synthetic. In order to facilitate such a study, the beginner will first be given contrasting odors to smell, and later materials belonging to a same odor family. Following are two tables relating to olfactory studies according to such requirements. Learning to smell his smelling strips, to identify and to distinguish all odorous materials from one another, the beginner will soon notice that the odor of the products changes with time, that the rate of evaporation is not the same for all products as shown on the following table.

162

# OLFACTORY STUDY OF ESSENTIAL OILS AND ABSOLUTES

## STUDY BY CONTRASTING ODOURS

| | | 1st study | 2nd study | 3rd study | 4th study | 5th study | 6th study | 7th study | 8th study | 9th study |
|---|---|---|---|---|---|---|---|---|---|---|
| 10th study | CITRUS Notes | Lemon | Bergamot | Tangerine | Orange (Portugal) | Sweet Orange | Bitter Orange | Cedrat | Lime | Orange (Guinea) |
| 11th study | WOODY Notes | Sandalwood | Cedarwood | Vetyver Java & Bourbon | Patchouly | Oakmoss (Essence) | Oakmoss (Absolute) | Pine, Sylvestre & Maritime | Cypress | Guaiac wood |
| 12th study | SPICY Notes | Cloves Bourbon | Cinnamon China & Ceylon | Bay | Nutmeg | Pepper | Pimento | Juniper (berries) | Cascarilla | Coriander |
| 13th study | ORANGE Notes | Neroli Bigarade | Petitgrain fr. Grasse | Petitgrain fr. Paraguay | Absolute Orange Flowers | Absolute Orange Flowers (water) | Petitgrain ex Bergamot-tree | Petitgrain ex Lemon-tree | Petitgrain ex Tangerine-tree | Absolute Orange Leaves |
| 14th study | ANISE Notes | Anise | Badiane | Sweet Fennel | Bitter Fennel | Basil | Tarragon | Cumin | | Caraway |
| 15th study | ROSE Notes | Absolute Rose de Mai | | | Rose Bulgarian (Essence) | Geranium African | Geranium fr. Grasse | Geranium Bourbon | Geranium Palmarosa | |
| 16th study | RUSTIC Notes (camphor-like) | Lavender | Lavendin | Spike, Spanish & Provencal | Rosemary | Thyme | Eucalyptus | Laurel Noble | Hyssop | Myrtle Origanum Sage Spanish |
| 17th study | BALSAM & AMBER Notes | Balsam Peru (Absolute) | Balsam Tolu (Essence) | Vanilla (Resinoid & Infusion) | Tonka Beans (Absolute) | Styrax | Cistus-Labdanum | Sage Sclary | Balsam Copaiba | |
| 18th study | FLORAL Notes | Absolute Jasmine | Absolute Tuberose | Absolute Jonquil | Absolute Hyacinth | Absolute Narcissus | Absolute Violet (leaves) | Absolute Cassie | Absolute Mimosa | Absolute Orris |
| 19th study | RESIN Notes | Olibanum | Benzoin | Opoponax | Myrrh | Elemi | Galbanum | | | |
| 20th study | ANIMAL Notes | Absolute Civet | Musk Tonquin (Infusion) | Castoreum | Costus | Ambrette (seeds) | | | | |
| 21st study | CITRONELLA Notes | Citronella Java & Ceylon | Lemongrass | Verbena | Melissa | | | | | |
| 22nd study | MINT Notes | Peppermint | Spearmint | Pennyroyal | Marjoram | | | | | |
| 23rd study | MISCELLANEOUS Notes | Ylang-Ylang | Cananga Java | | Niaouli | Bois de Rose | Shiu | Wintergreen | Cajeput | |

# OLFACTORY STUDY OF CHEMICALLY DEFINED AND SYNTHETIC PRODUCTS

## STUDY BY CONTRASTING ODOURS

| | | 1st study | 2nd study | 3rd study | 4th study | 5th study | 6th study | 7th study |
|---|---|---|---|---|---|---|---|---|
| 8th study | AMBER Notes | PAM | Musk Ambrette | Hibiscolide | | | | |
| 9th study | ANISE Notes | Anisic aldehyde | Anethol | Aubepine crystals | Anisic alcohol | Anisyl formate | Anisyl acetate | |
| 10th study | ALDEHYDIC Notes | Aldehyde C.7 | Aldehyde C. 8 | Aldehyde C. 9 | Aldehyde C. 10 | Aldehyde C. 11 | Aldehyde C. 12 (lauric) | Aldehyde C. 12 (MNA) |
| 11th study | ANIMAL Notes | Indole | Skatole | | | | | |
| 12th study | BALSAM Notes | Cinnamyl acetate | Cinnamic alcohol | Ethyl cinnamate | Methyl cinnamate | Amyl salicylate | Isobutyl salicylate | |
| 13th study | WOODY Notes | Cedryl acetate | Vetyveryl acetate | Acetivenol | Cedrol | Ionone 100% | Ionone alpha | Methylionone Vetyverol |
| 14th study | CITRUS (Lemon) Notes | Citral | Citronellal | Citronellyl acetate | Citronellyl butyrate | | | |
| 15th study | SPICY Notes | Cinnamic aldehyde | Eugenol | Isoeugenol | Methyleugenol | Methylisoeugenol | | |
| 16th study | LEAFY (Green) Notes | Phenylpropyl alcohol | Phenylacetic aldehyde | Centifol acetate | Centifol | Methyl heptine carbonate | Bromostyrol | Diphenyl oxide |
| 17th study | FRESH Notes | Hydroxycitronellal | Nerol | Geraniol | | | | |
| 18th study | FLORAL Notes | Linalool | Terpineol | | | | | |
| 19th study | FRUITY Notes | Amyl acetate | Aldehyde C. 14 | Aldehyde C. 16 | Aldehyde C. 18 | Amyl benzoate | Amyl cinnamate | Amyl formate |
| 20th study | JASMINE Notes | Benzyl acetate | Amylcinnamic aldehyde | Benzyl formate | Benzyl propionate | Benzyl cinnamate | Benzyl phenylacetate | Benzyl salicylate |
| 21st study | LAVENDER Notes | Terpinyl acetate | | | | | | |
| 22nd study | HONEYED Notes | Phenylacetic acid | Ethyl phenylacetate | Linalyl phenylacetate | | | | |
| 23rd study | MINTY Notes | Menthol | Rhodeol | | | | | |
| 24th study | MUSK Notes | Musk xylol | Musk Ketone | | | | | |
| 25th study | NARCISSUS Notes | Paracresol acetate | Methylparacresol | Paracresol phenylacetate | | | | |
| 26th study | ORANGE (peel) Notes | Linalyl acetate | Methyl anthranilate | Argeol | Linalyl benzoate | Dimethylanthranilate | Nerolin crystals | Yara-Yara |
| 27th study | ROSE Notes | Geranyl acetate | Rhodinyl acetate | Citronellol | Geraniol | Geraniol P | Rhodinol | Rhodol |
| 28th study | ROSE (petals) Notes | Phenylethyl alcohol | Phenylethyl acetate | Phenylethyl phenylacetate | | Palmarol | | |
| 29th study | ROSE (fruity) Notes | Rhodinyl formate | Geranyl formate | Rhodinyl propionate | Rhodinyl phenylacetate | Geranyl benzoate | Rhodinyl benzoate | Geranyl butyrate |
| 30th study | VANILLA Notes | Vanillin | Vanillal | Heliotropine | Coumarin | | | |

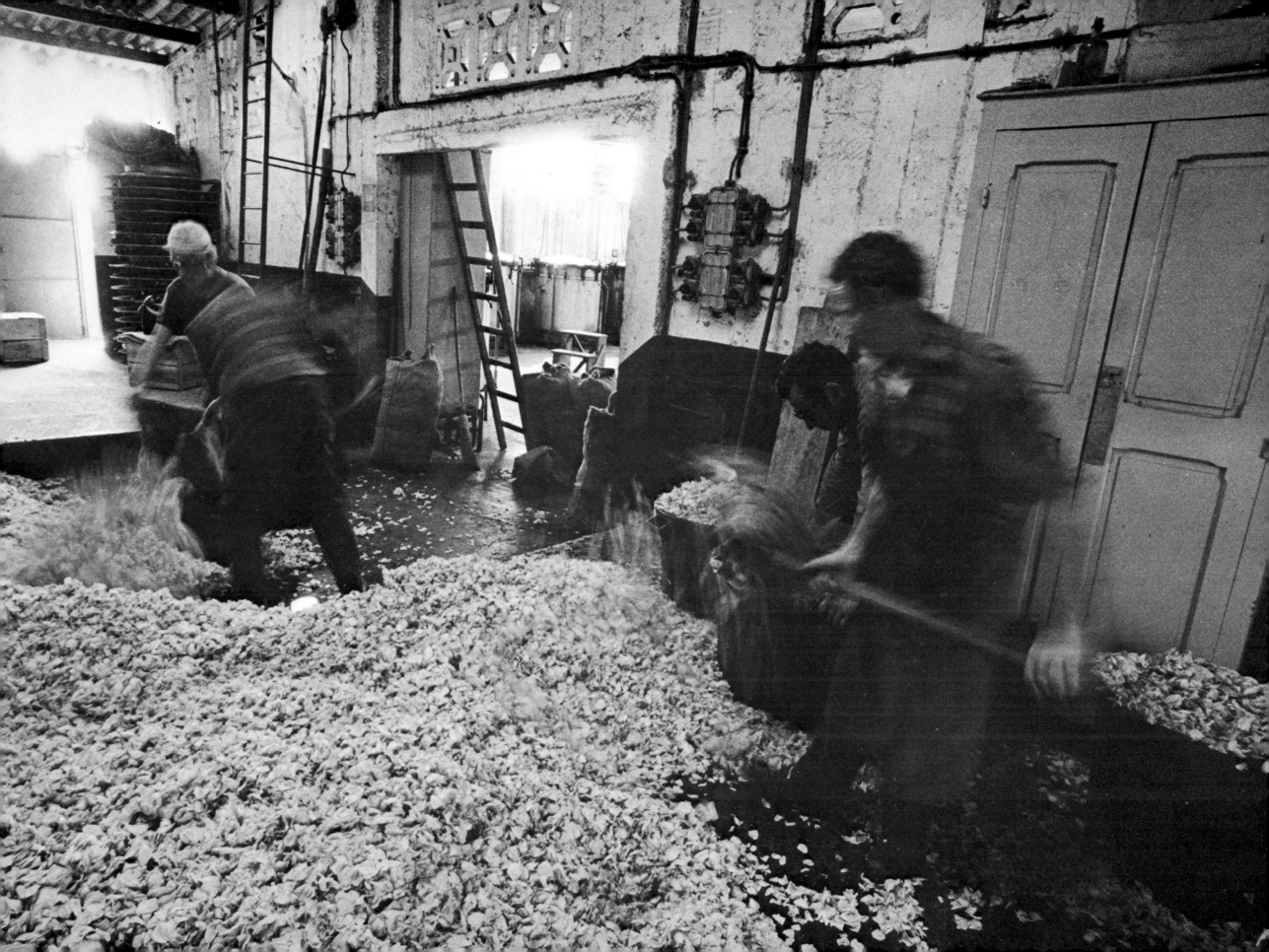

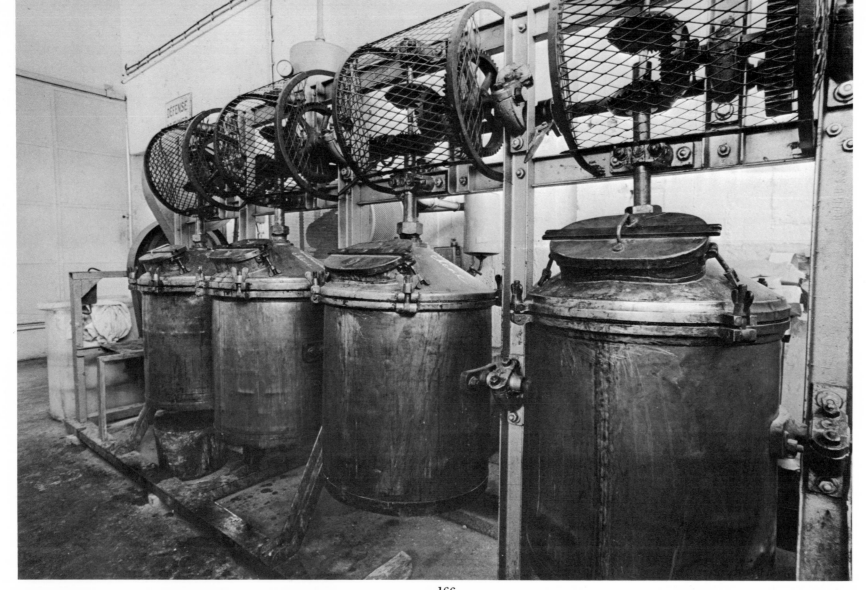

Therefore, the next step will be for him to establish *a classification of odorous materials according to their volatility.*

While such a classification could be established scientifically, the apprentice perfumer will soon attain unexpected proficiency by forgetting any technical information he may have, and by establishing "his" classification for himself, as I had to forty years ago.

On the smelling strip will first be inscribed the date and time at which a drop of the odorous material was deposited thereon, and later the date and time at which the product on the strip will begin to lose its main characteristic, its typical odor. When proceeding thus, no consideration should be taken of the ultimate off-odors, such as terpenic notes or the like. This technique will soon make it apparent for the student that while some products are very volatile and lacking in tenacity, others are of intermediate volatility and tenacity and others still are of low volatility and high tenacity.

Such data will then readily be set forth in tabular form, all available odorous materials being listed under three headings, as follows:

| Very volatile products lacking tenacity | Products of intermediate volatility and tenacity | Products of low volatility and high tenacity |
|---|---|---|
| *Top notes* | *Modifiers of base notes* | *Base notes* |
| Amyl acetate | Basil | Methylionone — Ionones |
| Bois de Rose | Terpineol | Absolute Orange Flower |
| Linalool | Petitgrain from Paraguay | Sage Sclary |
| Phenylethyl acetate | Galbanum | Amyl salicylate |
| Lemon | Verbena | Absolute Jasmine |
| Lavender | Thyme | Benzyl salicylate |
| Bergamot | Geranyl acetate | Cedarwood |
| Orange | Juniper | Aldehyde C.16 |
| Coriander | Tansy | Aldehyde C.18 |
| Tarragon | Phenylethyl alcohol | Sandalwood |
| Laurel noble | Geraniol | Artificial musks |
| Petitgrain from Lemontree | Absolute Lavender | Absolute Oakmoss |
| etc., etc. | Citronellal | Vetyver and derivatives |
| | Neroli | Patchouly |
| | Rose, Bulgarian | Celery |
| | Ylang | etc., etc. |
| | Geraninum | |
| | Aldehydes C.8 C.9 C.11 C.12 | |
| | Cloves | |
| | etc., etc. | |

The student will then have to be taught how to use this table. As set forth above, I have termed:

—very volatile products lacking tenacity . . . . *Top Notes*
—products of intermediate volatility and tenacity . *Modifiers*
—products of low volatility and high tenacity . . *Base Notes*

The reasons for this choice of terms are the following:

As indicated by their name, the *base notes* will serve to determine the chief characteristic of the perfume, the scent of which will last hours on end and will be essentially responsible for the success of the perfume, if any.

Anyone even remotely familiar with perfume materials is aware that all products of low volatility and high tenacity such as vetyver, oakmoss, patchouli, the methylionones and the like give off a rather unpleasant smell when freshly deposited on a smelling strip, but, on the other hand, that the scent given off during the subsequent stages of evaporation is excellent. This is the reason for the use of the *modifiers* of intermediate volatility and tenacity that will serve to change the unpleasant top note of the base products. Finally, the very volatile *top notes,* lacking tenacity, will serve to impart to the perfume composition a very pleasant odor on opening the bottle.

At the time of their first olfactory studies, therefore, the students should establish individually, for future personal reference, a table giving a classification of the rate of evaporation of all the materials they will eventually come to use. This will prevent them from using a modifier in place of a base note, or a top note instead of a modifier, or conversely. *No perfumer can afford not to be thoroughly familiar with this classification which is the sole available means for rationally creating perfumes.*

Too many perfumers still proceed by trial and error, in the hope that chance will lend a helping hand. A good perfumer should actually "smell" his perfume prior to the actual blending of the formulation, and start out by writing down in itemized form his complete selection of components.

My method reduces almost to nil the difficulties of perfume creation. Aware of the various stages of the odor development of perfumes, our students establish their formulations according to the rate of volatility of the products used; such formulations are therefore readily legible and easy to understand. They are, in a way, *olfactorily legible.* Always starting out with the top notes, they list, in logical succession, the modifiers and finally the base notes which will impart the chief characteristic of the perfume. Any of my formulas are written down according to this method which makes it possible to *pass a first judgment on a formula merely by reading it.*

Thus actual blending and scenting of a perfume formulation is not necessary at this stage; a careful appraisal of the written formula makes possible an effective readjustment which will unfailingly improve both its scenting power and its quality. Last but not least, the reasons for the adjustments can readily be explained to the students and understood by them. All those who were trained by us or who spent some time in our laboratory are familiar with this method and have successfully applied it since to their own students.

*For illustrative purposes, let us take as an example the creation of a Chypre note.*

I. *The "accord" between bases.* Absolute Oakmoss is the basic raw material for the Chypre note. It belongs to the series of products of low volatility and high tenacity, or base notes. Others of the more common materials belonging to this series are products such as the Ionones and Methylionones, Vetyver, Patchouli, Acetivenol, Cistus labdanum SIS, Althenol, Selvone, Ambergris 162 B, and the like. Therefore, we must choose among them the products which will blend with Absolute Oakmoss and impart an original characteristic to our perfume. We shall begin our study of this "accord" in the following manner:

We shall select a second product belonging to the series of base notes, whichever will seem most appropriate for blending with Absolute Oakmoss. In the present case, we shall use, for example, Absolute Cistus colorless or a similar product such as Ambergris 162 B, and we shall prepare a series of accords containing both constituents in the following ratios:

| Absolute Oakmoss | 9 8 7 6 5 |
|---|---|
| Ambergris 162 B | 1 2 3 4 5 |

We shall not test combinations beyond the 5:5 ratio, since the following ratios of materials:

| Absolute Oakmoss | 4 3 2 1 |
|---|---|
| Ambergris 162 B | 6 7 8 9 |

would no longer produce an accord based on Oakmoss, but an accord based on Ambergris. We shall then choose between the five accords based on Oakmoss and, for example, shall decide on the following:

6 Absolute Oakmoss
4 Ambergris 162 B

Since any Chypre note should also have a musklike character, we shall add a certain amount of Musk ketone or of Musk ambrette to the above accord. Thus, the base of the desired Chypre note will be as follows:

6 Absolute Oakmoss
4 Ambergris 162 B
1 Musk ketone

When smelling this blend on a smelling strip, we shall notice that its immediate effect is rather unpleasant, although this will fairly rapidly disappear and be replaced by a pleasant long-lasting note essentially characteristic of the personality of the ultimate perfume.

II. *The Modifiers.* How can we subdue or, rather, adjust this unpleasant note? We shall immediately find a solution to the problem by studying the table giving the classification of odorous materials according to volatility. Among the products of intermediate volatility and tenacity, we shall find which product, or products, will be best suited for blending with our accord between bases.

We shall choose a floral note, a Rose note, for example (Absolute Rose or Rose d'Orient 2644 JD). This Rose note will subdue the immediate effect of our accord between bases and make it more pleasant. It will play its part as a modifier of base notes, and this is the reason we have termed the products of intermediate volatility and tenacity "modifiers" (of base notes). To the Rose note we shall add a trace of Absolute Civet, so as to impart a slight animal note to the Chypre note. At this stage, the formula is as follows:

| *Modifiers* | 3 *Absolute Rose* or *Rose d'Orient* 2644 |
|---|---|
| | 1 *Absolute Civet, 10 per cent sol.* |

| *Bases* | 6 *Absolute Oakmoss* |
|---|---|
| | 4 *Ambergris* 162 B |
| | 1 *Musk ketone* |

III. *The top note.* Our formula, however, is not yet complete. We must add to it a top note, which will produce the immediate effect one smells on opening the bottle. This note is fairly important, since the potential buyer is easily influenced by it—with or without reason, as in no case can the top note be the characteristic note of the perfume.

This study is far easier than the study of the accord between bases, since the series of very volatile products lacking tenacity contains many odorous products, most of which possess very pleasant notes. The study of the accord between top notes can be carried out as set forth above for base notes, but with much more freedom and fantasy. Combinations, in this case, are countless and may be left entirely to the perfumer's initiative.

As with base notes, we may study several accords between two or three notes, or even four. Let us, for example, after testing various combinations, decide upon the use of Sweet Orange and Bergamot in the following amounts:

4 Sweet orange
1 Bergamot

Thus, the extremely simple formulation of our Chypre note may be written down as follows:

| Top Notes 25 per cent | 4 Sweet Orange 1 Bergamot |
|---|---|
| Modifiers 20 per cent | 3 Absolute Rose or Rose d'Orient 2644 1 Absolute Civet, 10 per cent sol. |
| Bases 55 per cent | 6 Absolute Oakmoss 4 Ambergris 162 B 1 Musk ketone |

It is understood that the above is not a complete formula, but that it is merely given for the purpose of illustrating the method set forth in this paper.

IV. *Proportions. Percentages of the three groups of products: bases, modifiers, and top notes.* This percentage is extremely important: it is, for the major part, responsible for the tenacity of the perfume. A perfume containing 20 per cent of bases, 30 per cent of modifiers, and 50 per cent of top notes would lack tenacity, since the percentage of bases would be relatively too low as compared to that of the more volatile modifiers and top notes. Therefore, the proportions are selected so as to obtain a balanced evolution during evaporation.

V. *Extension of the above formulation.* We shall now examine how this Chypre note formula could be completed or modified. Let us first consider the base notes. We have already realized the accord:

*Absolute Oakmoss*
*Ambergris 162 B*
*Musk ketone*

We might, for example, add to it Vetyver Bourbon, or Java, which will result in the following accord:

*Absolute Oakmoss*
*Ambergris 162 B*
*Vetyver Bourbon*
*Musk ketone*

and we shall endeavor to find the proper ratios of ingredients, as follows:

| | A | B | C | D |
|---|---|---|---|---|
| Absolute Oakmoss | 4 | 6 | 3 | 3 |
| Ambergris 162 B | 4 | 3 | 6 | 3 |
| Vetyver Bourbon | 4 | 3 | 3 | 6 |
| Musk ketone | 1 | 1 | 1 | 1 |

Thus, when studying the above accord, the main characteristic will be imparted by Oakmoss in experiment B, by Ambergris in experiment C and by Vetyver in experiment D.

The student perfumer will also be able to choose between the following accords:

| | | |
|---|---|---|
| *Absolute Oakmoss* | *Absolute Oakmoss* | *Absolute Oakmoss* |
| *Ambergris 162 B* | *Ambergris 162 B* | *Patchouli* |
| *Patchouli* | *Methylionone* | *Vetyver* |

*Absolute Oakmoss*
*Methylionone*
*Vetyver*
etc.,

according to his preferences with respect to the main odorous characteristic of the base of the Chypre note he wishes to create. Obviously, these accords could be increased to contain four, five, or six notes; for example:

| *Absolute Oakmoss* | *Absolute Oakmoss* | *Absolute Oakmoss* |
|---|---|---|
| *Ambergris 162 B* | *Methylionone* | *Ambergris 162 B* |
| *Patchouli* | *Vetyver* | *Vetyver* |
| *Vetyver* | *Patchouli* | *Patchouli* |
|  | *Ambergris 162 B* | *Aldehyde C. 14* |
| *Musk ketone* |  | *Absolute Jasmine* |
|  | *Musk ketone* |  |
|  |  | *Musk ketone* |

It is therefore apparent that this method offers endless possibilities for creating new notes and new perfumes, the perfumer being entirely free to use any odorous material in these accords, provided, however, that such materials are selected from the series of base notes; such complete freedom in the choice of the starting odorous materials may also be given to the beginner. Whatever the type of formulation, once we feel the accord between bases is complete and fully satisfactory, we shall have to reconsider our first selection of modifiers. In our first tentative Chypre note formula, we might, in place of the Rose note, use an Orange note, a Jasmine note, or any other floral note such as Lily of the Valley or Carnation. Again, top notes should also be similarly adjusted.

For the purpose of illustrating the procedure used for such adjustments, see the following series of modifications:

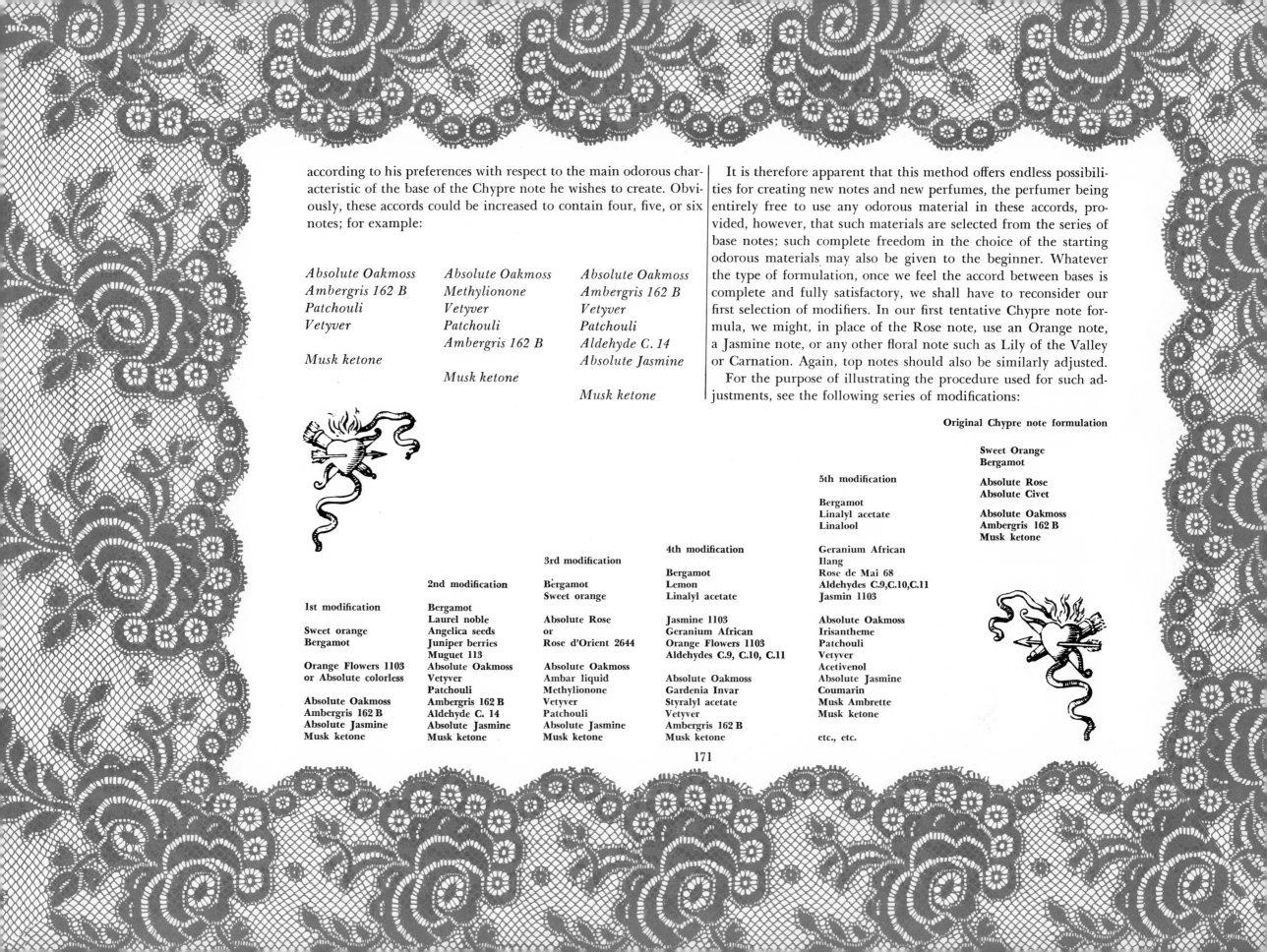

**Original Chypre note formulation**

Sweet Orange
Bergamot

Absolute Rose
Absolute Civet

Absolute Oakmoss
Ambergris 162 B
Musk ketone

**5th modification**

Bergamot
Linalyl acetate
Linalool

Geranium African
Ilang
Rose de Mai 68
Aldehydes C.9,C.10,C.11
Jasmin 1103

Absolute Oakmoss
Irisantheme
Patchouli
Vetyver
Acetivenol
Absolute Jasmine
Coumarin
Musk Ambrette
Musk ketone

etc., etc.

**4th modification**

Bergamot
Lemon
Linalyl acetate

Jasmine 1103
Geranium African
Orange Flowers 1103
Aldehydes C.9, C.10, C.11

Absolute Oakmoss
Gardenia Invar
Styralyl acetate
Vetyver
Ambergris 162 B
Musk ketone

**3rd modification**

Bergamot
Sweet orange

Absolute Rose
or
Rose d'Orient 2644

Absolute Oakmoss
Ambar liquid
Methylionone
Vetyver
Patchouli
Absolute Jasmine
Musk ketone

**2nd modification**

Bergamot
Laurel noble
Angelica seeds
Juniper berries
Muguet 113
Absolute Oakmoss
Vetyver
Patchouli
Ambergris 162 B
Aldehyde C. 14
Absolute Jasmine
Musk ketone

**1st modification**

Sweet orange
Bergamot

Orange Flowers 1103
or Absolute colorless

Absolute Oakmoss
Ambergris 162 B
Absolute Jasmine
Musk ketone

171

Thus modifications of the original formulation may be carried out endlessly; although the resultant blend is always within the scope of Chypre notes, an entirely different perfume is obtained each time. However, this result can be achieved only provided the original formula is written down as suggested above in the following order:

*Top notes*
*Modifiers*
*Base notes*

The specific example given above of the successive steps of perfume formulation shows how any particular type of perfume may be endlessly varied. But the method applies just as well when the perfumer wishes to obtain novel perfumes from a basic formula established to contain accords of which he is especially fond.

In this respect, I shall describe an experiment with which our former students are well familiar and which might be called "a brief lesson in perfumery." I first write down with a black pencil a very simple formula containing, let us say, about eight products and which results in a very acceptable perfume. To this formula, I then add new products, the names of which I write down with a red pencil: thus a second perfume is produced *while the proportions and the constituents of the first formulation remain unchanged.* Pursuing this amusing experiment, I add a new series of products to the second formula just obtained, writing down their names with a blue pencil; it is understood that these new products contain top notes, modifiers, and base notes. Again, without effecting any change in the products making up the first two formulations, a third perfume is produced which is also entirely different from the others . . . and the experiment might go on, endlessly, by mere addition of products.

At this point I feel the subject of accessory products should be mentioned. What are "accessory products"? As far as I am concerned, to this series belong products which, owing to their typical odor or to their high scenting power, cannot be used in large amounts in an accord between bases or between modifiers, but whose more or less trace presence in a formulation results in a complete change in the character of the latter and imparts to it a unique cachet. Examples of such products are aldehydes C.12 MNA and C.14, styralyl acetate, isobutylquinoline, galbanum, cascarilla. However, although I have just recommended the use of such products with moderation, this is not to be taken as a standing rule. Aldehyde C.12 MNA, for example, proves to be an exception, and it should be known that some products such as Geranium give most successful blends with as much as 50 per cent of it. The advantages that may be derived from the use of accessory products are therefore readily apparent.

But such considerations bring me quite naturally to mention an error that is quite common in young perfumers. Our eager would-be perfumers seem to feel that they are under the obligation to produce "well-rounded" perfumes—in other words, that they should subdue or hide any predominating odorous material. I believe this is actually the worst mistake a perfumer could be guilty of, since this desire for attaining maximum equilibrium in a perfume results in a subdued characterless ultimate composition.

One should never believe, before actual experimenting, that a formulation contains an excess of a given product. Such "excess" may quite possibly be due to the lack of some other product. Dominantly effective notes in perfumes should be neither feared nor deliberately avoided. They are a perfumer's own secret, and such "faults" have quite often been responsible for a tremendous commercial success. As a matter of fact, when a perfumer feels the amount of a basic product should be increased in a formulation, he should increase this original amount twofold, threefold, and even tenfold. This will afford him the almost unhoped-for opportunity of hitting on an outstanding accord. This amount can always be reduced at a later stage, but the perfumer will know at once what results can be expected from the use of an excess of Absolute Oakmoss, of Vetyver, of Methylionone, and the like in the ultimate formulation, an excess whch, sometimes, will pay.

At present, to meet with success, perfumes should actually explode all over, so to speak. Modern perfumery requires contrasts, sharply characterized olfactory values. The perfumer should be totally unprejudiced, should entirely disregard his own taste. Woe to him if he hates Vetyver, if he cannot stand Aldehydes! He should be aware that *there are no incompatibilities in perfumery,* that apparently clashing materials will blend successfully on addition of another product playing the part of a binding agent making their odors compatible. The creative perfumer should, above all else, consider the clientele's tastes. The commercial success of a new perfume, of a novel accord, is essentially dependent on his brain waves.

I have often been asked the question: "What is the latest fashion in perfumery?" There is no fashion in perfumery. Only actual sales success dictate the fashion. A good perfumer is a perfumer who knows how to create a best seller.

Great perfumers, like great concert pianists, should make it a strict rule to practice scales—in other words, to study possible accords between bases, since only therefrom can they derive the necessary technique conductive to virtuosity. While this is an overwhelming, all-embracing task, an effort should be made to reduce it to less gigantic, more readily accessible proportions. It is not necessary, when studying accords based on Chypre notes, for example, to consider the combinations of Absolute Oakmoss with all existing odorous products. The perfumer will first select the odorous raw materials he will see fit to use in his creation of a Chypre note, and it is only from such materials that he will study the satisfactory accords between bases.

The very selection a perfumer makes of the raw materials to be used as ingredients in a new formulation is the best of all possible standards for appraising his originality, his initiative, and his genius, on which the success of a new perfume is entirely dependent. And while it is possible to devise a method that will enable the apprentice perfumer to understand and to acquire some sort of technique, in perfumery as in many other fields many will be called but few will be chosen, since the essential qualities that lead to success cannot be taught, any more than can be taught enthusiasm, the joy of living and of creating, and the love for one's calling. These are innate qualities without which there is no great perfumer.

I think there is not much more I can say about the method I devised for my work, and it is up to young perfumers to take over where we left off. If willing, on the basis of the method I have set forth, they may *study accords with products other than Absolute Oakmoss,* that is accords with Vetyver, Patchouli, Sandalwood, Methylionone, and so on. Unless they find the work deadly dull from the start, they will enjoy many months of systematic research from which they will draw many useful lessons. My own experiments with Absolute Oakmoss have already passed the one thousand mark, and at least as many, if not more, remain to be carried out, since such investigations are endless. To facilitate their work, I recommend proceeding as follows: Let us assume the study of all possible accords with the natural products listed under the base notes heading of the table relating to a classification of products with respect to the evaporation rate is complete. The accords with synthetic or defined products can then be studied.

It will be advantageous to work systematically, taking into consideration, where accords are concerned, various suitable combinations of the great variety of constituents offered to the perfumer's choice. In these various accords the proportions between products will vary according to our young perfumer's inspiration and originality, so that an accord already set forth, e.g.,

6 *Absolute Oakmoss*
3 *Ambergris 162 B*

173

3 *Vetyver Bourbon*
1 *Musk ketone*

might very well become

5 or 4 *Absolute Oakmoss*
3 or 2 *Ambergris 162 B*
4 or 6 *Vetyver Bourbon*
1    1 *Musk ketone*


The same is true where selection of the products is concerned. When so desiring, the perfumer may vary his choice somewhat less systematically and use whatever materials appeal to his taste. Free scope is given him in this respect, and there is no absolute rule to be followed in the search for accords, since any modifications *deemed useful* will serve to produce very characteristic novel notes.

The olfactory evaluations of such working formulations will be effected desirably *on evaporation* because their starting notes might appear somewhat surprising due to the lack of modifier products. The bottles containing these accords will be filed in boxes, and their labels will show the number corresponding to the formula. After completion and adequate selection of the accords, the student perfumer will advantageously practice olfactory evaluation of their constituents. This will prove the best possible olfactory training and will provide a constant checking means of the student's familiarity with perfumery raw materials. Thus any research work undertaken will be greatly facilitated. As already stated, miracles in perfumery are few and far between, and the perfumer will never be able to identify the accord

*Absolute Oakmoss*
*Methylionone*
*Vetyver*
*Musk Ambrette*

unless thoroughly trained to do so. Considerable and very rapid improvement of the student's know-how will follow, resulting in a wonderful aptitude for identifying the constituents of perfumes he will wish to study.

Although fully aware of the difficult monotonous work involved, I feel the long years devoted to it are *absolutely necessary*. In no other way can a creative perfumer expect to attain proficiency. Could a musician write a symphony without ever having practiced solfeggio, scales, harmony? It should be emphasized, time and time again, that olfactory studies alone will open the way to true mastery and, hence, to success. Should freakish chance play into your hand and make a sales success of some early attempt, do not believe, by any means, that you have become a master of your art. Emphatically not. Rest satisfied only when the day comes when you can boast of a number of successful creations to your credit *and feel assured that many more will follow.*

All my colleagues have noted the self-complacency of some very green perfumers who have not yet created anything worthwhile, and never will, because they do not work. They take laboratory life easily, smelling strip close to the nose all day long, feeling entirely open to some miraculous, perpetually elusive inspiration. Others are entirely lacking in imagination and never even try to create something of their own, bearing no resemblance whatever to perfumes already on the market; they restrict their efforts to the imitation of successful perfumes, with some not always happy modifications! They apparently delude themselves into the belief they have created something bearing the mark of their personality.

What a pity that the time of truly original creations—where great craftsmen relentlessly pursued their search for novel notes—may seem a thing of the past. This deplorable state of affairs cannot be said to be specific to perfumery, since similar erring ways seem to have become the rule in music, where rank imitations are even more frequent. Young composers appear to seek inspiration from successful tunes, distorting them to suit their purpose, modifying their rhythm, and seem convinced that their amateur music will become as great a commercial success as the original. The same is true at present in our industry. It is in this respect that, in my opinion, there is actually no particular fashion in perfumery; it is a fact that *the perfumes with sales appeal derive for the major part from perfumes dating back thirty years or more* and still foremost in the best-seller list. It could very easily be demonstrated that many of the more recently successful perfumes fall into this category. Obviously, young perfumers with a good "nose" find it much easier to seek inspiration from some acknowledged good perfume than to devote themselves to a search for novel original notes.

Let our future perfumers meditate upon the subject and discover the zest of true creative effort. Means for such achievements have been made available to them. Let them persevere in their task, in spite of disappointing results, even if such efforts may seem unrewarding at first. Perfume-creating is far from easy. But what pride once they have created a perfume they can call entirely their own! Only then will they understand that it is *better to be imitated than to imitate*. There lies the sign of success.

The task of our young perfumers should be facilitated. Therefore, I advise them once again to establish for each floral or fancy note a table corresponding to said note and giving in tabular form the top notes, modifiers, and base notes compatible with the perfume they wish to create. Such tables are valuable memoranda.

Having undertaken a study of Chypre notes, I shall give below, as an example, a table relating to such notes; although incomplete, it is illustrative of the method and can be used by students as a starting basis for a similar table of their own, established according to their personal tastes, since I have limited my own choice to substantially conventional materials.

Quite obviously, such accords are endless. But many can be eliminated and the student's choice limited to those he considers really worthwhile.

How should the actual smelling test be carried out? Although

## CHYPRE

| TOP NOTES | MODIFIERS | BASE NOTES |
|---|---|---|
| Sweet orange | Absolute Rose | Absolute Oakmoss |
| Bergamot | Bulgarian Rose | Patchouly |
| Linalyl acetate | Geraniums | Vetyver and derivatives |
| Geranyl acetate | Nerolis, Petitgrains | Acetivenol |
| Rhodol acetate | Absolute Civet, 10 % sol. | Sandalwood |
| Geraniol | Absolute Orange Flowers | Absolute Cistus colorless |
| Linalool | Rhodol | Ambergris 162 B |
| Lemon | Rhodinol | Ambar Liquid JD |
| Bois de Rose | Phenylethyl alcohol | Methyleugenol |
| Etc. | Phenylethyl acetate | Olibanum |
| | Pine, maritime, sylvester | Ionones, Methylionones |
| | Cinnamic alcohol | Orris concrete |
| | Styrax | Sage sclary |
| | Absolute Styrax colorless | Opoponax |
| | Argeol | Absolute Jasmine |
| | Coriander | Absolute Ambrette |
| | Ylangs | Ambrette oil |
| | Cinnamon, China | Musks |
| | Cinnamon, Ceylon | Etc. |
| | Muguet 113 or Invar | |
| | Jasmine 1103 | |
| | Orange Flowers 1103 | |
| | Œillet 25 | |
| | Cloves, Eugenol, Isoeugenol | |
| | Etc. | |

| ACCESSORY PRODUCTS | BASES OR SPECIALITIES |
|---|---|
| Caraway | Althenol, Selvone or Corona |
| Galbanum | Bouvardia 198 |
| Costus | Corional |
| Juniper berries | Cuir de Russie 18-167 |
| Laurel noble | Daltonia 1096 |
| Angelica seeds | Tobacco Flower |
| Hyssop | Myrisia |
| Aldehydes C 9, C 10, C 11, C 12, C 14 | Mousse 32, Mousse 1026 |
| | Mousse Sylvestre |
| | Mousse de Chypre |
| | Mousse poivrée |
| Celery | Mousse JD Base |
| Etc. | Mousse R |
| | Pimenal 44 |
| | Etc. |

such a question may seem quite bizarre, it is nevertheless most important. Above all, *do not use a smelling strip*. Why? Because, when smelling a perfume or some accord from a smelling strip, one does not in the least obtain even an approximation of the *true scent* of the perfume.

The following anecdote will explain why I abandoned the use of the smelling strip for appraising new perfumes. I happened to be visiting Lisbon, some thirty years ago, and was lunching with our agent and his wife. I felt intrigued by the excellent scent of her perfume and finally asked for its name, since I had no recollection of it. She laughed and answered that this was a sample of one of my latest creations I had given her husband during my last visit. Paradoxically, I had not recognized my own perfume, being unfamiliar with its true full scent since I had always appraised it from a smelling strip. This served to convince me that the smelling strip can in no way be used for effecting an over-all evaluation of a perfume's true full scent. I became quite concerned with the problem and, when back in Grasse, inquired about the sales of the product I had just discovered . . . and found out that sales orders represented substantial amounts. From this time on, I gave up using smelling strips for the evaluation of my own creations and used *vaporization*.

How should one vaporize a perfume undergoing olfactory evaluation? Many suitable devices are available, but I obtained the best results with a very simple cheap spraying device of the type commonly used by artists for spraying a very thin coating of clear varnish on charcoal or sanguine drawings. Thus, the perfume is vaporized for between five and seven seconds, in the center of a room, care being taken not to direct the perfume cloud onto the walls. The room is then closed, and the experimenter returns to it after two or three minutes and can then effect olfactory evaluation of the resulting scented atmosphere. *The immediate and precise sensation produced by the character of the perfume and especially by its fully developed scent*, as it will be released under

actual use conditions, is thus obtained; this achievement would not have been possible with a smelling strip. In addition to this significant advantage, the perfumer will gain precious time with such tests, in contrast to the long hours necessary for full development of the perfume on the smelling strip before a perfumer can properly appraise the main character of his new creation. Such vaporization produces the true, fully developed scent, without any possible error, and permits immediate rearrangement of working formulas. A large number of olfactory evaluations are thus made possible, in contrast to the slow results obtained with the smelling strip. I have found this procedure fully satisfactory for almost thirty-five years.

*On the other hand, it goes without saying that the smelling strip is indispensable and irreplaceable for the olfactory evaluation of perfumery raw materials.*

This means of carrying out olfactory evaluations also has another advantage: I found out that certain perfumes offered to a potential buyer were sometimes rejected when smelled from a smelling strip, whereas vaporization of the same perfumes resulted in a sale. I wish to insist that student perfumers carry out this experiment when evaluating their creations. Surprising results will probably ensue, and many will be disappointed by perfumes they had rated good when using a smelling strip and which appear rather indifferent on vaporization, but the contrary will also occur.

It should always be kept in mind that it is the true, fully developed scent of a perfume that is responsible for its sales appeal and that is the best of all advertising for your creations. It is because of it that a woman purchases a perfume. As a matter of fact, *perfumes are not selected but are adopted by women*. Various reasons can be found for this attitude. One of the chief reasons a woman buys a specific perfume is that it is "all the rage," being the latest creation of a fashionable couturier, and thus she will be able to answer any inquiry with "It is X's new perfume!" But should no one react to her new perfume, should it be disregarded by her husband, her friends, or her hairdresser, she will promptly discard it for good. If in contrast, from the day of the purchase, all compliment her on her good taste and ask for the name of the perfume, she will feel flattered and will make it hers. Women will also adopt a perfume they have smelled on a friend, having been able to appreciate its scented trail, or a perfume that has long been held in high repute.

I have seen women refuse a high-grade perfume offered to them by the salesgirl at the perfume counter of a department store, and return to purchase the same perfume a few minutes later. What are the reasons for such sudden change of opinion?

1. They may have evaluated the perfume on opening the perfume bottle. This was a gross error, since they could smell only the very volatile top notes which in no way permitted one to detect the principal character of the perfume; the women remained ignorant of its fully developed scent.

2. They may have evaluated the perfume by putting a drop on their ungloved hand, just as they would have tested a cream or a lipstick, omitting to take into account the odor due to their skin or that imparted by the glove. This too rapid evaluation, carried out under poor conditions, has not made possible the perception of the scent characteristic of the perfume.

3. They have smelled the perfume on some friend, and this has settled their choice, having appreciated its true character. Such cases are frequent. As a matter of fact, I have often remarked how incapable a woman was to pass judgment on a perfume. Early in my career, I used to make the great mistake of giving samples of my newly created perfumes to women chosen among the more fashionable and clever of my friends and then requesting their advice on the olfactory value of my gift. As a result, I often had to listen to utterly senseless criticism. Faced by such incompetence, I decided to stop asking for advice on the value of my creations. I merely offered a bottle of my new perfume and quietly waited for any reactions that might come unsolicited. If after a few days noth-

ing came of it, I decided my perfume was a frost and merely wrote it off. But if, on the contrary, as soon as the perfume was tried, I was told, "My dear, this perfume is wonderful, sensational—they are all asking for its name," then I felt sure my perfume was good and could become a success. And ninety-nine times out of a hundred it was a success. *Vox populi*. This is the reason I am entirely opposed to panel tests which are so extensively used in the United States when a perfume is to be evaluated. The panel test, just like the smelling strip, should be used only for the evaluation of raw materials.

My conclusion is this: never ask a woman for her opinion of the perfume you have just created. She will feel embarrassed and you will leave yourself open to great disappointment. In the early stages of my career I was full of great illusions and firmly believed all my wishes would come true. Far too often was I sure of having created wonders which, in fact, were nothing to speak of. The only sure guide is vaporization, which will provide true information on the olfactory value of perfumes.

We have shown how beginners in the art of perfumery could undertake their apprenticeship in a most simple and lively manner that makes it possible for them to formulate well-balanced basic accords at an early stage in their studies, and to trim such accords with materials selected according to their own taste and imagination.

It is quite apparent that here, again, all conceivable combinations are possible, or almost possible, since in perfumery, as in many other fields, everything is a matter of discrimination, of selection, and, essentially, of proportions. Since the study of top notes and of modifiers has led us to define more accurately the conditions under which floral notes and fast-evaporating essential oils or chemicals should be used, we shall consider the broader aspects of the formulation of colognes which are more commonly and more readily used and possess the not-to-be-ignored advantage of being less expensive.

# COLOGNES

Colognes are predominantly toilet goods that should have an odor lacking in tenacity, either because the odor should be just sufficient to add to the over-all pleasant feeling of cleanliness, or because it should not detrimentally affect one's regular perfume. It is understood that modifiers and base notes may be added to Cologne formulations, for the purpose of imparting more lasting properties to such compositions, but such materials should always be used with moderation in Colognes.

The main constituents used in the formulation of Colognes are set forth below in tabular form, the table being given only for

## RAW MATERIALS FOR COLOGNE FORMULATIONS

| Top notes | Modifiers | Base notes |
|---|---|---|
| Bois de rose | Basil | Sage sclary |
| Linalool | Petitgrain, ex Bergamot-tree | Ionones |
| Tangerine | *Petitgrain, fr. Paraguay* | Methylionones |
| Bitter Orange | *Petitgrain ex Lemon-tree* | Orris concrete |
| Citron | Petitgrain ex Tangerine-tree | Sandalwood |
| *Lemon* | *Verbena* | Cinnamon, fr. China and Ceylon |
| *Lavenders* | *Petitgrain bigarade* | Nerolin crystals |
| *Bergamot* | Tansy | Yara-Yara |
| Lavandin | *Petitgrain fr. Grasse* | Benzyl salicylate |
| Coriander | *Géraniums, African and Bourbon* | Resinoid No. 1 Benzoin |
| *Sweet Orange* | Hyssop | Resinoid No. 1 Balsam Tolu |
| Sweet Fennel | Lemongrass | Resinoid No. 1 Balsam Peru |
| Bitter Fennel | Cloves Bourbon | Bromstyrol |
| Citral | Pine | Methylnaphthylketone |
| Tarragon | Wild thyme | *Artificial musks* |
| Lime | *Neroli bigarade petals* | Coumarin |
| Marjoram | Isoeugenol | Vanillin |
| Linalyl acetate | Methyl cinnamate | Absolute Tonka Beans |
| Terpinyl acetate | Ylang-Ylang | Vetyveryl acetate |
|  | Ethyl cinnamate | Vetyver, fr. Java and Bourbon |
| etc., etc. | Methylisoeugenol | Acetivenol |
|  | Methyleugenol | Absolute colourless Cistus Labdanum |
|  | *Rosemary* | Olibanum |
|  | Phixia (Hydroxycitronellal) | Opoponax |
|  | Aldehydes C9, C10, C11, C12, | Argeol |
|  | Methylnonylacetaldehyde | Indolene |
|  | Bay | Hibiscolide |
|  | Thyme | Lactone MC 15 |
|  | Absolute Orange Flowers |  |
|  | Phenylethyl alcohol | etc., etc. |
|  | Geranyl acetate |  |
|  | Geraniol |  |
|  | Citronellol |  |
|  | Citronellal |  |
|  | Cinnamyl acetate |  |
|  | etc., etc. |  |

illustrative purposes and as an indication of the work that can be undertaken by any student in perfumery.

In spite of the pleasant note of most constituents, it is difficult to create a "good" Cologne, that is, a Cologne that will have sales appeal. Again—I beg to be forgiven but cannot help repeating myself!—the personal touch of the perfumer-creator will be determining. A perfumer's technical know-how and olfactory memory will serve to produce a well-balanced formulation. But the perfumer's fancy, his sense of humor sometimes, his desire to promote some flash of interest and amusement, and his deep-rooted love for his art will lead him more safely than any so-called recipe to hit unerringly on an immediately popular formulation . . . popularity being the mark of a "good" Cologne.

Types of accords with two, three, and four products are given below. These are given only as an indication, and may serve as a basis for more elaborate studies. It goes without saying that top notes and modifiers may be included in the accords set forth and, thus, increase the already large scope of possibilities offered in this field.

The last accord set forth below leads us to a much more rapid

### Accords with two products

| | | | |
|---|---|---|---|
| 7 | Bergamot | 9 | Bergamot |
| 3 | Lemon | 1 | Lavender |
| 7 | Bergamot | 6 | Bergamot |
| 3 | Neroli bigarade petals | 4 | Petitgrain fr. Grasse |
| 9 | Bergamot | 9 | Bergamot |
| 1 | Wild thyme | 1 | Argeol |
| 4 | Lemon | 9 | Sweet Orange |
| 6 | Bois de Rose | 1 | Neroli bigarade petals |
| 9 | Neroli bigarade petals | 4 7 | Bergamot |
| 1 | Verbena | 6 1 | Verbena |
| 5 9 | Lemon | | etc. |
| 5 1 | Sweet Orange | | |

### Accords with three products

| | | | |
|---|---|---|---|
| 6 | Bergamot | 3 | Lemon |
| 3 | Sweet Orange | 3 | Sweet Orange |
| 3 | Lavender | 3 | Petitgrain fr. Grasse |
| 6 | Lemon | 6 | Lemon |
| 3 | Lavender | 3 | Tangerine |
| 3 | Sweet Orange | 3 | Petitgrain fr. Grasse |
| 6 3 3 | Bergamot | | etc. |
| 3 6 3 | Lemon | | |
| 3 3 6 | Sweet Orange | | |

### Accords with four products

| | | | |
|---|---|---|---|
| 6 | Lemon | 6 | Lemon |
| 2 | Lavender | 2 | Petitgrain fr. Grasse |
| 2 | Bergamot | 2 | Bergamot |
| 2 | Neroli bigarade petals | 2 | Bois de Rose |
| 2 | Petitgrain fr. Grasse | 3 | Bergamot |
| 6 | Geranium African | 3 | Lavender |
| 2 | Bois de Rose | 3 | Sweet Orange |
| 2 | Verbena | 3 | Geranium African |
| 2 | Bergamot | 2 | Bergamot |
| 2 | Lemon | 6 | Lemon |
| 6 | Sweet Orange | 2 | Lavender |
| 2 | Tangerine | 2 | Bois de Rose |
| 2 6 | Bergamot | 2 2 | Bergamot |
| 2 2 | Lemon | 6 2 | Lemon |
| 2 2 | Sweet Orange | 2 2 | Sweet Orange |
| 6 2 | Lavender | 2 6 | Bois de Rose, etc. |

### Accords with five products

| | |
|---|---|
| 6 2 2 | Bergamot |
| 2 2 2 | Lemon |
| 2 6 2 | Sweet Orange |
| 2 2 2 | Petitgrain Grasse |
| 2 2 6 | Lavender |
| | etc. |

method of research that makes it possible to dispense with the long, tedious search for accords which, in Colognes, seem to be inexhaustible.

In addition to conventional-type Colognes, there are also fancy-type so-called Imperial, Russian, Royal, Amber Colognes that are merely conventional Colognes modified with additional components such as those listed below.

For a better understanding of the method used, a general table is given to show how, starting from formulation (d), many modifications of a same formula can be obtained.

These are only a few samples of the fascinating discoveries that can be made in the practice of our art and that are so numerous that an entire chapter should be devoted to them. They are vivid proof of how encouraging this type of research may be, although it may appear tedious to the uninitiated.

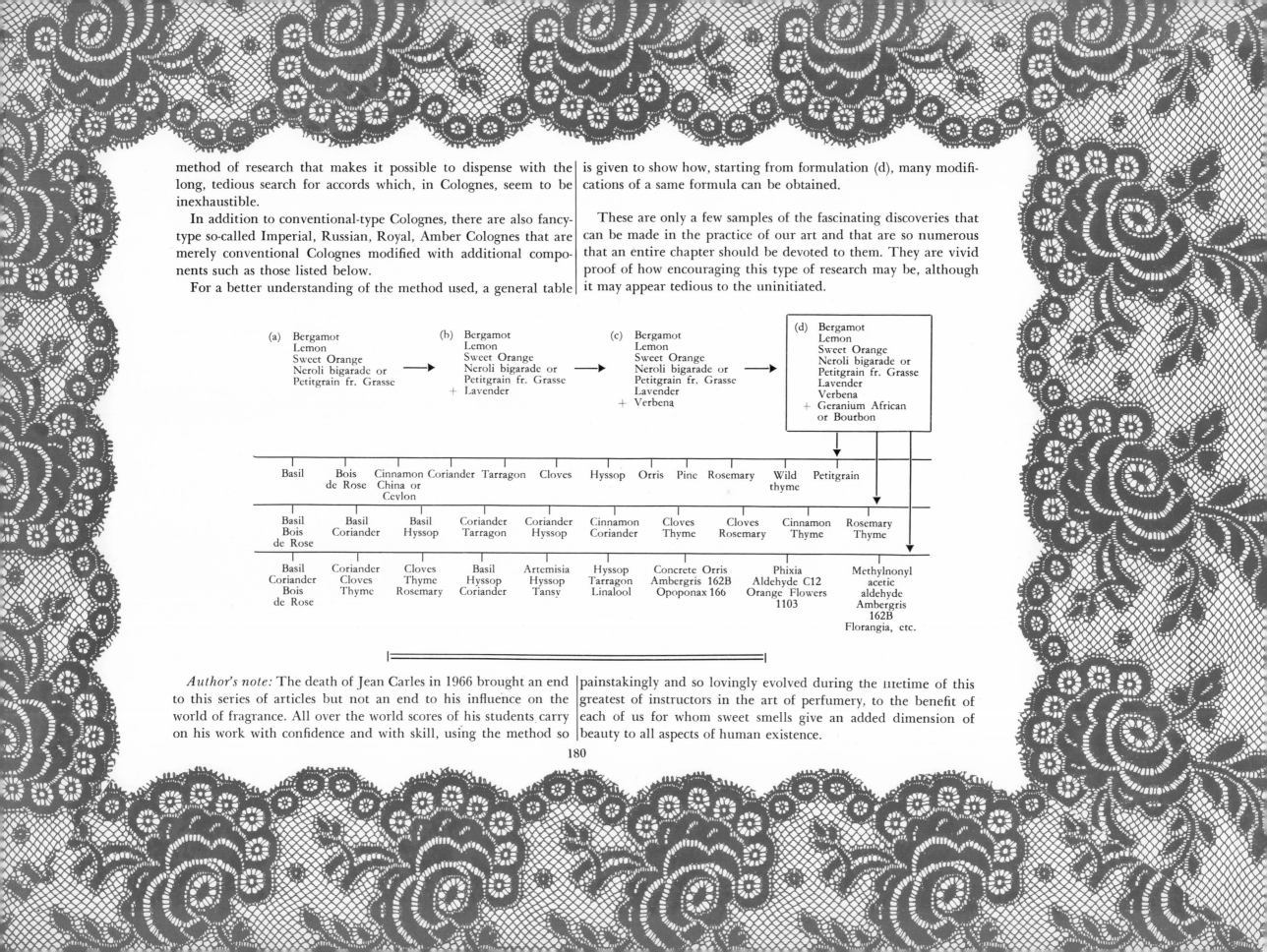

(a) Bergamot / Lemon / Sweet Orange / Neroli bigarade or Petitgrain fr. Grasse →

(b) Bergamot / Lemon / Sweet Orange / Neroli bigarade or Petitgrain fr. Grasse + Lavender →

(c) Bergamot / Lemon / Sweet Orange / Neroli bigarade or Petitgrain fr. Grasse / Lavender + Verbena →

(d) Bergamot / Lemon / Sweet Orange / Neroli bigarade or Petitgrain fr. Grasse / Lavender / Verbena + Geranium African or Bourbon

| Basil | Bois de Rose | Cinnamon China or Ceylon | Coriander | Tarragon | Cloves | Hyssop | Orris | Pine | Rosemary | Wild thyme | Petitgrain |
|---|---|---|---|---|---|---|---|---|---|---|---|
| Basil Bois de Rose | Basil Coriander | Basil Hyssop | Coriander Tarragon | Coriander Hyssop | Cinnamon Coriander | Cloves Thyme | Cloves Rosemary | Cinnamon Thyme | Rosemary Thyme | | |
| Basil Coriander Bois de Rose | Coriander Cloves Thyme | Cloves Thyme Rosemary | Basil Hyssop Coriander | Artemisia Hyssop Tansy | Hyssop Tarragon Linalool | Concrete Orris Ambergris 162B Opoponax 166 | Phixia Aldehyde C12 Orange Flowers 1103 | Methylnonyl acetic aldehyde Ambergris 162B Florangia, etc. | | | |

*Author's note:* The death of Jean Carles in 1966 brought an end to this series of articles but not an end to his influence on the world of fragrance. All over the world scores of his students carry on his work with confidence and with skill, using the method so painstakingly and so lovingly evolved during the lifetime of this greatest of instructors in the art of perfumery, to the benefit of each of us for whom sweet smells give an added dimension of beauty to all aspects of human existence.

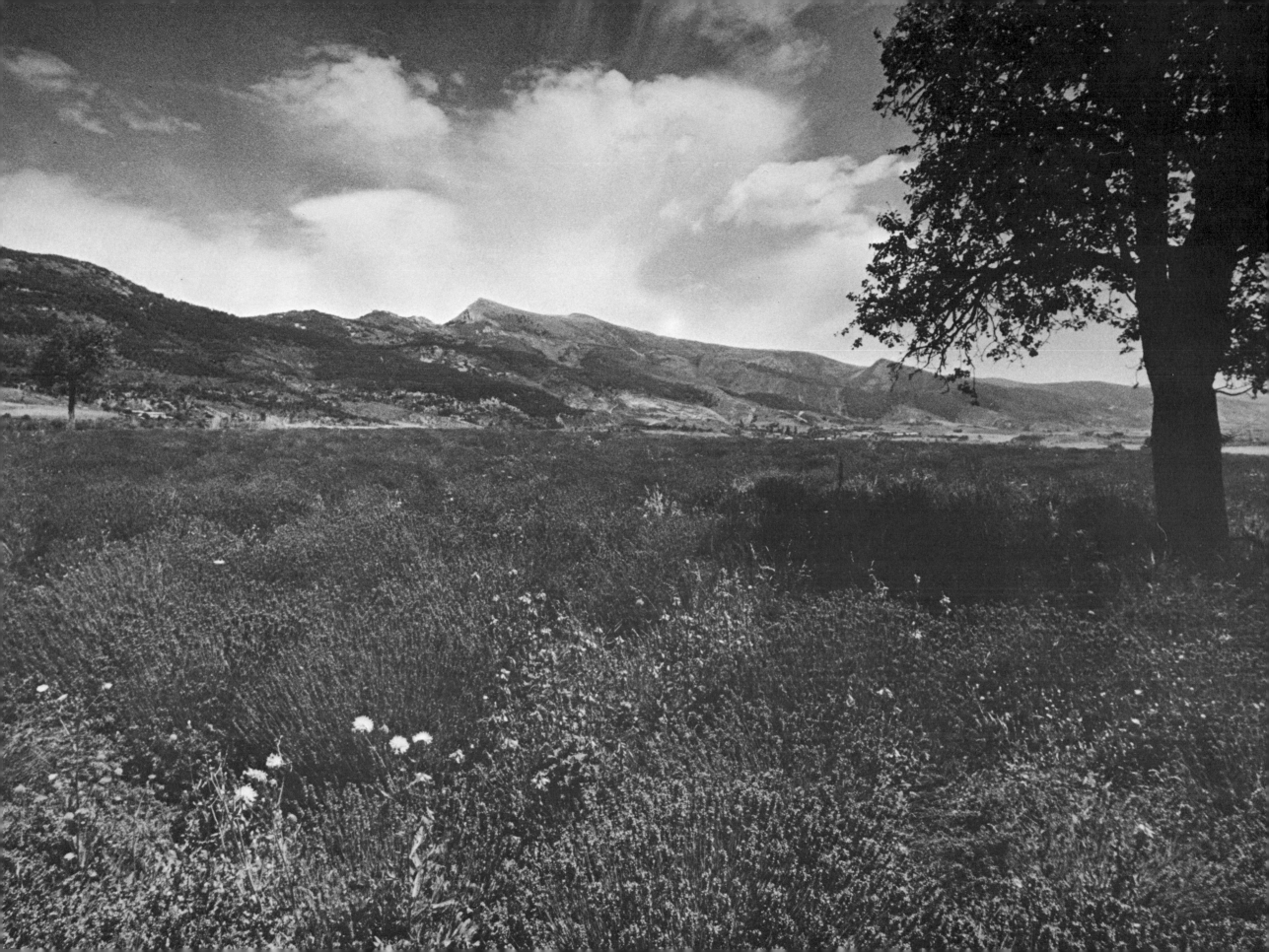

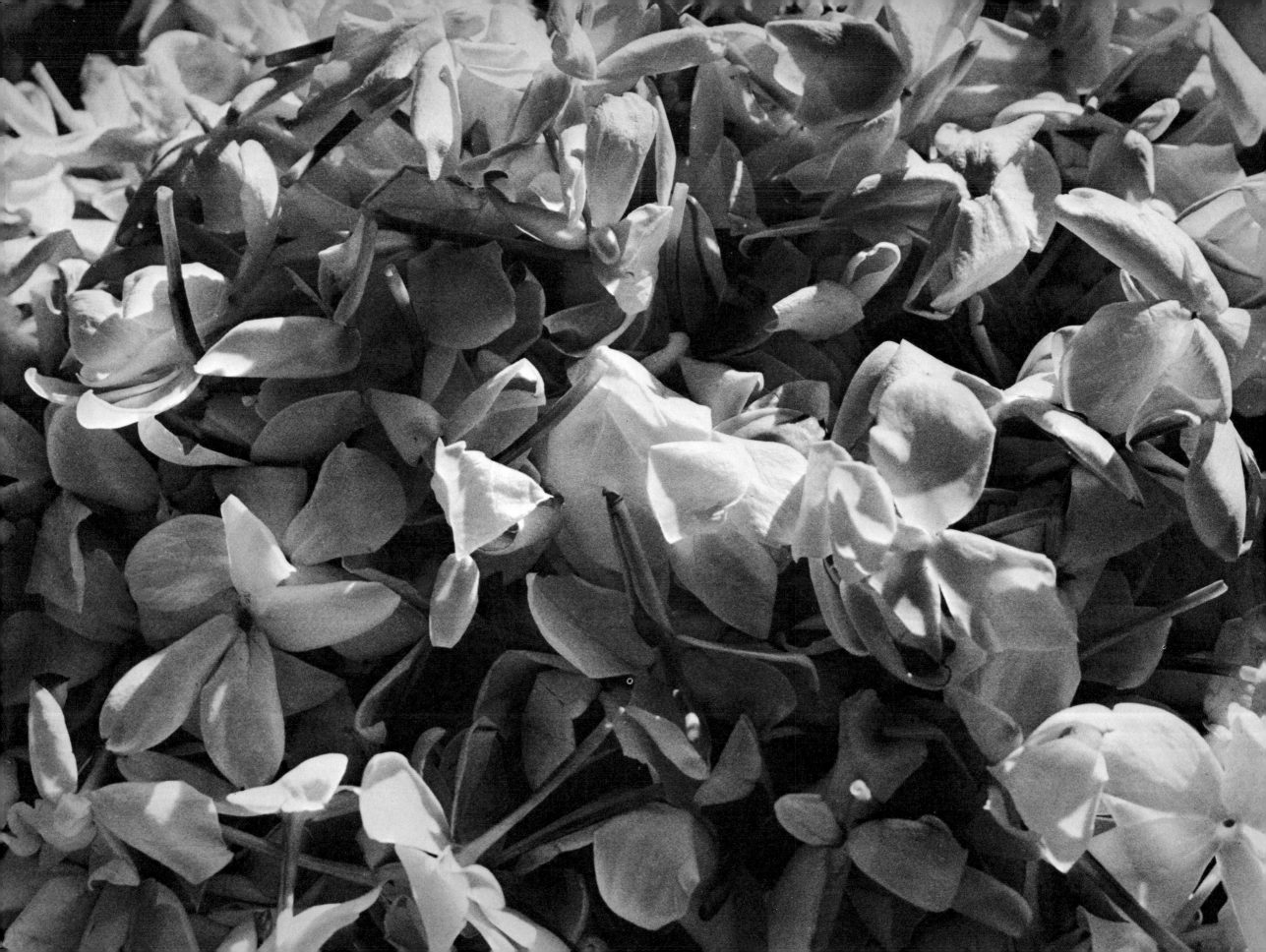

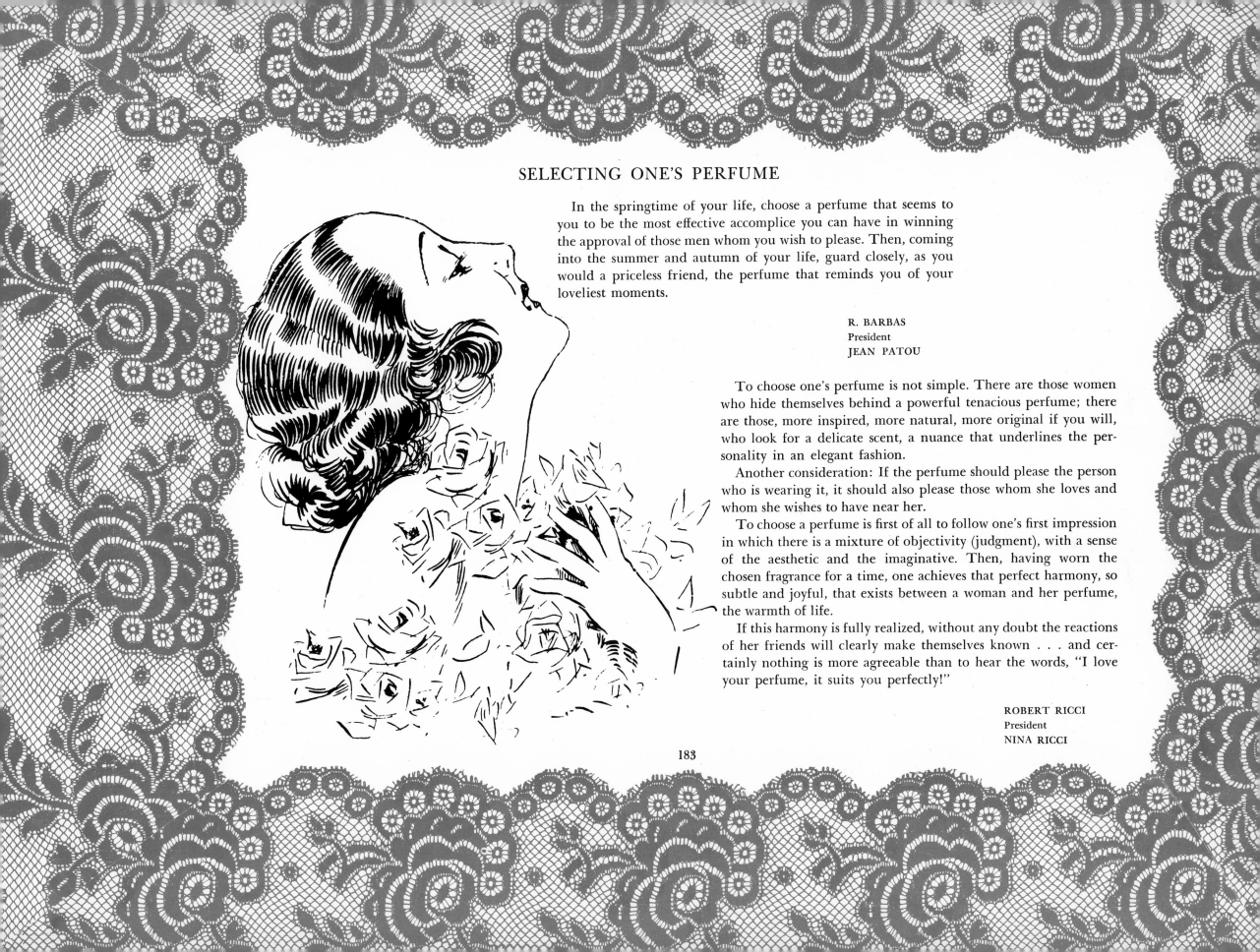

## SELECTING ONE'S PERFUME

In the springtime of your life, choose a perfume that seems to you to be the most effective accomplice you can have in winning the approval of those men whom you wish to please. Then, coming into the summer and autumn of your life, guard closely, as you would a priceless friend, the perfume that reminds you of your loveliest moments.

R. BARBAS
President
JEAN PATOU

To choose one's perfume is not simple. There are those women who hide themselves behind a powerful tenacious perfume; there are those, more inspired, more natural, more original if you will, who look for a delicate scent, a nuance that underlines the personality in an elegant fashion.

Another consideration: If the perfume should please the person who is wearing it, it should also please those whom she loves and whom she wishes to have near her.

To choose a perfume is first of all to follow one's first impression in which there is a mixture of objectivity (judgment), with a sense of the aesthetic and the imaginative. Then, having worn the chosen fragrance for a time, one achieves that perfect harmony, so subtle and joyful, that exists between a woman and her perfume, the warmth of life.

If this harmony is fully realized, without any doubt the reactions of her friends will clearly make themselves known . . . and certainly nothing is more agreeable than to hear the words, "I love your perfume, it suits you perfectly!"

ROBERT RICCI
President
NINA RICCI

September 1973

Women always choose their perfumes marvelously well.

Perfume is, above all, created to enhance the attractiveness of the female. All the "Great Perfumes" are extremely sensual and voluptuous; they are perfumes that stimulate an emotion.

Women have a deep instinct for self-preservation; a woman doesn't take the risk of alienating her husband by using a perfume that he finds disagreeable.

In making a choice, one is wise not to smell too many fragrances at the same time. Certainly there are no perfumes for blondes and perfumes for brunettes, inasmuch as the tinting of hair obviates such a distinction. For the most part, one chooses a perfume that complements the personality.

. . . there are distinguished perfumes

. . . sensual, provocative perfumes

. . . perfumes that are becoming to mysterious, enigmatic women,

. . . perfumes that are discreet, perfumes for the youthful, and perfumes that are very female, very assertive and haunting.

PARFUMS GUERLAIN

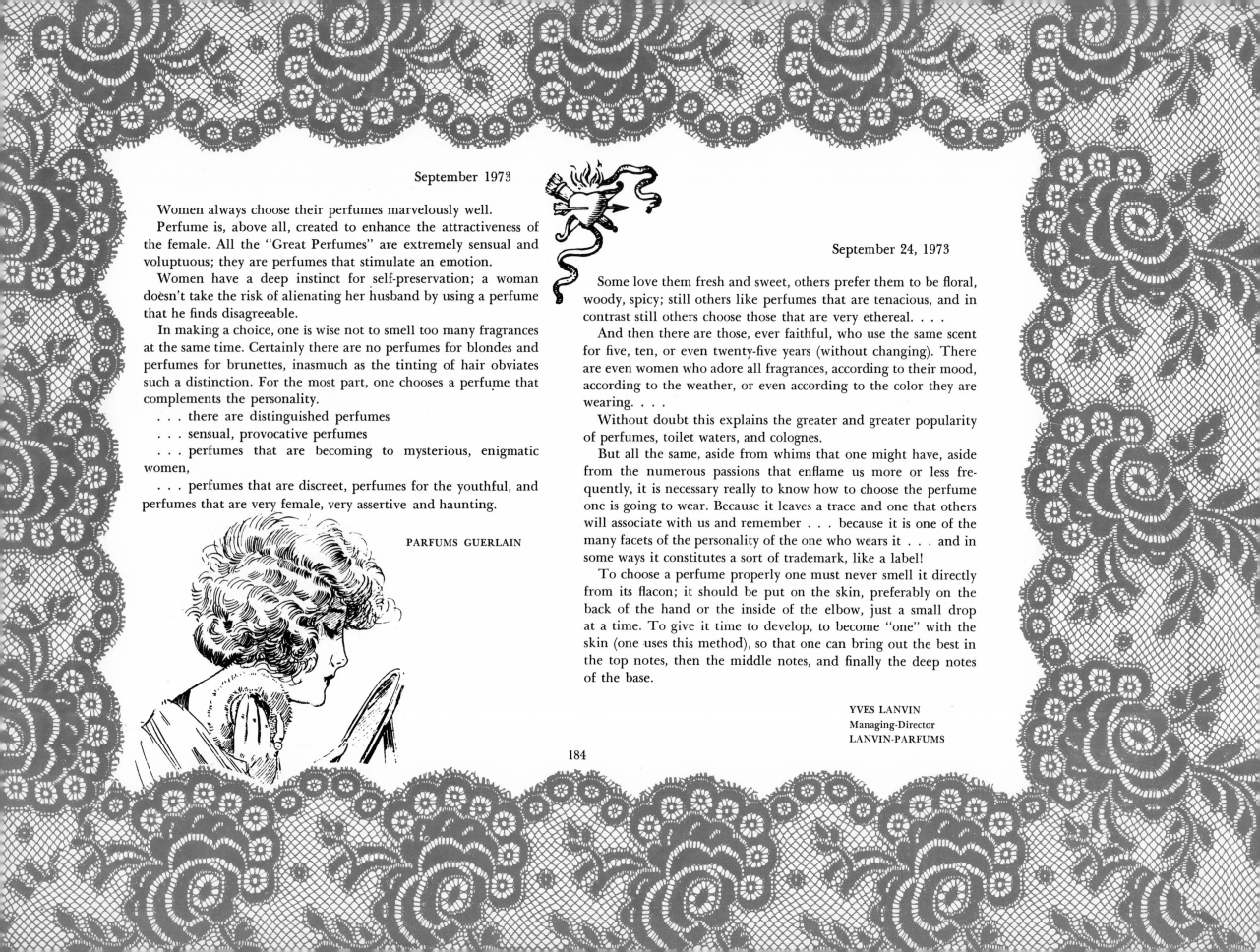

September 24, 1973

Some love them fresh and sweet, others prefer them to be floral, woody, spicy; still others like perfumes that are tenacious, and in contrast still others choose those that are very ethereal. . . .

And then there are those, ever faithful, who use the same scent for five, ten, or even twenty-five years (without changing). There are even women who adore all fragrances, according to their mood, according to the weather, or even according to the color they are wearing. . . .

Without doubt this explains the greater and greater popularity of perfumes, toilet waters, and colognes.

But all the same, aside from whims that one might have, aside from the numerous passions that enflame us more or less frequently, it is necessary really to know how to choose the perfume one is going to wear. Because it leaves a trace and one that others will associate with us and remember . . . because it is one of the many facets of the personality of the one who wears it . . . and in some ways it constitutes a sort of trademark, like a label!

To choose a perfume properly one must never smell it directly from its flacon; it should be put on the skin, preferably on the back of the hand or the inside of the elbow, just a small drop at a time. To give it time to develop, to become "one" with the skin (one uses this method), so that one can bring out the best in the top notes, then the middle notes, and finally the deep notes of the base.

YVES LANVIN
Managing-Director
LANVIN-PARFUMS

184

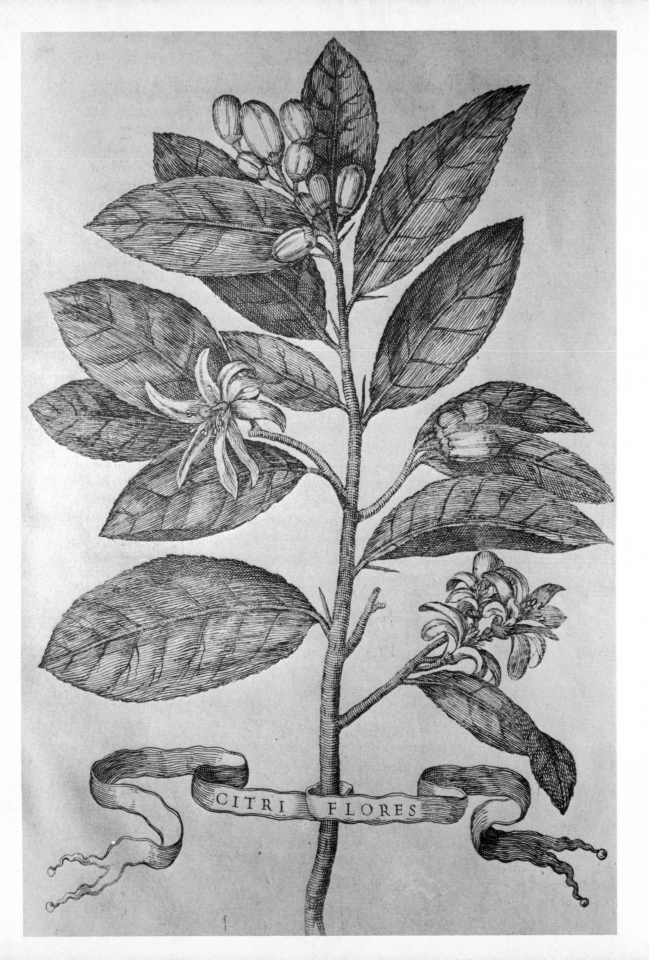

CITRI FLORES

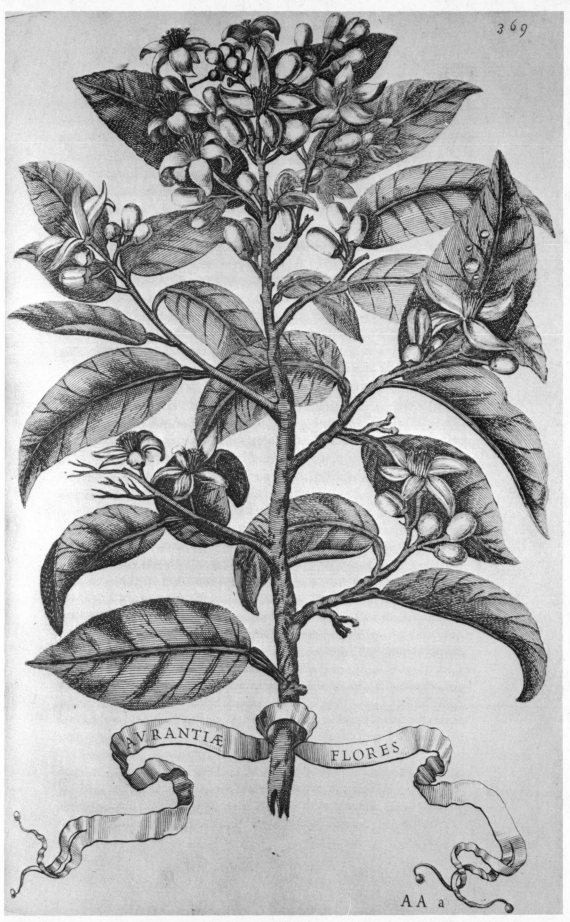

AVRANTIÆ FLORES

AA a

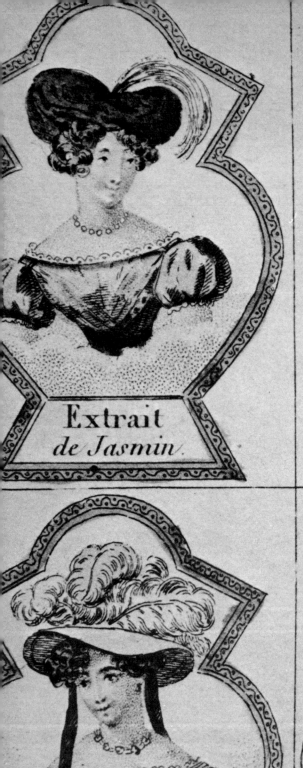

Extrait
de Jasmin.

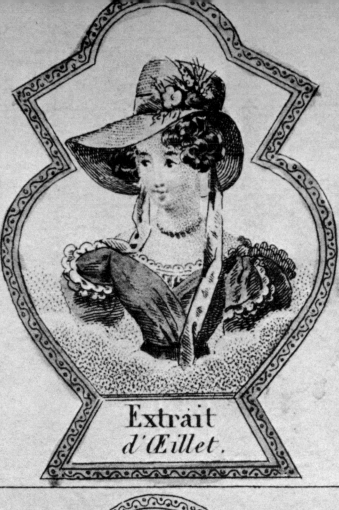

Extrait
d'Œillet.

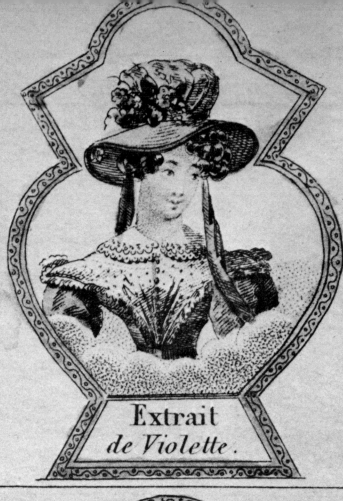

Extrait
de Violette.

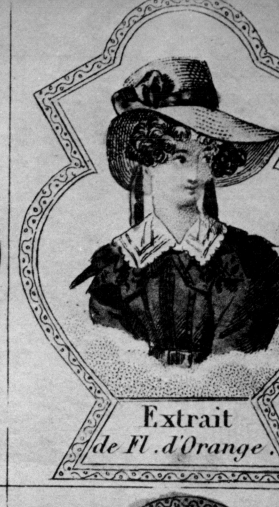

Extrait
de Fl. d'Orange.

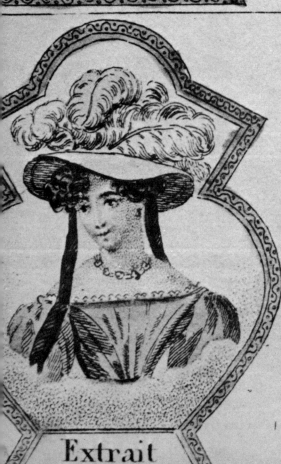

Extrait
de Vanille.

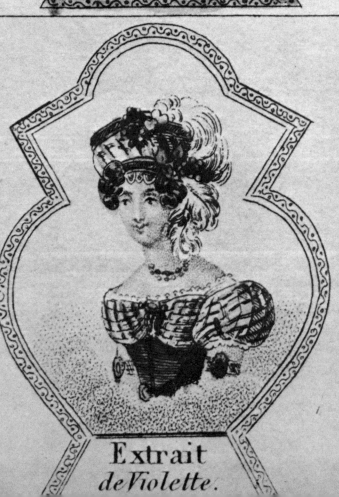

Extrait
de Violette.

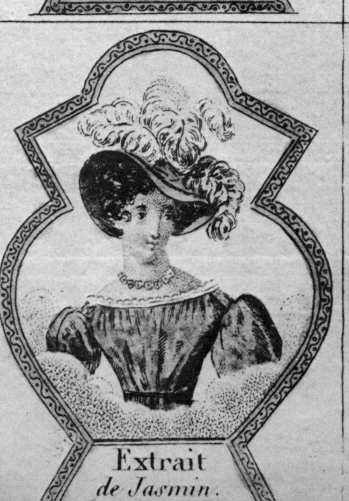

Extrait
de Jasmin.

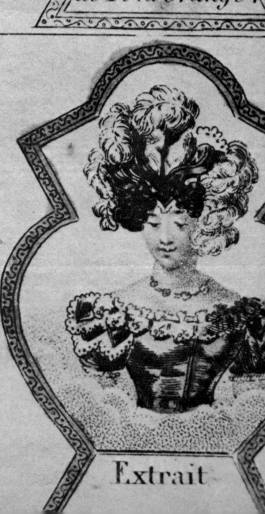

Extrait

December 1973

For a woman, choosing a perfume is both a delightful and difficult task.

Let us first be very precise. The choice concerns what we, in the business, call "the perfumage." It should not be compared or rather confused (mistaken) with "hygiene" that is choice of products aiming at toiletry, bath, or other skin care products.

With all this in mind, it is possible to give three steps and one helpful suggestion to help a woman choose the perfume of her choice.

1. A woman has to choose her perfume *for herself* before anything else.
2. She should choose what she prefers, even if her choice seems a little aloof to her, but with one condition: the fragrance she chooses has to give her a limited "aura." In this field, discretion is synonym of elegance.
3. A woman should not hesitate to have fun, to change and to try to live with different perfumes before making a definite choice.

*The recommendation:*

The "parfums de toilette," real perfumes but slightly lighter, created by many well-known French perfume houses, seem to be the best way for a woman to try a perfume, and to initiate herself to different fragrances.

A. GOSSET
*Chairman of the Board of
Parfums Rochas*

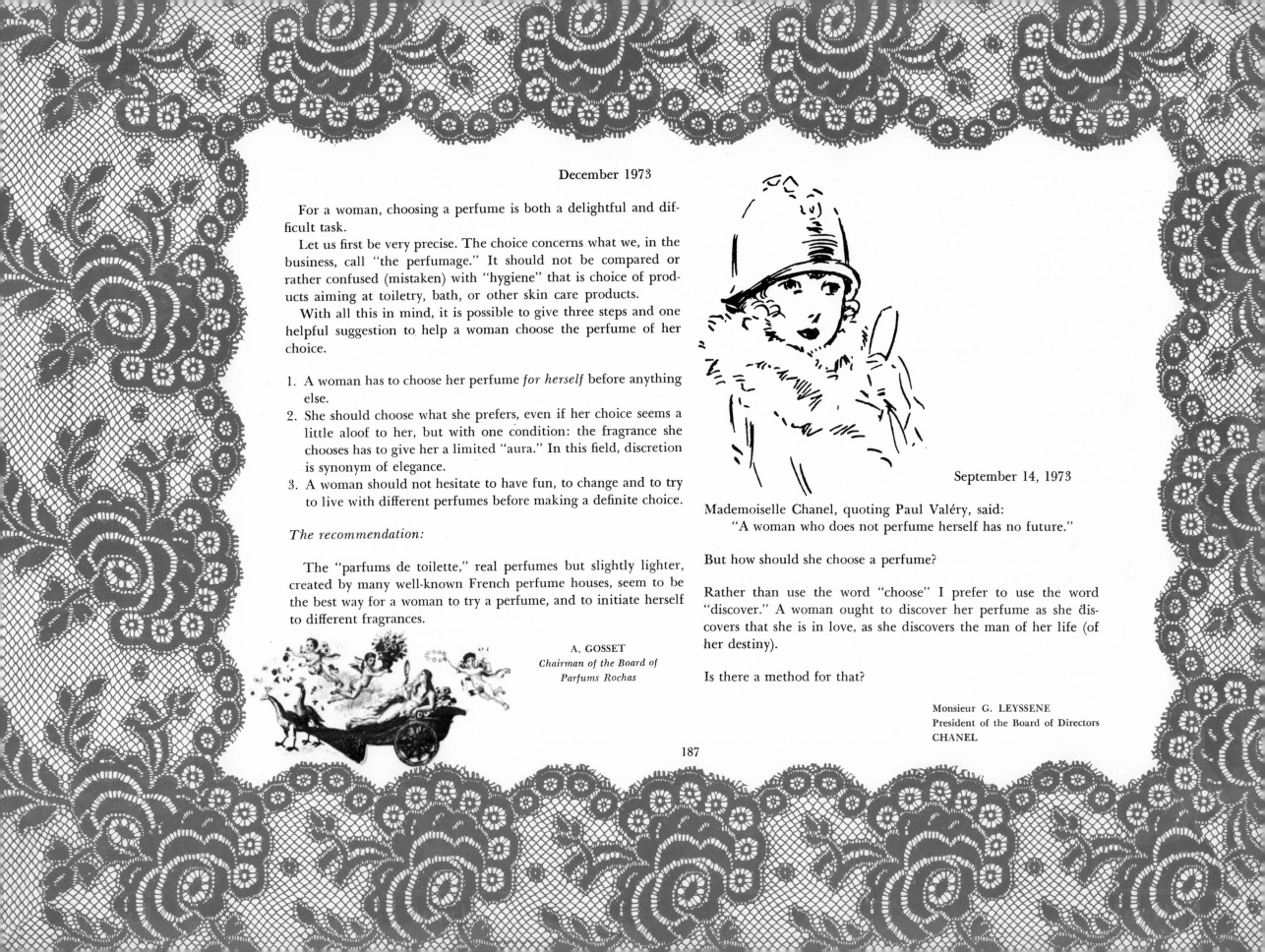

September 14, 1973

Mademoiselle Chanel, quoting Paul Valéry, said:
    "A woman who does not perfume herself has no future."

But how should she choose a perfume?

Rather than use the word "choose" I prefer to use the word "discover." A woman ought to discover her perfume as she discovers that she is in love, as she discovers the man of her life (of her destiny).

Is there a method for that?

Monsieur G. LEYSSENE
President of the Board of Directors
CHANEL

187

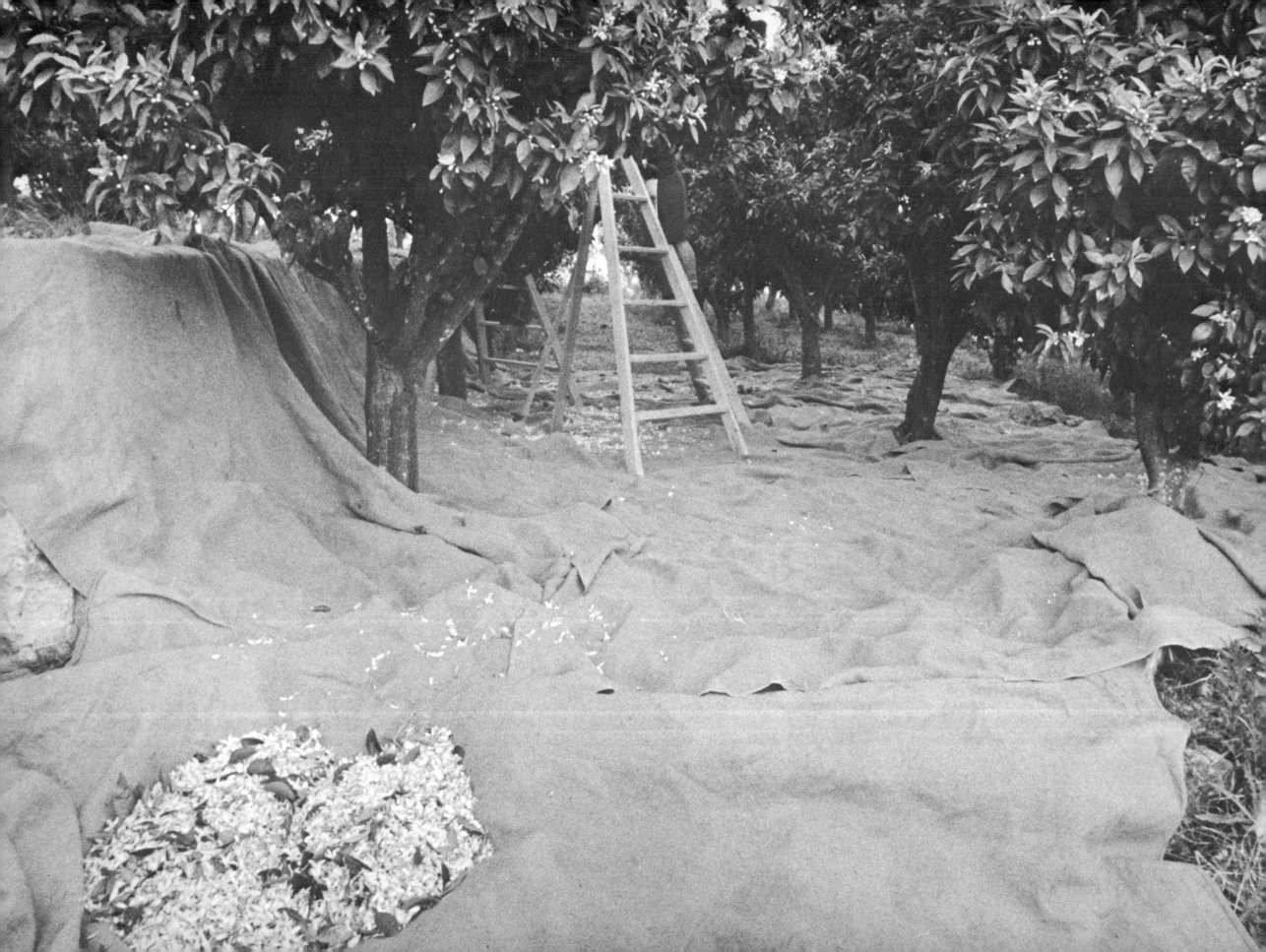

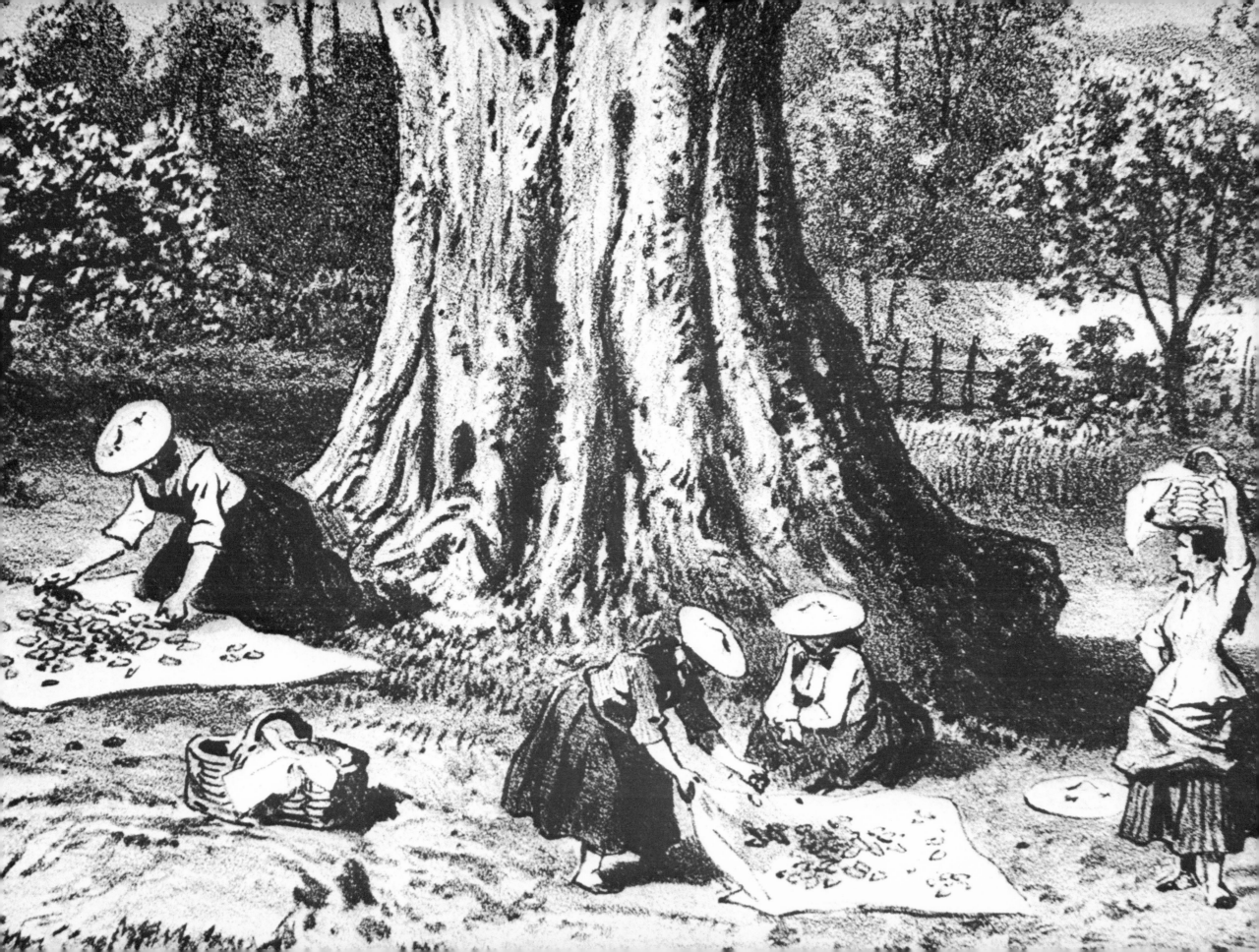

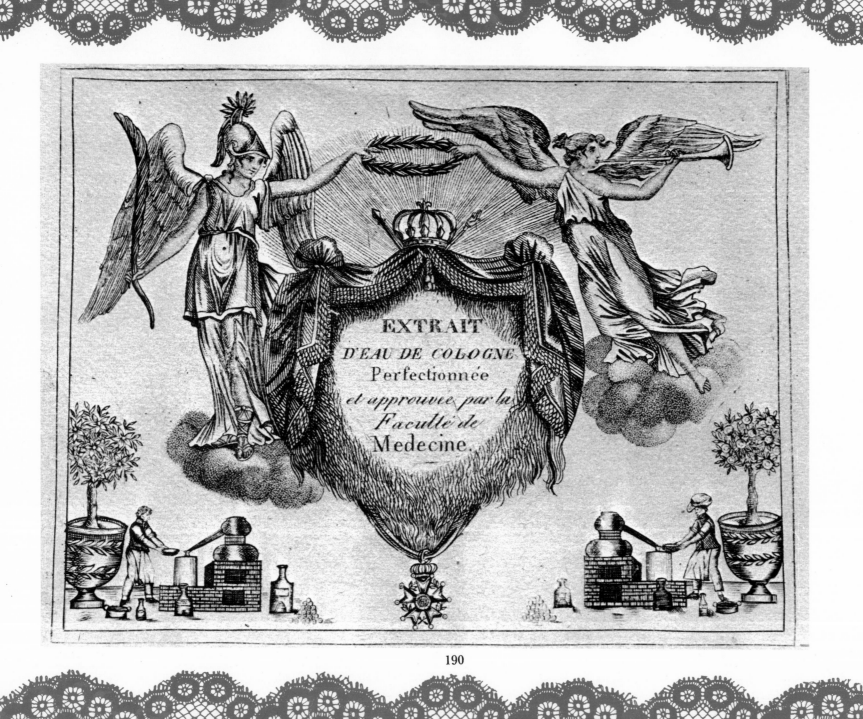

EXTRAIT
D'EAU DE COLOGNE
Perfectionnée
et approuvée par la
Faculté de
Medecine.

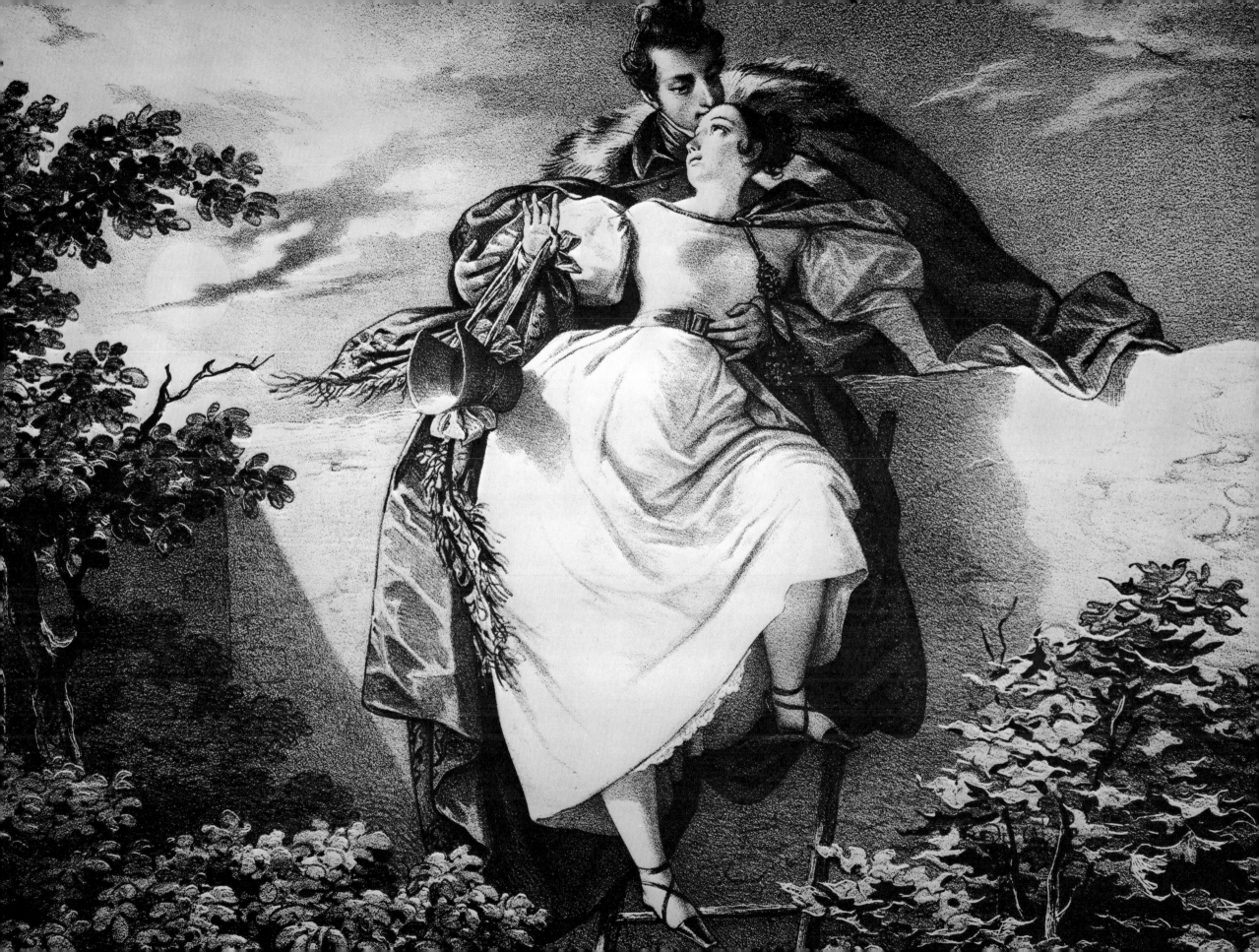

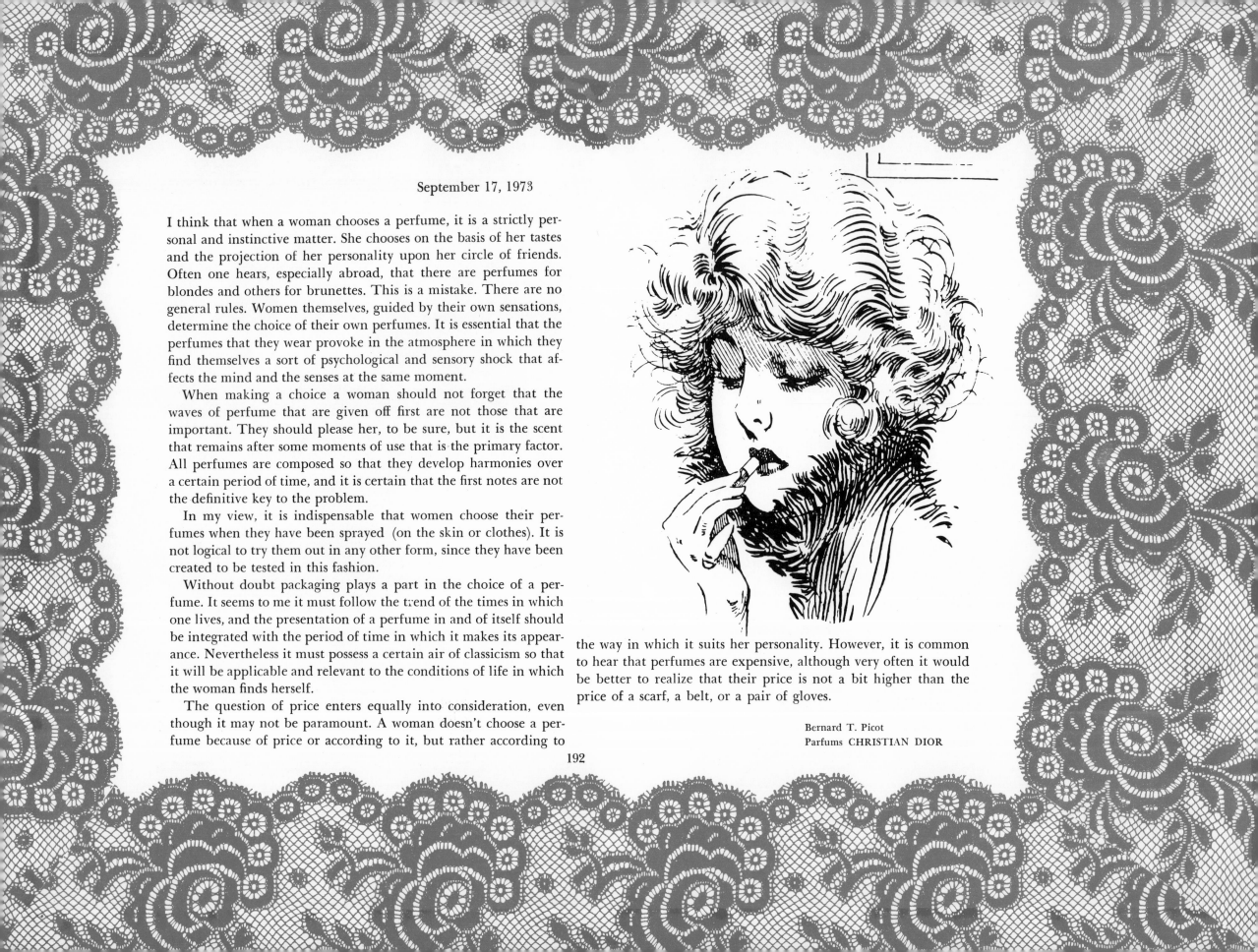

September 17, 1973

I think that when a woman chooses a perfume, it is a strictly personal and instinctive matter. She chooses on the basis of her tastes and the projection of her personality upon her circle of friends. Often one hears, especially abroad, that there are perfumes for blondes and others for brunettes. This is a mistake. There are no general rules. Women themselves, guided by their own sensations, determine the choice of their own perfumes. It is essential that the perfumes that they wear provoke in the atmosphere in which they find themselves a sort of psychological and sensory shock that affects the mind and the senses at the same moment.

When making a choice a woman should not forget that the waves of perfume that are given off first are not those that are important. They should please her, to be sure, but it is the scent that remains after some moments of use that is the primary factor. All perfumes are composed so that they develop harmonies over a certain period of time, and it is certain that the first notes are not the definitive key to the problem.

In my view, it is indispensable that women choose their perfumes when they have been sprayed (on the skin or clothes). It is not logical to try them out in any other form, since they have been created to be tested in this fashion.

Without doubt packaging plays a part in the choice of a perfume. It seems to me it must follow the trend of the times in which one lives, and the presentation of a perfume in and of itself should be integrated with the period of time in which it makes its appearance. Nevertheless it must possess a certain air of classicism so that it will be applicable and relevant to the conditions of life in which the woman finds herself.

The question of price enters equally into consideration, even though it may not be paramount. A woman doesn't choose a perfume because of price or according to it, but rather according to the way in which it suits her personality. However, it is common to hear that perfumes are expensive, although very often it would be better to realize that their price is not a bit higher than the price of a scarf, a belt, or a pair of gloves.

Bernard T. Picot
Parfums CHRISTIAN DIOR

192

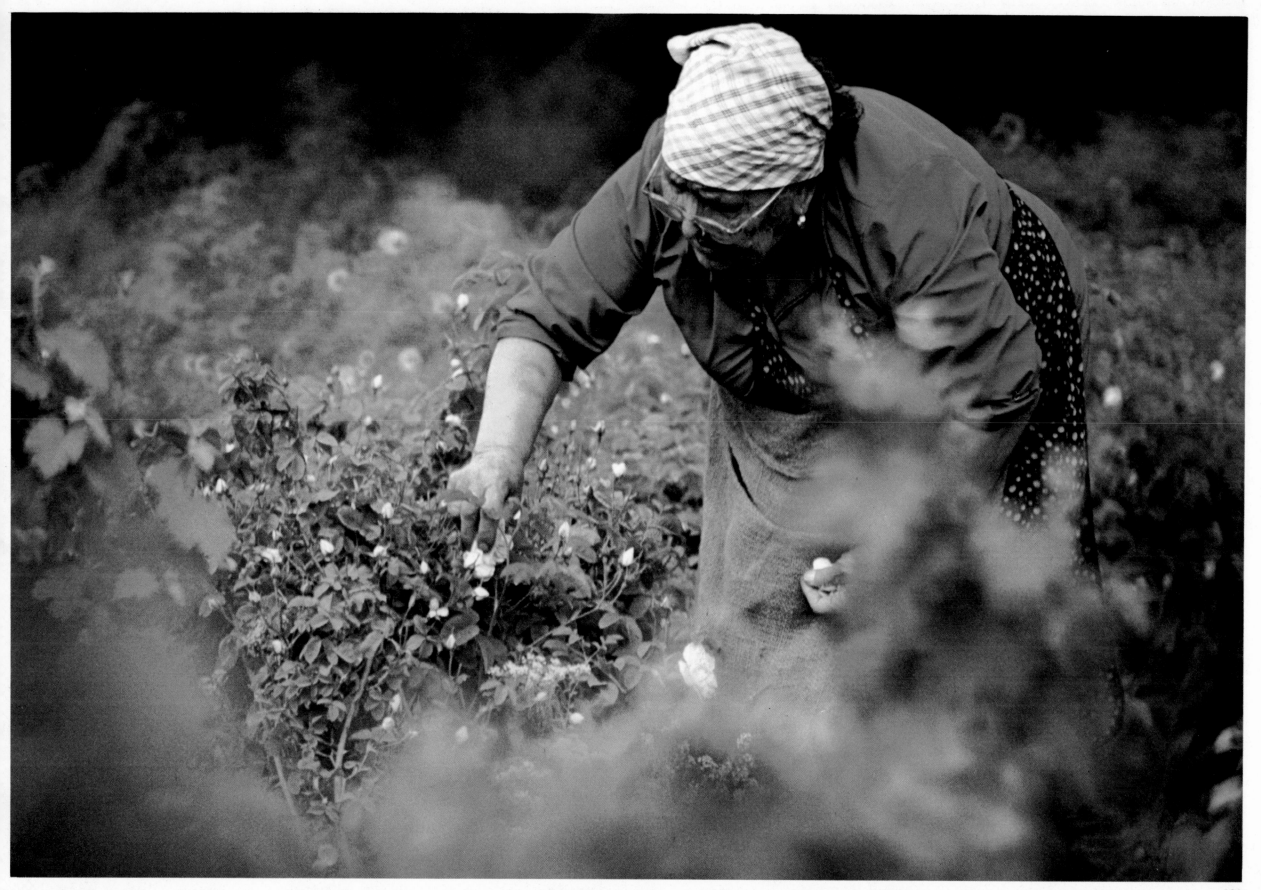

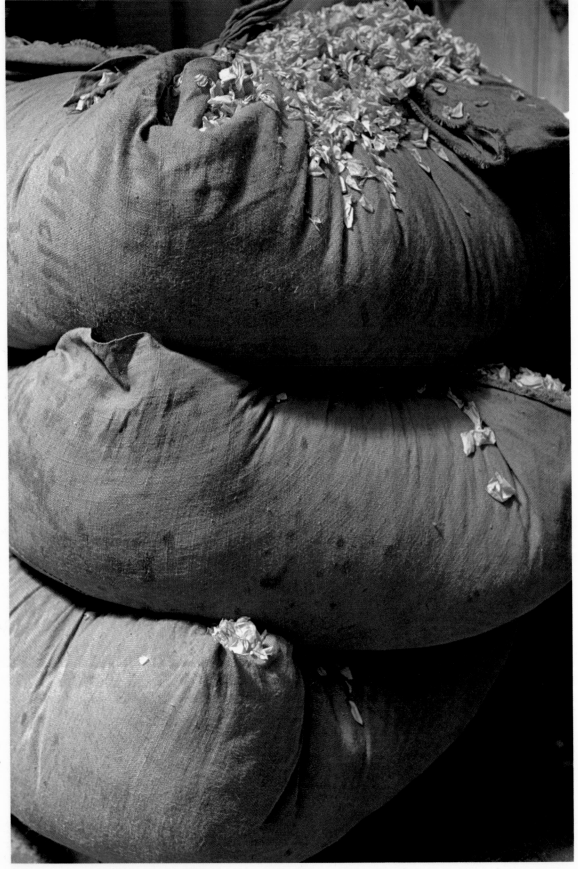

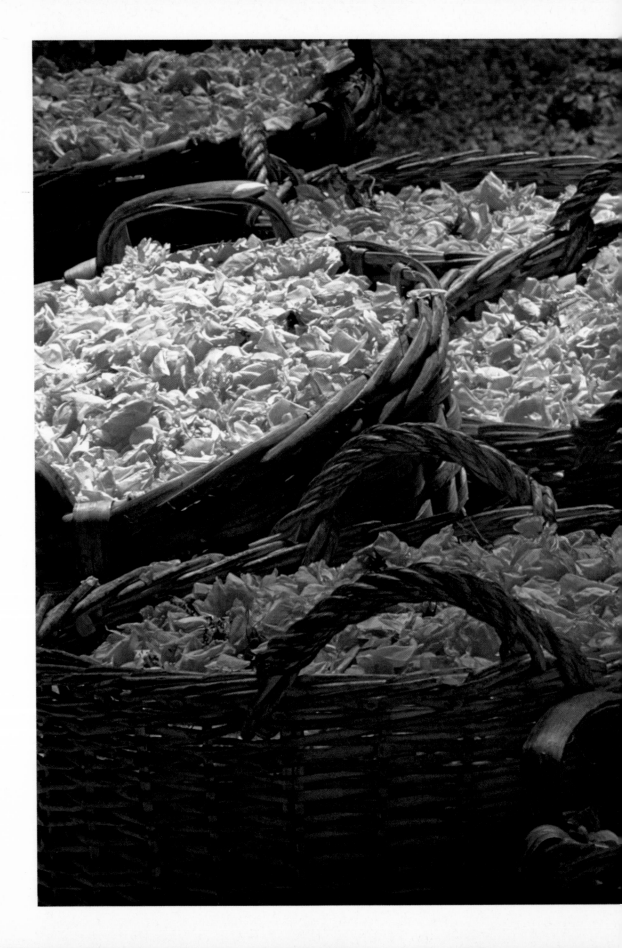

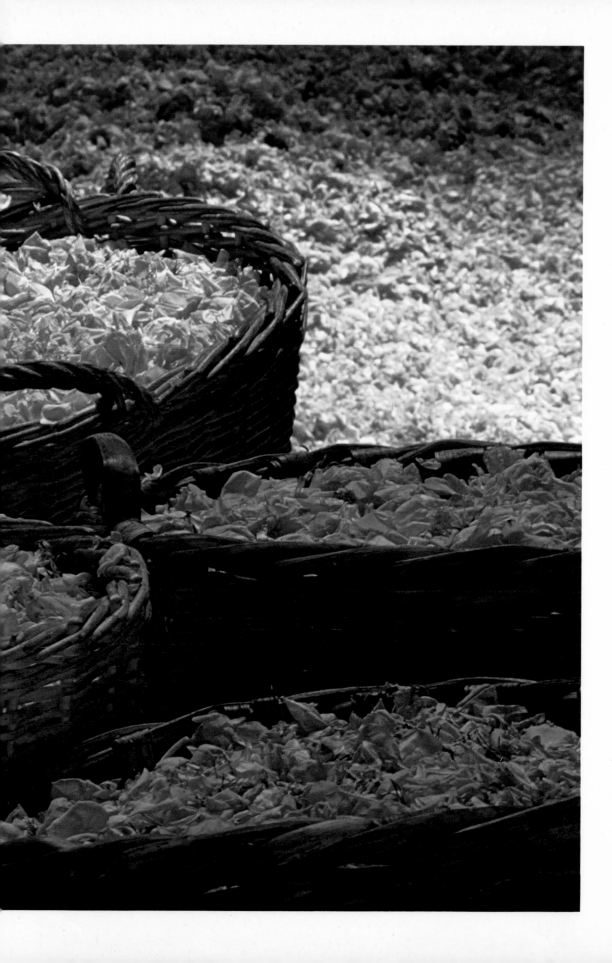
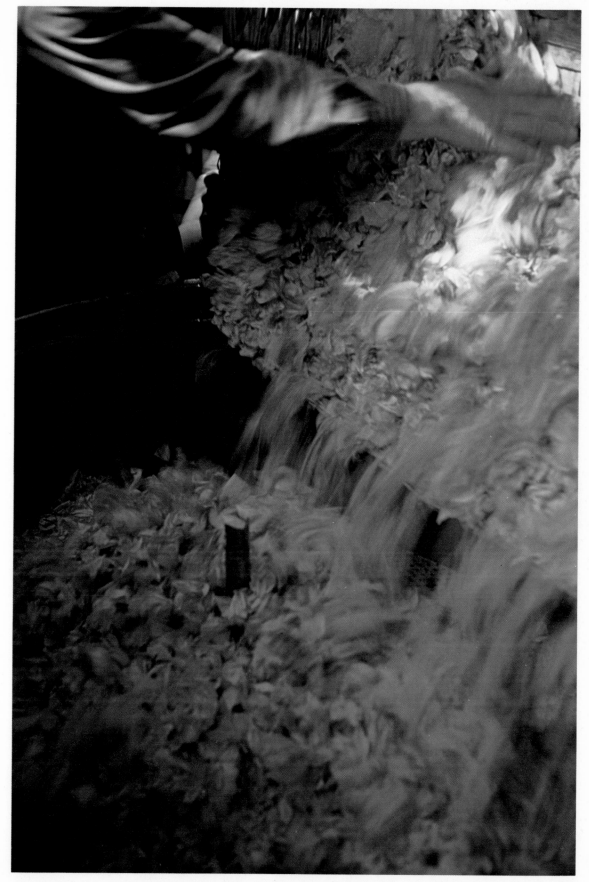